Pain Care Essentials and Innovations

Pain Care Essentials and Innovations

Edited by

SANJOG PANGARKAR, MD
Professor
Department of Medicine
David Geffen School of Medicine at UCLA
Los Angeles, California, United States

Director, Inpatient & Interventional Pain Service
Department of Physical Medicine & Rehabilitation
VA Greater Los Angeles Healthcare System
Los Angeles, California, United States

QUYNH G. PHAM, MD
Professor
Department of Medicine
David Geffen School of Medicine at UCLA
Los Angeles, CA, United States

Program Director
Pain Medicine Fellowship
Department of Physical Medicine and Rehabilitation
VA Greater Los Angeles Healthcare System
Los Angeles, CA, United States

BLESSEN C. EAPEN, MD
Associate Professor
Department of Medicine
David Geffen School of Medicine at UCLA
Los Angeles, CA, United States

Chief
Physical Medicine and Rehabilitation Service
VA Greater Los Angeles Healthcare System
Los Angeles, CA, United States

ELSEVIER

Notices

The views expressed in this text are those of the authors and do not reflect the official policy of the Department of Veterans Affairs, Department of Army, Department of Defense, or U.S. Government. The editors are employees of the U.S. government and do not have any conflicts of interest.

Publisher: Cathleen Sether
Acquisitions Editor: Humayra Rahman
Editorial Project Manager: Mona Zahir
Production Project Manager: Kiruthika Govindaraju
Cover Designer: Matthew Limbert

3251 Riverport Lane
St. Louis, Missouri 63043

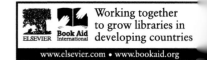

Working together
to grow libraries in
developing countries

www.elsevier.com • www.bookaid.org

To our colleagues at the Greater Los Angeles VA Healthcare System, we thank you for your continued dedication to patients, to teaching, and your passion toward the field of Pain Medicine. To our current and former medical students, residents, and fellows, we thank you for the questions that kept us on our toes!

To our families, we thank you for providing unrelenting support, unconditional love, and much needed patience to make this text possible.

This text would not have been possible without the hard work and dedication of our many contributors, who sacrificed valuable time and effort to impart their wisdom and knowledge, so we can all learn from their expertise.

Blessen Eapen, MD
Quynh Pham, MD
Sanjog Pangarkar, MD

List of Contributors

Dixie Aragaki, MD
Professor
Department of Medicine
David Geffen School of Medicine at UCLA
Los Angeles, CA, United States

Program Director
PM&R Residency
Department of Physical Medicine and Rehabilitation
VA Greater Los Angeles Healthcare System
Los Angeles, CA, United States

Brian Boies, MD
Associate Professor
UT Health San Antonio
Department of Anesthesiology
San Antonio, TX, United States

Christopher Brophy, MD
Resident Physician
Department of Physical Medicine and Rehabilitation
VA Greater Los Angeles Healthcare System
Los Angeles, CA, United States

Kelly Bruno, MD
Associate Professor
Center for Pain Medicine
University of California San Diego
San Diego, CA, United States

Lindsay Burke, MD
Resident Physician
Department of PM&R
Rutgers New Jersey Medical School
Newark, NJ, United States

George C. Chang Chien, DO
Director
Pain Management & PM&R
Ventura County Medical Center UCLA
Ventura, CA, United States

Director
Regenerative Medicine GCC Institute
Newport Beach, CA, United States

Allen S. Chen, MD, MPH
Assistant Professor
Chief, Interventional Spine Service
Department of Orthopaedic Surgery
David Geffen School of Medicine at UCLA
Los Angeles, CA, United States

Kathy Chou, DO
Resident Physician
Department of PM&R
Rutgers New Jersey Medical School
Kessler Institute for Rehabilitation
Newark, NJ, United States

Nathan Clements, MD
Resident Physician
UT Health San Antonio
Department of PM&R
San Antonio, TX, United States

Briana Cobos, MA
UT Health San Antonio
Department of Psychiatry
San Antonio, TX, United States

Chanel Davidoff, DO
Resident Physician
Department of PM&R
Donald and Barbara Zucker School of Medicine
Hofstra Northwell Health
New Hyde Park, NY, United States

Jesse Doolin, MS
UT Health San Antonio
Department of Psychiatry
San Antonio, TX, United States

Kelly A. Eddinger, BS, RVT
Senior Technician
Department of Anesthesiology
University of California San Diego
La Jolla, CA, United States

Kenneth Finn, MD
Attending Physician
Springs Rehabilitation, PC
Colorado Springs, CO, United States

Casey J. Fisher, MD
Attending Physician
Interventional Spine and Pain Medicine
Pain Relief Solutions
Poway, CA, United States

Brett Gerstman, MD
Clinical Assistant Professor
Department of PM&R
Rutgers New Jersey Medical School
Newark, NJ, United States

Pain Medicine & Physical Medicine and Rehabilitation
New Jersey Spine Center
Chatham, NJ, United States

Adam Hintz, MD
Pain Medicine Fellow
Department of Physical Medicine and Rehabilitation
VA Greater Los Angeles Healthcare System
Los Angeles, CA, United States

Patricia Jacobs, MD
Palliative Care Program
Department of Medicine
David Geffen School of Medicine at UCLA
Los Angeles, CA, United States

Hyung S. Kim, MD
Associate Professor
Department of Medicine
David Geffen School of Medicine at UCLA
Los Angeles, CA, United States

Eric Leung, MD
Assistant Professor
Department of Rehabilitation and Regenerative
   Medicine
Columbia University College of Physicians & Surgeons
New York, NY, United States

Donald D. McGeary, PhD
Associate Professor
UT Health San Antonio
Department of Psychiatry
Department of PM&R
San Antonio, TX, United States

Ambereen K. Mehta, MD
Assistant Professor of Medicine
Hospice and Palliative Care
Department of Medicine
David Geffen School of Medicine at UCLA
Los Angeles, CA, United States

Stephen A. Mudra, MD
Chief
Primary Care Pain Management
Board Certified Internal Medicine & Addiction
NF/SG Veterans Healthcare System
Gainesville, FL, United States

Paul Nabity, PhD
UT Health San Antonio
Department of Psychiatry
San Antonio, TX, United States

Ameet S. Nagpal, MD, MS, MEd
Associate Professor
UT Health San Antonio
Department of Anesthesiology
San Antonio, TX, United States

Udai Nanda, DO
Clinical Instructor
Department of Medicine
David Geffen School of Medicine at UCLA
Los Angeles, CA, United States

Rebecca Ovsiowitz, MD
Associate Professor
Department of Medicine
David Geffen School of Medicine at UCLA
Los Angeles, CA, United States

Edward K. Pang, DO
Clinical Instructor
Department of Medicine
David Geffen School of Medicine at UCLA
Los Angeles, CA, United States

Eric Prommer, MD, FAAHPM, HMDC
Associate Professor
David Geffen School of Medicine at UCLA
Department of Medicine
Hospice and Palliative Medicine
Los Angeles, CA, United States

David E. Reed, II, PhD
Postdoctoral Fellow
UT Health San Antonio
Department of Psychiatry
San Antonio, TX, United States

Ilene Robeck, BA, MD
Director
Virtual Pain Care
Telehealth
Veterans Health Administration
Richmond, VA, United States

Gabriel Rudd-Barnard, MD
Clinical Instructor
Department of Medicine
David Geffen School of Medicine at UCLA
Los Angeles, CA, United States

Associate Director: Center for the Rehabilitation of
    Pain Syndromes (CRPS)
California Pain Medicine Center
Santa Monica, CA, United States

Gaurav Sunny Sharma, MD
Assistant Professor
UT Southwestern Medical Center
Department of PM&R
Dallas, TX, United States

Joseph Solberg, DO
Assistant Professor
Department of Rehabilitation and Regenerative
    Medicine
Columbia University College of Physicians & Surgeons
New York, NY, United States

Agnes Stogicza, MD
Chief Pain Physician
Anesthesiologist
MOM Saint Magdolna Private Hospital
Budapest, Hungary

Kirsten Tillisch, MD
Professor
Digestive Diseases Medicine
David Geffen School of Medicine at UCLA
Los Angeles, CA, United States

Center for Neurobiology of Stress
David Geffen School of Medicine at UCLA
Los Angeles, CA, United States

Chief
Integrative Medicine
Veterans Health Administration
Los Angeles, CA, United States

Hunter Vincent, DO
Pain Medicine Fellow
Department of Physical Medicine and Rehabilitation
VA Greater Los Angeles Healthcare System
Los Angeles, CA, United States

Darrell Vydra, MD
Resident Physician
UT Health San Antonio
Department of PM&R
San Antonio, TX, United States

William White, DO
Resident Physician
UC Davis Department of PM&R
Sacramento, CA, United States

Tony L. Yaksh, PhD
Professor of Anesthesiology
Professor of Pharmacology
University of California San Diego
San Diego, CA, United States

Mauro Zappaterra, MD, PhD
Director
Multidisciplinary Care and Clinical Research
Synovation Medical Group
Pasadena, CA, United States

Teaching Consultant/Staff Physician
Department of Physical Medicine and Rehabilitation
VA Greater Los Angeles Healthcare System
Los Angeles, CA, United States

Preface

The field of Pain Medicine is constantly evolving. From the Cartesian theory of pain described by Descartes in the 17th century to Melzack and Wall's theory of pain modulation in the 1960s, our current knowledge of the exact mechanism and treatment of pain continues to evolve. In the 1990s, we learned that pain was not adequately recognized and addressed. This deficiency in assessment started a movement to educate clinicians on the recognition and treatment of pain. Unfortunately, the increasing awareness of the need to treat pain and the misleading marketing of opioid safety contributed to the opioid epidemic that soon followed. In attempts to reduce opioid-related deaths, the Centers for Disease Control established guidelines for opioid use. Given the climate and debate on effectiveness of opioid therapy, new treatment options have emerged but many lack evidence and efficacy.

Furthermore, the difficulty of managing these conditions arises from the complex nature of pain, lack of reliable objective measures, and the variability of response to these treatments. In this text, we present the current theories on pain mechanisms and evidence-based treatments for common pain conditions. In addition to reviewing treatment options (opioids, cannabis, complementary integrative health, regenerative medicine), the text will review up-to-date management guidelines (medication, interventional, behavioral, etc.), current views, and resources for opioid use disorders, and emerging research that may shape the future of the field. This book can be used as a reference by clinicians to assist them in optimizing individualized treatment plans, using current, evidence based-treatment options and management guidelines. It can also be used by trainees in the course of studying for specialty boards.

We are grateful to our contributing authors for sharing their knowledge and expertise in this field. Their continued dedication to the field of Pain Medicine and to their patients continues to push the boundaries of our understanding in this field. We hope that the future of Pain Medicine focuses on patient-centered care and biopsychosocial approaches that improve patient outcomes and function.

Acknowledgments

We wish to express special thanks to our young medical illustrators, Vanessa Tran, Calvin Nguyen, Nancy Dinh, Spencer Tran, and Elaina Truong, who spent countless hours drawing and refining many of the illustrations presented.

We are grateful to Quinn Wonders, PharmD, BCPS, for updating the Inpatient Pain chapter with the latest medications and tables, and for her valuable advice with patient care.

Contents

CHAPTER 1

Basic Science of Pain

CASEY J. FISHER, MD • TONY L. YAKSH, PHD • KELLY BRUNO, MD •
KELLY A. EDDINGER, BS, RVT

INTRODUCTION

Clinically, the most commonly referenced definition of pain initially described by Harold Merskey in 1964, and as adopted by the International Association in the Study of Pain in 1979, defines pain as "an unpleasant sensory and emotional experience associated with actual or potential tissue damage, or described in terms of such damage."[1] In this chapter, we will give an overview of the pathways involved in pain processing as it occurs in both the central and peripheral nervous systems as is currently conceived. This overview will include: anatomy involved in the processing of nociceptive stimuli; the fundamentals of systems underlying acute nociception and persistent pain states; and the linkage to chronic pain and how the immune system plays a role in this processing.

PERIPHERAL ANATOMY
Primary Afferents[2-4]

The signal of acute nociceptive pain is propagated along sensory neurons, which have cell bodies (somas) that lie in the dorsal root ganglia (DRG) and send one of their axon projections to the periphery and the other to the dorsal horn of the spinal cord in the central nervous system. The axons of peripheral afferents can be classified by anatomical characteristics (Erlanger-Gasser), Conduction Velocity (Lloyd-Hunt), and by their respective thresholds for activation. Most commonly, they are known by anatomical classification into two types of A fibers (β and δ) and C fibers.

C fibers are small, unmyelinated, and therefore, slow conducting fibers (<2 m/s). These primary sensory afferent neurons represent the majority of afferent fibers found in the periphery and are most commonly high threshold fibers, meaning they are not activated unless the stimulus (thermal, mechanical, or chemical) is at an intensity sufficiently high enough to potentially cause tissue injury. As nociceptors, or receptors that

detect noxious stimuli, they are triggered to discharge when the range of temperature or pressure corresponds to what would be considered painful. The distal terminals of these small C fibers display large branching dendritic trees and are characterized as being "free" nerve endings. These nerve endings can be activated further by many specific agents in the periphery in response to tissue injury, inflammation, or infection in a concentration-dependent fashion. Table 1.1 depicts the source and nature of these agents as well as the eponymous receptor on C fibers that is activated with each agent. The fact that there are multiple stimulus modalities for these C fibers that can lead to a signal of pain is the reason they are known as C-polymodal nociceptors. In fact, C fibers can be characterized further by what provokes them to fire. There are some C fibers that do not respond to mechanical stimulation. These so-called silent nociceptors, or mechanically insensitive afferents (MIAs), only respond to very high levels of nonphysiologic mechanical stimulation and/or heat. However, they can acquire sensitivity in the face of pathology, such as inflammation, which leads to a sensitized state and activation by relatively low-intensity mechanical/thermal stimuli.

Like C fibers, A-δ fibers are small and can be high threshold. But, A-δ fibers are myelinated, and therefore, faster, with conduction velocity between 10 and 40 m/s. As such, A-δ fibers act as nociceptors and mediate "first" or "fast" pain, whereas C fibers are responsible for "second" or "slow" pain. To put this in context, consider what happens when you touch a hot object. Your immediate reaction is to pull your hand away, which is mediated by noxious thermal sensation activating fast conducting A-∂ afferents. Typically, there is also a slower sensation of pain traveling over the slowly conducting C fibers, which relay tissue damage in the form of a burning sensation. Some populations of A-δ fibers can also be lower threshold at times, meaning they begin to discharge

TABLE 1.1
Summary of Agents, Tissue Source, and Receptors Found at C Fibers[12].

Agents	Tissue Source	Receptors
Amines	Mast cells (histamine) Platelets (serotonin)	H1 5HT3
Bradykinin	Clotting factors (bradykinin)	BK 1, BK2
Lipidic acids	Prostanoids (PGE2), leukotrienes	EP
Cytokines	Macrophages (interleukins, tumor necrosis factor)	IL-1, TNFR
Primary afferent peptides	C fibers [substance P (SP), calcitonin gene-related peptide (CGRP)]	NK1, CGRP
Proteinases	Inflammatory cells (thrombin, trypsin)	PAR3, PAR1
Low pH or hyperkalemia	Tissue injury [(H+), (K+), adenosine]	ASIC3/ VR1, A2
Lipopolysaccharide (LPS), formyl peptide	Bacteria (LPS, formyl peptide)	TLR4, FPR1

when the range of temperature or pressure corresponds to what would be nontissue damaging. In the case of thermal stimulus, it would be considered a mildly noxious warm/hot sensation. In the case of mechanical stimulus, it would be considered touch or pressure that is borderline painful. A-δ fibers also differ from C fibers in that they express specialized nerve endings that serve to define their response characteristics. This relationship will be delineated further in the peripheral physiology section.

In contrast, A-β fibers are large, myelinated fibers with the fastest conduction velocity (>40 m/s) of primary afferent neurons. They are low threshold afferent fibers that fire in response to low threshold mechanical stimulation, such as touch or pressure. Under normal physiologic states, activation of these afferents does not generate a noxious sensation. However, there are certain conditions in which these afferents initiate a pain sensation, or allodynia. The definition of allodynia is low-intensity tactile or thermal stimuli causing a pain state. This can occur in scenarios where there is nerve damage (for example, carpal tunnel or sciatic nerve lesions).

All of the afferent nerve fibers share the following important characteristics related to the pattern in which they respond to a stimulus and the manner in which they fire:

i)   Afferent nerve fibers display little or no spontaneous firing. They do not spontaneously discharge like other nerve cells of the brain or heart;

ii) Peripheral afferents typically display a monotonic increase in discharge frequency that covaries with stimulus intensity. This means that if the thermal or mechanical intensity increases, there will be a monotonic increase in discharge frequency because there will be a greater depolarization of the terminal, which will increase frequency of axon discharge; and

iii) Afferents serve to encode modality by being able to transduce thermal, mechanical, and/or chemical signals into a depolarization based on their individual nerve ending transduction properties. For the larger A-β fiber afferents, the nerve endings are highly specialized, e.g., Pacinian corpuscle, and only respond to specific low threshold stimuli, whereas the free nerve endings of the small C fibers respond to a more diverse array of signals at higher threshold.

Somatic and Visceral Afferents[4,5]

The location of peripheral afferents is also important when it comes to the type of pain sensation. Peripheral afferent axon projections to the periphery are found throughout the body. The axon projections to the skin, joints, and muscles are involved in somatic pain. The axon projections to the organs are involved in visceral pain. The main functional differences between afferents in the viscera and somatic systems are that there is little distinction between nociceptive afferents and nonnociceptive afferents, and there is significant prevalence of MIAs in the viscera. The visceral afferents only exist as high threshold and low threshold afferents, the latter of which responds to a range of stimulation intensities. The main anatomical difference between afferents in the viscera and afferents in the somatic system is that there are significantly fewer afferents in the viscera. Less than 10% of the total spinal cord afferent input comes from the visceral afferents. This often means that visceral input travels to its more central projections along with somatic input. The concept of referred pain, whereby organ pathology causes a

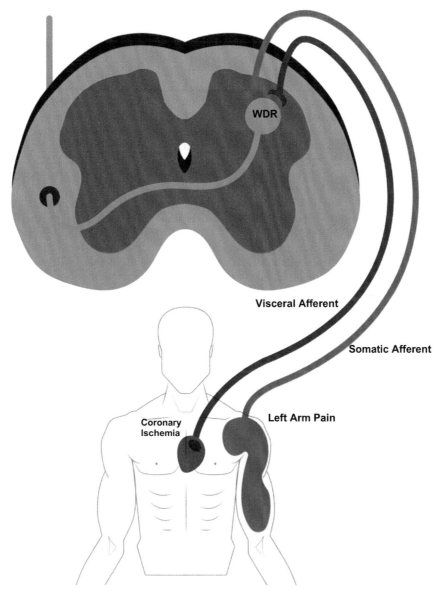

FIG. 1.1 Viscerosomatic convergence. (Credit: Kelly A. Eddinger.)

concomitant dermatomal spread of pain, is thought to be caused by convergence of somatic and visceral afferents onto the same wide dynamic range neurons (WDRs) at the dorsal horn level (see Fig. 1.1). This leads to the message generated by a visceral afferent being conflated with the input generated by a particular somatic region, thereby accounting for the "referred pain" profile of a visceral stimulus. WDR neurons will be discussed further in the central anatomy section.

CENTRAL ANATOMY

First-Order Neurons: Spinal Dorsal Horn Projections[6,7]

If the signal generated by an acute nociceptive stimulus is followed anatomically, from distally to proximally, the peripheral afferents extend through the DRG, where the afferent cell body lies, to the axon terminals of the spinal cord. Then, they terminate at the dorsal horn, where the dorsal root entry zone (DREZ) is found. The smaller afferents tend to enter the DREZ more laterally, and the larger afferents tend to enter the DREZ more medially. The small and large afferents collectively enter the dorsal horn as the fascicles that make up the nerve root. Nerve roots are divided into cervical, thoracic, lumbar, and sacral segments in a rostrocaudal distribution and enter on the ipsilateral side of the dorsal horn.

High threshold, small, unmyelinated afferents (C fibers) project to the more superficial regions of the dorsal horn: Lamina I (marginal layer), Lamina II (substantia gelatinosa), and the central canal (Lamina X). These segmental penetrating axons also send axons rostrally and caudally, traveling in the lateral tract of Lissauer, up to the level at which they enter the dorsal horn. This collateralization can be up to several segments above or below the entry point into the dorsal horn. Low threshold, large, myelinated afferents (A-β fibers) project deeper into the dorsal horn (Laminae IV, V, and VI), a region known as the nucleus proprius. Smaller myelinated afferents (A-δ fibers) project to the marginal layer and substantia gelatinosa layers (Laminae I and II) as well as the deeper layer of the nucleus proprius (Lamina V). Larger A type fibers also collateralize up to 1 to 2 segments rostral or caudal to their entry point, but they collateralize in the dorsal columns to travel up to the dorsal column nuclei (see Fig. 1.2).

Second-Order Neurons: Dorsal Horn Anatomy and Functional Organization[8,9]
The dorsal horn is made up principally of second-order neurons that will send projections into the ascending spinal tracts to transmit sensory information to the brainstem and cortex. These second-order neurons can be classified according to their functional characteristics as well as their anatomic location within the dorsal horn itself. Cross-sectional anatomy of the gray matter of the dorsal horn has been well characterized and is

a way to organize the types of second-order neurons that give rise to the tracts of the spinal cord (See Fig. 1.2). As discussed earlier, specific sensory afferents project to specific locations within the dorsal horn.

The most superficial, dorsal level of the dorsal horn is known as the marginal zone or Lamina I, according to the Rexed Lamina(e) classification. The marginal zone is where C fibers and A-δ fibers terminate. As such, neurons in this layer respond selectively to high threshold stimulation and send projections into the spinal tracts located in the ventrolateral (or anterolateral) section of the cord on the contralateral side of entry. These tracts will eventually project to the various nuclei in the contralateral brainstem and thalamus, more formally known as the spinothalamic tracts. As discussed before, some of the neurons in the marginal zone project ipsilaterally for a few segments in the white matter along the dorsolateral tract of Lissauer before entering the gray matter on the contralateral side and joining the tracts in the ventrolateral quadrant of the spinal cord. These projections are otherwise known as part of the intersegmental system.

Lamina II, also known as the substantia gelatinosa, is where C fibers and A-δ fibers terminate. However, it is also where many local interneurons are located. Interneurons are second-order neurons that project from the more superficial dorsal horn layers to the deeper layers of the Nucleus Proprius (Laminae III, IV, V, and VI). These interneurons are classified as excitatory or inhibitory and serve to locally regulate the excitability of dorsal horn projection neurons. The complexity of this layer is due in part to the fact that second-order interneurons are in direct communication with second-order neurons, which make up the ascending spinal tracts that are all in communication, either directly or indirectly, with the original primary afferents, including C fibers and A-δ fibers.

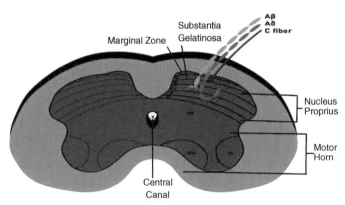

FIG. 1.2 Dorsal horn cross section. See text for further discussion. (Credit: Kelly A. Eddinger.)

The nucleus proprius (Laminae III, IV, V, and VI), where large, myelinated, primary afferents (A-β fibers) terminate, has large-soma neurons, which send their dendrites up into the upper lamina to make contact with small, high threshold afferent input. Large, low threshold afferents make synaptic contact on the cell bodies and the ascending dendrites. Thus, they receive convergent low and high threshold input. This enables them to respond to low threshold and show increasing discharge rates with increasing stimulus intensities as small afferents are engaged. Accordingly, these cells are referred to as WDR neurons.

The central canal (Lamina X) is the deepest layer of the dorsal horn. This location is where a large amount of visceral afferent input occurs and where smaller somatic afferents (C fibers and A-δ fibers) also terminate. Signals received here are high threshold temperature and noxious mechanical stimulation. The tracts located here are the second-order neurons that are crossing midline and ascending to form the anterolateral portion of the spinothalamic tracts.

Organization of the dorsal horn is not strictly based on anatomic location of the second-order neurons. Second-order neurons can also be organized by how they respond to stimuli and, therefore, by their function. There are high threshold neurons in Lamina I and II that are nociceptive specific and respond only to highly intense stimulation. The other type of second-order neuron, described above, which is based on how it responds is the WDR neuron (see Table 1.2). As the name suggests, these neurons respond to a wide range of stimulus intensities and they are able to respond with increased frequency based on how intense the stimulation is that they are receiving. This concept of a graded response to stimulation is how innocuous light touch is differentiated from a noxious pinch or squeeze. The location of these neurons is principally in the nucleus proprius (Laminae III, IV, V, and VI).

WDR neurons are also known as modality convergent neurons because they do not necessarily discriminate between the source of the primary afferent from which they receive input. As mentioned previously, the somatic and visceral afferents can cause a referred pain due to viscerosomatic convergence. This explains why pain caused by coronary artery occlusion during a myocardial infarction can cause a concomitant dermatomal pattern of pain. This convergence can also occur between deeper and more superficial somatic structures, which explains why deep muscle or bone pain can also show a pattern of dermatomal spread of pain similar to the referred pain of coronary artery ischemia.

Another characteristic of WDR neurons is that they can be prompted to exist in a state of ongoing discharge by low frequency, repetitive stimulation of C fiber primary afferents. This continuous discharge has been termed "wind-up" by Mendell and Wall in 1965. Wind up, also known now as central sensitization, will be discussed in detail later in the physiology section of this chapter.

Third-Order Neurons: Ascending and Descending Spinal Tracts and Supraspinal Projections[9–11]

In order to understand where the third-order neurons project, it is first necessary to understand the different individual ascending projections that make up the ascending sensory spinal tracts. The four major projections identified in the ventrolateral quadrant of the spinal cord are the spinothalamic, the spinoparabrachial, the spinoreticulothalamic, and the spinomesencephalic projections. A fifth ascending projection that transmits sensory information, but not necessarily pain unless

TABLE 1.2
Organization of Primary, Secondary, and Tertiary Neurons.

Primary Afferents	Secondary Projections	Tertiary Projections	Results
C fibers	Dorsal horn—Laminae I and II	Spinothalamic tracts to mediodorsalis nucleus of thalamus	Anterior cingulate cortex—emotional pain response
A-δ fibers	Dorsal horn—Laminae II and V	Spinothalamic tracts to ventrobasal thalamus	Somatosensory cortex—precision mapping of pain response
A-β fibers	Dorsal columns collateralization	Dorsal columns to medial lemniscus	Somatosensory cortex—tactile sensation and proprioception

the system is in a state of evoked hyperpathia, is the dorsal column medial lemniscal pathway. These projections terminate in three main brainstem regions: the diencephalon, the mesencephalon, and the medulla. The third-order neurons in these regions then project further to the cortex or within the diencephalon or mesencephalon.

The spinothalamic projections consist of both WDR neurons coming from the Lamina V portion of the dorsal horn and high threshold, pain-specific Lamina I neurons. The pain-specific, high threshold neurons make up the ascending tracts that will project into the posterior ventral medial nucleus (VMpo) and the medial dorsal nucleus of the thalamus. The third-order neurons in the medial dorsal nucleus then project to the anterior cingulate cortex. The third-order neurons in the VMpo then project to the insula. These pathways are both known to be less precise about the actual intensity and localization of the pain and more involved in the emotional and affectual aspects of pain. In contrast, the third-order neurons in the ventrobasal nucleus of the thalamus, where the WDR neurons from Lamina V terminate, are more precise about intensity and localization of the pain (see Fig. 1.3 and 1.5). Third-order neurons in the ventrobasal nucleus project to the somatosensory cortex and input in these areas follows a strict pattern that is consistent with the sensory homunculus in the cortex. In other words, input in this area can be interpreted over a range of intensities with precision as to what part of the body is affected somatotopically and what is the modality of the injury.

The spinoparabrachial projections start as ascending tracts in the contralateral ventrolateral section of the dorsal horn and they terminate in the parabrachial nucleus of the pons (see Fig. 1.4). Third-order neurons in this area then project to the amygdala and the VMpo. As noted earlier, the VMpo also projects to the insula, meaning that these projections appear to have a role in the "affective" aspect of pain. Previous animal and human studies of lesions in the areas of the temporal lobe and amygdala show a dysfunction in the association of the stimulus intensity of pain with its affective component (suffering).

The spinoreticulothalamic projections start as ascending tracts in the ipsilateral dorsal horn just like the WDR neurons of the spinothalamic tract, but these tracts ascend to the reticular formation of the medulla. Here, the third-order neurons project to the intralaminar nucleus of the thalamus that further relays

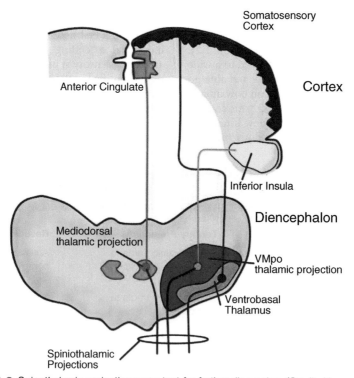

FIG. 1.3 Spinothalamic projections: see text for further discussion. (Credit: Nancy Dinh.)

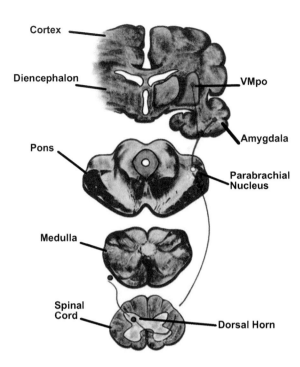

Cortex

Diencephalon

VMpo

Amygdala

Pons

Parabrachial
Nucleus

Medulla

Spinal
Cord

Dorsal Horn

FIG. 1.4 Spinoparabrachial projections: see text for further discussion. (Credit: Calvin Nguyen.)

information to many areas of the cortex. The reticular formation and its projections to the cortex are a part of the reticular activating system, which is in part responsible for regulating wakefulness and sleep-wake transition. This serves as a plausible pathway for pain interpretation to effect sleep and the sleep-wake pattern (see Fig. 1.5).

The spinomesencephalic projections start as ascending tracts as a part of the anterolateral system but terminate at the periaqueductal gray (PAG) matter and the reticular formation of the mesencephalon. From there, third-order neurons project to the lateral thalamus. The PAG is not well understood, but it does play a role in descending inhibition of pain through the bulbospinal pathway and it also causes autonomic responses in humans when stimulated (see Fig. 1.5).

While the transmission of the pain signal is known to be produced by the ascending tracts, there is some evidence that there are descending tracts that can facilitate the signal. The bulbospinal projections are descending tracts that transmit a signal in from the nucleus raphe magnus of the medulla to the dorsal horn that is excitatory in nature, but it serves to modulate the central sensitization at the WDR neuron level using serotonergic receptors.

As mentioned previously, the dorsal column projections are made up, in large part, due to the collateralization of the large, low threshold, primary afferents, A-β fibers (see Table 1.2). These ascending tracts stay ipsilateral and ascend along the dorsal columns to the nuclei in the medulla, where they then project to second-order neurons, which will cross over and continue to ascend as a part of the medial lemniscus to the thalamus. The third-order neurons there then project to the cortex. This system is not responsible specifically for pain, but it is responsible for tactile sensation and limb proprioception which can be painful in certain pathologic states that will be considered in the next sections (see Fig. 1.6).

PHYSIOLOGY OF NOCICEPTION
Acute Pain[12,13]

The initial report of pain and the physical movement to avoid a certain stimulus are responses that stem from activity that is initiated at the peripheral sensory terminal. This activity, in the form of a signal, sent via terminal depolarization of small unmyelinated (C fibers) and myelinated (A-δ fibers) primary afferent sensory neurons is due to the presence of potential damaging stimuli. This noxious stimulus, which can be thermal, chemical, or mechanical, creates a signal that the body identifies as pain.

In most cases, acute pain is considered to be protective, with the intention to remove the body from further harm. The initial noxious stimulus is sensed by peripheral nociceptors that communicate with the spinal cord and ultimately send the signal to cortical regions of the brain. The most immediate and direct response to a noxious stimulus is the flexor withdrawal reflex. When a nociceptor is activated by a noxious stimulus, the signal travels through the primary sensory neuron to the dorsal horn where it synapses with an interneuron. The interneuron synapses with an alpha motor neuron. Once the signal passes to the motor neuron, a motor command is sent from the ventral horn of the spinal cord to the flexor and extensor muscles resulting in removal of the body part from the noxious stimulus. This reflex does not require processing at the cortical level, allowing for a rapid response to avoid further injury.

The signal of nociception in this case is activation of C fibers. Activation of C fibers occurs with tissue pathology in the form of injury, inflammation, or infection. These disease states cause increase in inflammatory mediators including protons, prostaglandins (PGE2), thromboxanes, leukotrienes, growth factors, cytokines, chemokines, and neuropeptides

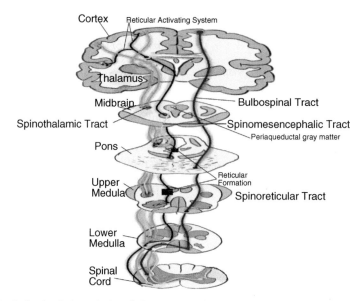

FIG. 1.5 Spinothalamic, Spinoreticular, Spinomesencephalic, and Bulbospinal projections. See text for further discussion. (Credit: Nancy Dinh.)

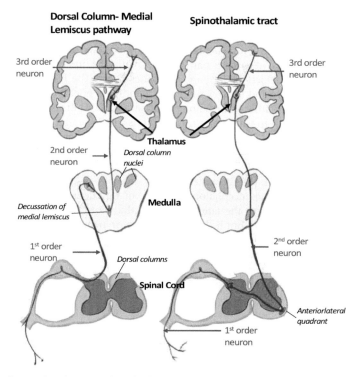

FIG. 1.6 Comparison between dorsal column and spinothalamic tracts. (Credit: Vanessa Tran.)

(see Table 1.1). The presence of inflammatory mediators in the periphery causes sensitization of the primary afferents and leads to hyperexcitable states. This hyperexcitable state can occur in all innervated tissues.

Persistent Pain[12]

For all intents and purposes, the hyperexcitable state in the periphery resolves when the inflammatory process resolves, except in certain cases where it does not resolve. Persistent pain states do occur due to sensitization in the periphery and at the dorsal horn, which is known as peripheral sensitization. When the sensitization occurs at the dorsal horn level or above, it is referred to as central sensitization.

Peripheral Sensitization[12,14]

In physiological states, the activation and firing of sensory nerve endings in response to nonnoxious stimuli occurs at a defined range. In states of chronic pain, the sensory nerve endings become sensitized such that they exhibit a reduced firing threshold and/ or an increased response to activation. This hyperexcitable response to noxious and nonnoxious stimuli is termed peripheral sensitization. Following tissue injury, cell damage occurs with activation of afferent nociceptive neurons and the aggregation of inflammatory cells at the site of injury. Activated nociceptors and nonneuronal cells release chemical mediators including protons, prostaglandins (PGE2), thromboxanes, leukotrienes, growth factors, cytokines, chemokines, and neuropeptides that mediate peripheral sensitization. Each of these extracellular products interacts with specific receptors found on the small afferent nerve ending (see Table 1.1).

Binding of these mediators to the respective receptor on the sensory afferent terminal leads to cellular depolarization, increased intracellular calcium, and activation of protein kinases (e.g., protein kinase C and mitogen-activated protein kinases). These kinases serve to alter transducer molecules (e.g., TRPV1) and ion channels (e.g., voltage-sensitive sodium channels) causing increased excitability of the nociceptor. In some cases, the nociceptors are sensitized in such a way to become spontaneously active (as initiated by the local chemical milieu). When this occurs, the nociceptor may be activated by a less intense physical stimulus resulting in an allodynic state. Peripheral sensitization leads to ongoing pain and primary hyperalgesia.

Dorsal Root Ganglia[15]

It has become increasingly apparent that the DRG is a complex local neural network. Aside from the presence of neuronal cell body of the afferent, the DRG is composed of astrocyte-like satellite cells that invest each cell body. The innervation provided by postganglionic sympathetic axons reflects the fact that the DRG lies outside the conventional blood-brain barrier and has a sympathetically innervated vasculature. They also have a large population of macrophages that are activated by neuroinflammatory stimuli, blood vessels, and of note, significant axon collaterals which arise from the DRG cell body to release neurotransmitters in the DRG (see Fig. 1.7). The importance of this complexity is that the DRG neuron can be the initiator of ectopic activity which drives action potentials down the glomerulus (connecting the cell body to its axon) and generate an action potential traveling both orthodromically as well as antidromically. The DRG also express the same receptors and channels that are

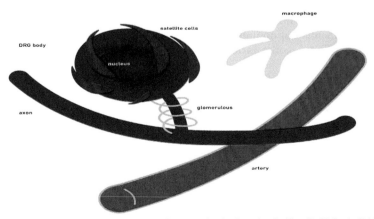

FIG. 1.7 Dorsal root ganglion structure. See text for further detail. (Credit: Kelly A. Eddinger.)

expressed on the afferent neuron terminals and correspondingly respond to the same mediators that act on these terminals. Following peripheral tissue injury, the DRG may initiate upregulation of voltage-gated Na and Ca channels as well as an increase in macrophages that release proinflammatory mediators that drive ectopic DRG activity.

Central Sensitization[12,16,17]

Central sensitization is the amplification and/or maintenance of peripheral nociceptive input at the spinal and supraspinal levels. Sensitization occurs due to increased excitation or reduced inhibition of excitatory primary afferent neurons. This occurs in response to persistent nociceptive input resulting in increased release of glutamate, calcitonin gene-related peptide (CGRP), brain-derived growth factor (BDGF), and substance P from primary afferent terminals in the spinal cord and trigeminal nucleus that results in activity-dependent changes in dorsal horn spinal function.

Second-order neurons receive input from both low and high threshold primary afferents. The input is received in a stimulus intensity-dependent manner so that an increase in discharge of WDR neurons results in an increase in output frequency. Repetitive stimulation of C fibers causes progressive and sustained partial depolarization of the cell making it more susceptible to future afferent input. Under normal conditions, the WDR neuron may be activated by a natural stimulus at a discrete location. After C fiber conditioning, a natural stimulus applied over a larger area now displays the ability to activate the same WDR neuron. As previously mentioned, this exaggerated discharge of WDR neurons evoked by repetitive stimulation of primary afferent neurons was termed "wind-up" by Mendell and Wall.

The result of central sensitization is an increased receptive field of the second-order neuron known as secondary hyperpathia by which pain can be evoked by a nonnoxious stimulus in adjacent noninjured tissue. Two mechanisms contribute to the increase in receptive field:

i) As reviewed above, primary sensory afferent neurons collateralize upon entering the spinal cord, sending segments rostrally and caudally up to several segments; and

ii) The facilitation of central sensitization is greatly dependent on phosphorylation of the glutamate-activated n-methyl-D-aspartate (NMDA) receptor. In physiological conditions, the NMDA channel remains quiescent due to continuous blockage by magnesium (Mg). However, when the membrane undergoes progressive depolarization as produced in response to repetitive stimulation via activation of AMPA and neurokinin 1 (NK1) receptors by glutamate and substance P, respectively, the Mg blockade is removed, and glutamate is able to activate the receptor. In response, there is an influx of Ca that activates voltage-gated Ca channels and phosphorylating enzymes including protein kinases A and C (PKA, PKC) and mitogen-activated protein kinases (MAPK). Thus, excitation of afferent input along the collaterals of distal segments is insufficient to cause the neuron to fire, but once neurons in that distal segment become sensitized (as with "wind-up") after injury, the input is sufficient to allow that distant segmental neuron to fire.

Specifically, PKC activates the NMDA receptor and Na channels, causing further depolarization contributing to "wind up." P38 MAPK phosphorylates enzymes including phospholipase A2, which initiates release of arachidonic acid and provides the substrate for cyclooxygenase (COX) to synthesize prostaglandins (PGE). PGE acts presynaptically to enhance opening of voltage-gated Ca channels and postsynaptically to block glycinergic inhibition at the interneuron level. The activation of afferent input and second-order neurons is regulated by local inhibitory interneurons containing inhibitory amino acids including GABA and glycine. When high frequency afferent input occurs, inhibition is reduced leading to increased response of WDR neurons. The loss of inhibition via GABA or glycine input augments the response of WDR neurons leading to facilitation of dorsal horn excitability (see Fig. 1.8).

Neuropathic Pain[18-21]

Neuropathic pain, defined as damage to the peripheral afferent nerve axon itself as opposed to other structures in the periphery around the primary afferent, causes an initial retrograde degeneration of the nerve axon in a process called Wallerian degeneration. This degeneration leads to axon sprouting, whereby the axons will attempt to reconnect causing a neuroma formation. This injury can cause peripheral and central sensitization just like injury in other areas, but it also causes a reorganization in the central processing of pain which should be differentiated from central or peripheral sensitization because it is specific to nerve cell damage.

The reorganization of central processing that occurs with neuropathic injury and pain is seen clinically with the phenomenon of tactile allodynia. This anomaly whereby large, low threshold, sensory primary afferents (A-β fibers) that are normally only activated causing a sensation of light touch can produce a nociceptive signal giving the sensation of pain reflects several events in two main areas of pain transmission:

i) Injured afferent axons will develop spontaneous activity. This ectopic activity arises both at the site of injury and from the DRG of the injured afferent neuron.

ii) The dorsal horn, following injury, will also show reorganization through multiple mechanisms including spinal glutamate release, microglia and astrocyte activity increase, loss of GABAergic and glycinergic control, and increased sympathetic input. As discussed earlier, glutamate is responsible for increased NMDA activation causing neuronal excitability. Astrocyte and microglia activation lead to increased COX, NOS, and glutamate, which contribute to a hyperexcitable state.

Normally, glycine agonism and GABA antagonism serve to regulate the excitatory potential of A-β fibers in the dorsal horn. Loss of that regulatory inhibition causes A-β fibers to produce an aggressive depolarization of the WDR neurons. Of note, after nerve injury, there does not appear to be a loss of GABA/glycine

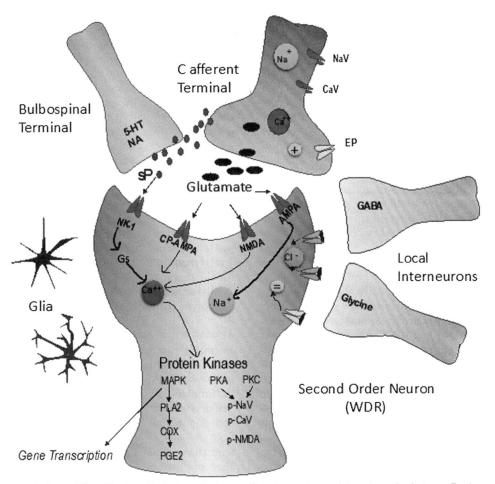

FIG. 1.8 Central Sensitization: Excitation of primary afferents produces glutamate and substance P release, which acts post synaptically on second-order neurons and excitation increases intracellular Calcium and activates a myriad of protein kinases. See text for further discussion. Sp, substance P; MAPK, mitogen-activated protein kinase; PLA2, phospholipase A2; PGE2, prostaglandin E2; Gs, stimulatory signaling protein; NA, noradrenalin, Ca^{++}, calcium; 5-HT, serotonin; Na^+, sodium; COX, cyclooxygenase; PKA, protein kinase A; PKC, protein kinase C; EP, prostaglandin receptor; CaV, voltage-gated calcium channel; NaV, voltage-gated sodium channel; NK-1, Neurokinin 1 receptor; AMPA receptor, a-amino-3-hydroxy-5methyl-4-isoxazolepropionic acid receptor; CP-AMPA, calcium permeable AMPA receptor; NMDA, N-methyl-D-aspartate receptor; WDR, wide dynamic range neuron. (Credit: Vanessa Tran.)

content release of receptors. However, it is now appreciated that after nerve injury, the chloride (Cl) gradient is altered due to the loss of cellular chloride transporters. As a result, at this point, GABA or glycine receptor activation results in an increased permeability to Cl, and in contrast to the normal state, Cl in the nerve injury animal will flow out carrying negative charge and resulting in a paradoxical depolarization. Hence, GABA and glycine release become an excitatory linkage rather that an inhibitory linkage.

Additionally, the presence of a neuroma will cause sympathetic postganglionic afferents to sprout and be present at the neuroma site and in the DRG. Stimulation of these sympathetics will drive ectopic activity at both the neuroma and at the DRG at that level.

Immune and Inflammatory Mechanisms[12,22-24]

It has been well established that the process of neuropathic and inflammatory pain not only involves neuronal pathways that transmit signals from peripheral tissue via the spinal cord to the brain but also immune cells that release and modulate a range of inflammatory mediators. Interestingly, evidence suggests that proinflammatory cytokines are able to act directly on nociceptors in the periphery as well as the dorsal horn of the spinal cord resulting in increased afferent input and subsequent peripheral and central sensitization, respectively. The immune system is comprised of two independent, but intricately connected systems—the innate immune system and the adaptive immune system. The innate immune system is continuously active and monitoring for foreign pathogens or injury to which it mounts a generalized response. Alternatively, the adaptive immune system is an acquired and specific immunity that retains memory from prior exposures. Emerging evidence has implicated both of these systems in the development of and maintenance of chronic pain.

Injury and inflammation give rise to the release of a variety of products that can activate sensory components of the innate immune system, through recognition sites such as the Toll-like receptors (TLRs). While classically expressed on inflammatory cells (macrophages), it became appreciated that they were also present on microglia and astrocytes in the neuraxis. Further, these signaling receptors are present on DRG neurons and of course on macrophages that are widely expressed in the DRG. Activated macrophages release inflammatory mediators, most notably tumor necrosis factor-α (TNF-α), interleukin-1β (IL-1β), nerve growth factor (NGF), nitric oxide (NO), and prostanoids as well as complement proteins that initiate the innate inflammatory cascade. Neutrophils are the predominant recruited cell type in an acute and early inflammatory response causing proinflammatory effects through the release of lipoxygenase products, prostaglandins, NO, cytokines, and chemokines as well as possible antinociceptive effects through the expression of opioids. The inflammatory mediators released by innate immune cells modulate peripheral and central sensitization that contributes to pain hypersensitivity.

Recent evidence suggests that adaptive immunity may also play a role in chronic pain; however, this role is less clear. The adaptive immune system is comprised of B and T cells. Although some recent data suggest that B cells may play a role through antibody production, the majority of recent literature has focused on the involvement of T cells in the production and resolution of chronic pain. Studies have found that infiltration of T cells occurs days to weeks postinjury, first at the site of injury and distal end of the nerve, then within the DRG, and last within the dorsal horn of the spinal cord. T cells have been found to both suppress and promote pain via multiple mechanisms and variations in expression. T cells may indirectly modulate neuroinflammation via the antiinflammatory reflex. In response to norepinephrine, β2-adrenergic receptor-expressing T cells release acetylcholine, which signals macrophages to switch from producing proinflammatory to antiinflammatory products causing dampening of the immune system. T cells present in the periphery also express receptors for glutamate, substance P, and CGRP, which regulate T-cell adhesion, migration, and immunological phenotype that drives neuroinflammation.

Transition of Acute to Chronic Pain[12,25-28]

Normally, pain resolves with termination of the acute noxious stimulus and resolution of tissue injury. In some cases, pain persists after the resolution of the acute inflammatory response. There is increased appreciation that development of persistent pain after an acute injury or inflammation may reflect a mechanistic transition from an acute to a chronic pain state reflecting long-term changes that sustain and amplify pain signaling. The mechanisms underlying this transition are complex and at present poorly understood. However, this process has been demonstrated in a variety of clinical pain states including after tissue injury, nerve damage, and inflammatory pain. Studies performed using experimental pain models such as K/BxN serum-transfer arthritis and collagen antibody-induced arthritis (CAIA) have found that the animals experience tactile allodynia that persists long after the localized swelling and inflammation has resolved. This process appears to involve discrete pathophysiological changes that are mediated by a combination of localized inflammatory mediators that drive peripheral and central sensitization and neuroimmune mechanisms.

As mentioned earlier, following tissue injury, damaged cells release factors that attract mast cells, macrophages, and neutrophils that release proinflammatory mediators and NGF. Proinflammatory molecules activate primary afferent neurons, including A-β fibers and C fibers, that initiate a process resulting in increased expression of Na channels that are thought to play a key role in spontaneous ectopic activity and increased peripheral sensitization. NGF, a neurotrophic factor that promotes the growth of damaged neurons, is also thought to play a role in sensitizing peripheral nociceptors through activation of TrkA receptors.

Meanwhile, similar changes occur in dorsal horn neurons with upregulation of Na and TRPV1 receptors contributing to a hyperexcitable state. Continuous stimulation also results in prolonged slow depolarization and activation of NMDA receptors that drive "wind-up" and neuroplastic changes that enhance signal transduction. Activation of intracellular signal transduction cascades lead to posttranslational changes of receptors and ion channels present on primary sensory and central neurons.

Although peripheral and central sensitization appears necessary for the transition from acute to chronic pain, recent studies suggest that immune mechanisms likely also play a role.

As reviewed above, small afferent input due to local injury produces ongoing molecule changes. Such changes occur at two levels. First, at the terminal (activation of kinases, increased expression of channels and receptors) leading to sensitization. Second in models of chronic inflammation, early inflammation leads to a postinflammation pain state where the animal displays enhanced peripheral afferent and postganglionic sympathetic sprouting in the joint and the DRG. It is interesting that many of these changes observed in chronic inflammatory states develop a phenotype (sprouting, glia activation) which resembles that of a nerve injury. Microglia provide the primary neuroimmune response and migrate to the central terminals of afferent peripheral nerves where they undergo activation in response to pain signals. Activated microglia signal the secretion of cytokines, chemokines, and neurotrophic factors that contribute to the development and maintenance of central sensitization. Notably, proliferation of microglia has been found in the ipsilateral dorsal horn after injury.

Recent studies have also identified Toll-like receptor 4 (TLR4) as a potential driver of the transition from acute to chronic pain. Using the K/BxN model of arthritis, researchers found that TLR4 knockout mice showed a resolution in pain that corresponded with the resolution of inflammation. Further work has demonstrated that administration of a TLR4 antagonist can prevent the development of persistent pain state in wild-type mice suggesting that spinal TLR4 signaling plays a significant role in mediating the transition from acute to chronic pain. There are undoubtably other regulatory systems that may have a similar impact.

REFERENCES

1. Cohen M, Quintner J, van Rysewyk S. Reconsidering the IASP definition of pain. *Pain Rep.* 2018;3.
2. Raja SN, Meyer RA, Campbell JN. Peripheral mechanisms of somatic pain. *Anesthesiology.* 1988;68:571.
3. Koltzenburg M. Neural mechanisms of cutaneous nociceptive pain. *Clin J Pain.* 2000;16(Suppl 3):S131.
4. Weidner C, Schmelz M, Schmidt R, Hansson B, Handwerker HO, Torebjörk HE. Functional attributes discriminating mechano-insensitive and mechano-responsive C nociceptors in human skin. *J Neurosci.* 1999;19(22):10184–10190.
5. Sikandar S, Dickenson AH. Visceral pain: the ins and outs, the ups and downs. *Curr Opin Support Palliat Care.* 2012; 6(1):17–26.
6. Willis Jr WD, Westlund KN. The role of the dorsal column pathway in visceral nociception. *Curr Pain Headache Rep.* 2001;5:20.
7. Ralston HJ. Pain and the primate thalamus. *Prog Brain Res.* 2005;1(49):1–10.
8. Willis WD. The somatosensory system, with emphasis on structures important for pain. *Brian Res Rev.* 2007;55: 297–313.
9. Central pain pathways: the spinothalamic tract. In: Purves D, Augustine GJ, Fitzpatrick D, et al., eds. *Neuroscience.* 2nd ed. Sunderland (MA): Sinauer Associates; 2001. Available from: https://www.ncbi.nlm.nih.gov/books/NBK10967/.
10. Price DD. Psychological and neural mechanisms of the affective dimension of pain. *Science.* 2000;288(5472): 1769–1772.
11. Dostrovsky J. Role of thalamus in pain. *Prog Brain Res.* 2000;129:245.
12. Woller S, Eddinger K, Corr M, Yaksh T. An overview of pathways encoding nociception. *Clin Exp Rheumatol.* 2017;35(Suppl. 107):S40–S46.
13. Brennan T, Zahn P, Pogatzki-Zahn E. Mechanisms of incisional pain. *Anesthesiol Clin North Am.* 2005;23(1).
14. Gangadharan V, Kuner R. Pain hypersensitivity mechanisms at a glance. *Dis Model Mech.* 2013;6(4):889–895.
15. Ahimsadasan N, Kumar A. Neuroanatomy, Dorsal Root Ganglion [Updated October 27, 2018]. In:

StatPearls. Treasure Island (FL): StatPearls Publishing; January 2019.

16. Woolf C. Central sensitization: implications for the diagnosis and treatment of pain. *Pain*. 2011;152(Suppl. 3):S2−S15.

17. Harte S, Harris R, Clauw D. The neurobiology of central sensitization. *J Appl Behav Res*. 2018;23:e12137.

18. Woolf C, Mannion R. Neuropathic pain: aetiology, symptoms, mechanisms, and management. *Lancet*. 1999; 353.

19. Costigan M, Scholz J, Woolf CJ. Neuropathic pain: a maladaptive response of the nervous system to damage. *Annu Rev Neurosci*. 2009;32:1−32.

20. Zeilhofer HU. *Cell Mol Life Sci*. 2005;62:2027.

21. Tsuda M, Masuda T, Tozaki-Saitoh H, Inoue K. Microglial regulation of neuropathic pain. *J Pharmacol Sci*. 2013; 121(2):89−94.

22. Totsch S, Sorge R. Immune system involvement in specific pain conditions. *Mol Pain*. 2018;13:1−17.

23. Laumet G, Ma J, Robison A, Kumari S, Heijnen C, Kavelaar A. T cells as an emerging target for chronic pain therapy. *Front Mol Neurosci*. 2019;12:216.

24. Bruno K, Woller S, Miller Y, et al. Targeting toll-like receptor -4 (TLR-4)-an emerging therapeutic target for persistent pain states. *Pain*. 2018:1−8.

25. Feizerfan A, Sheh G. Transition from acute to chronic pain. Continuing education in anaesthesia. *Criti Care Pain*. 2015;15:98−102.

26. Vallejo R, Tilley D, Vogel L, Benyamin R. The role of glia and immune system in the development and maintenance of neuropathic pain. *Pain Pract*. 2010;10:167−184.

27. Chapman R, Vierck C. The transition of acute postoperative to chronic pain: an integrative overview of research on mechanisms. *J Pain*. 2017;18:359e1−359e38.

28. Peng J, Gu N, Zhou L, et al. Microglia and monocytes synergistically promote the transition from acute to chronic pain after nerve injury. *Nat Commun*. 2016;7.

CHAPTER 2

Headache

DONALD MCGEARY, PHD

INTRODUCTION

Headache is an extraordinarily common and disabling condition that, despite widespread attention in both the scientific literature and popular media, is still poorly understood. The Global Burden of Diseases, Injuries, and Risk Factors (GBD) studies identified headache as a "global public health concern" with an estimated 3 billion people worldwide experiencing a primary headache (migraine or tension-type headache [TTH]) in 2016.[1] GBD studies found that more people worldwide experienced TTHs compared to other common headache types (1.89 billion compared to 1.04 billion migraineurs), though migraine was significantly more disabling, especially among women. Although some may consider headache as less disabling than chronic musculoskeletal pain because of the episodic nature of headache presentation, it is important to note that headache-related disability often extends beyond discrete head pain episodes as patients seek to limit exposure to potential headache triggers. Unlike chronic musculoskeletal pain, headache is difficult to assess because it can differ across a number of dimensions including pain intensity, duration of headache episodes, and frequency of headache episodes (whereas musculoskeletal pain is often assessed as a continuous phenomenon focusing primarily on pain intensity). Classification of headache is generally broken into two categories: primary and secondary headache. Primary headaches (those that develop through their own mechanisms) include migraine, tension-type, and trigeminal neuralgia headaches. Secondary headache includes headache that develops as a result another physical condition including head injury, vascular/nonvascular cranial disorders, substance use, and psychiatric disorders (Fig. 2.1).

This chapter will describe the three primary headaches (because of their high prevalence) and their recommended treatments and will briefly touch on one of the more common secondary headaches (posttraumatic headache [PTH]: headache related to head or neck injury). Each section will also discuss headache assessment. Finally, this chapter will close with a discussion of *Medication Overuse Headache*, a subcategory of headache attributable to overuse of medication for headache control.

PRIMARY HEADACHES

Migraine Headache

Migraine headaches may occur in up to 12% of the US population with significantly higher prevalence among women (18%) compared to men (6%[2]). Both episodic (<15 headache days per month) and chronic migraine (≥15 headache days per month) are significantly disabling and are more likely to occur in individuals with chronic musculoskeletal pain, asthma, and mood disorders.[3,4] According to the third edition of the International Classification of Headache Disorders (ICHD-3[5]), migraine headache is characterized as headache lasting from 4 to 72 h (when untreated) during which nausea/vomiting and/or sensitivity to light or sound (photophobia, phonophobia) will occur. To be classified as migraine, headache must include at least two of the following characteristics: unilateral location, pulsating pain quality, moderate to severe intensity, and/or aggravation with activity. Migraine can be classified into two major "types" based on the presence or absence of aura symptoms (sensory, speech, motor, retinal, or head/neck pain symptoms). Although there is extensive extant studies of mechanistic differences between the two migraine types, there is little available information about how treatment could differ between the two groups (due to a paucity of comparative trials and the likelihood that many migraineurs experience both types of migraine[6]). (Table 2.1).

Pain Care Essentials and Innovations. https://doi.org/10.1016/B978-0-323-72216-2.00002-8

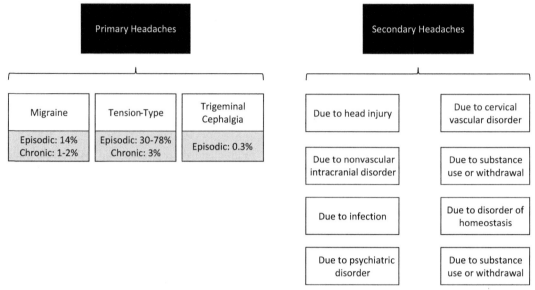

FIG. 2.1 ICHD-3 organization of headache diagnostic categories.

Despite extensive study, there is still some debate on the underlying putative mechanisms that drive migraine headache. There is strong evidence supporting the roles of genetics/epigenetics, hormones, neurological factors, nutrition, and vascular changes, but the evolution of migraine across time and situations makes it difficult to specify general risk factors for migraine. Fortunately, the broad range of causal factors makes migraine headache one of the most widely researched forms of head pain, resulting in numerous available treatments and a robust body of research literature assessing the efficacy of these treatments.

Migraine headache is best assessed using a headache diary (described in detail below) and measures of headache-related disability. Self-report measures of disability allow a treatment provider to assess the impact that headache experience has on an individual's functioning, in some cases with more precision than objective functional measures (i.e., functional capacity evaluation). Self-limiting and psychological disability are significant components of migraine experience. Migraineurs certainly limit activity (including socialization) during a migraine episode but may also do so between episodes in order to avoid environmental or stress-related triggers that may foster another headache. Thus, measures of self-reported disability are the most powerful tools for assessing the mechanisms and extent to which an individual with migraine is disabled by their headache. The Migraine Disability Assessment (MIDAS) questionnaire is perhaps the most commonly used self-report disability measure for migraine. MIDAS assesses disability across multiple life domains (school/work, housework, recreation) using five brief items asking patients to report the number of days over the last 3 months for which activity in a given domain was avoided or otherwise affected by headache. Total MIDAS scores correlate significantly with physician judgments about headache severity.[8] (Table2.2).

Prophylactic treatments: Migraine prophylactic agents are highly researched but underutilized in migraineurs.[7] These agents are designed to address biological trigger mechanisms for headache onset through various therapeutic channels including alteration of neurotransmitters, calcium channel blocking mechanisms, and direct action on peripheral and central pain networks. Although patients benefit from multiple options for migraine prophylaxis, which can be tailored to maximally benefit each individual migraineur, there is a paucity of comparative research that can be used to help providers choose which agents work best for certain types of migraine patients. Jackson and colleagues[7] meta-analyzed 53 different studies of over 10 different migraine prophylactic agent types and found that most agents resulted in a clinically significant decrease in headache days. The authors found that drugs like amitriptyline (an atypical antidepressant) produced consistently strong migraine prevention outcomes, though there was limited evidence supporting amitriptyline as superior to other agents. They did note that tailored migraine prevention is supported by the available research, especially when tailoring is done to accommodate comorbid health conditions (e.g., prescribing beta-blockers for migraineurs with comorbid hypertension). Some have cautioned that treating providers should first consider FDA-recommended

TABLE 2.1
ICHD-3 diagnostic criteria for migraine headache.

Core Features	Subtype Features	Duration
At least five attacks Duration between 4 and 72 h 2+ of these features: • Unilateral • Pulsating quality • Moderate/severe pain • Aggravation by activity	*With aura*: At least two headaches with fully reversible aura meeting three of the following: • Aura may spread • More than one aura symptom may present • Aura lasts 5–60 min • Aura is unilateral • Aura is positive • Headache follows aura within 1 hour	Headache on 15+ days/month for 3+ months
At least one of the following: • Nausea/vomiting • Photo/phonophobia	*Hemiplegic migraine*: Aura presents with fully reversible motor weakness, sensory and/or, speech symptoms	8 days/month, headache meets criteria for either type of migraine

frontline agents for migraine prophylaxis (e.g., divalproex, topiramate, metoprolol, etc.) followed by amitriptyline as a second-line option.[9]

Abortive treatments: While prophylactic agents are designed to prevent the onset of migraine headache, abortive medications are used to diminish and potentially stop migraine symptoms after the headache begins. Stopping migraine symptom cascade is more difficult than preventing onset, so outcomes of abortive treatments are likely less powerful than prophylactic outcomes. Unfortunately, because prophylactic agents are underutilized in migraine management, there is some evidence showing that migraine sufferers use abortive agents to control migraines at very high rates. For example, one study of prescription patterns for migraine from 1998 to 2006 found that anti-inflammatory analgesics were used (as an abortive agent) at much higher rates than prophylactic medications like triptans.[10] As with prophylactic medication, abortive agents should be tailored to everyone's headache presentation and clinical picture. Lucas[11] recommends using simple analgesics to address mild migraine symptoms, and stronger medications should be used for more severe symptoms (including tailored responses to address cooccurring nausea and vomiting). Al-Quliti and Assaedi[12] recommend distinguishing between nonspecific (analgesics, anti-inflammatory) and specific (ergots, triptans) abortive agents, with nonspecific agents recommended for children who can tolerate potential gastrointestinal side effects and specific agents like triptans recommended for more severe migraine when given early in migraine onset. Migraineurs use

opioid medications at higher rates than the general public, and opioid medications are frequently used to address patients with severe migraine symptoms (even children and young adults), especially when these patients present for care in Emergency Departments.[13,14] Most abortive agents are more effective in terminating severe migraine compared to opioids, and prolonged opioid use can result in increased head pain (due to opioid-induced hyperalgesia), opioid dependence, and gastrointestinal symptoms.[13,15,16] Generally, the evolving research literature warns against using opioid medications for headache control in any venue, and other treatment options are recommended. Finally, migraine treatment providers increasingly recommend botulinum toxin (e.g., BTX-A or Botox), a neurotoxic protein that can inhibit muscle spasms and hyperactivity, for the treatment of chronic migraine headache. Injection of BTX-A into pericranial muscles can significantly improve migraine headache and decrease reliance on medication for migraine control, which some investigators attribute to better control of muscle contraction migraine triggering.[17] A recent study of BTX-A for chronic migraine found a median decrease of 3.5 headache days per month as well as decreased analgesic medication use for up to 9 months, though the investigation did not detect a significant improvement in headache-related disability in this small and possibly underpowered study.[18] Larger controlled trials are needed to better affirm the short- and long-term benefits of botox for migraine.

Controversy: CGRP receptor antagonists and monoclonal antibodies: Recent studies have identified calcitonin

	Migraine disability assessment test	Six-item headache impact test
Headache diary	**MIDAS**	**HIT-6**
Various formats available	5 patient self-report items	6 patient self-report items
Assess:	Assess # of days migraine affected	Rate frequency of headache
Headache frequency	various activities over the past 3	symptoms severity over the past 4
Episode intensity	months	weeks
Episode duration	2 supplemental questions for	Numeric rating scale (6,8,10,11,13
Most common summary is headache	providers	points per item)
days/month	Score = sum of days across the 5	Score = sum of points across all 6
Can use headache index	patient self-report items	items

TABLE 2.2
Summary of common migraine headache assessment tools.

gene–related peptide as a possible mechanism for episodic migraine. These studies gave rise to an evolving clinical trial landscape assessing the safety and efficacy of CGRP monoclonal antibodies as a potential treatment for these debilitating headache. As described by Moriarty and colleagues,[19] CGRP is a neuropeptide with broad influence over multiple putative mechanisms of migraine including vasodilation and pain signaling pathways, and CGRP has been shown to upregulate during migraine headache events (cf.[20]). Experimental infusion of CGRP has been linked to migraine onset, cementing CGRP as a causal mechanism in migraine headache.[21] Growing interest in CGRP as a causative factor in migraine led to the emergence of pharmacological interventions that block CGRP effects. Unfortunately, small-molecule CGRP antagonists, though effective, have been linked to liver toxicity, slowing development of these agents in migraine clinical trials. Attention has now turned to CGRP monoclonal antibodies (mAbs) as an effective and safe alternative due to the specificity of mAbs treatment targets and lower potential liver toxicity compared to small-molecule CGRP antagonists.[22] To date, there are over 20 available CGRP monoclonal antibodies, studies of which have returned largely favorable outcomes. There is some equivocation in the extant body of available research at the time of this chapter regarding efficacy and safety of CGRP mAb (cf. [23]), and more research is likely needed to confirm their effectiveness compared to other migraine treatments.

Nonpharmacological migraine treatment: Numerous studies have confirmed both the benefit and safe side effect profile of nonpharmacological interventions (NPIs) for migraine, though these treatments are highly underutilized due to a lack of awareness among medical providers about the efficacy of these interventions and lack of availability of strong NPI in the

treatment community. Foremost among migraine NPIs, cognitive and behavioral therapies (CBT) have the strongest level of support. CBT approaches to migraine management combine behavior change, migraine trigger management, cognitive therapies to address alarming cognitions about stress and headache, and relaxation strategies to reduce headache interference in functioning and improve quality of life. Once engaged with CBT, treatment retention rates are comparable to standard medical care,[24] and patients report high levels of satisfaction with CBT-based migraine interventions.[25] A meta-analysis of CBT for migraine found nine times greater odds of significant improvement in migraine for pediatric samples, [26] and one of the largest studies of CBT for pediatric migraine to date found that the addition of CBT to amitriptyline doubled the improvement in headache days per months compared to amitriptyline alone.[27,28] Indeed, comparisons of pharmacological to NPIs for pediatric migraine conclude that CBT-based interventions should be a frontline option for children with migraine because of the minimal side effects and stronger outcomes for CBT in extant studies.[29] Some CBT treatments will offer stress management and/or relaxation using biofeedback. Biofeedback is not a "type" of treatment for migraine but serves as a treatment adjunct, often using thermal or electromyographic sensors to help the patient identify and manage physiological stress. Decreased physical stress is associated with better headache outcomes, but there is some debate about the added benefit of biofeedback as an adjunct to behavioral relaxation training and concerns about patient retention for biofeedback-assisted relaxation.[30] There is growing evidence that complementary and integrative health interventions like yoga and acupuncture are helpful for abortive migraine treatment, with preliminary outcomes showing decreased reliance on medication for migraine treatment with prolonged use of these interventions.[31] Physical therapy can improve some migraine symptoms particularly in patients with cervical or temporomandibular pain.[32,33] Massage therapy is often offered as a migraine intervention, though the research on massage for migraine is not yet well-developed and the putative mechanisms of benefit for massage in migraine are unclear (Fig. 2.2).

Conclusion: Migraine headaches represent one of the most prevalent and debilitating pain conditions worldwide. Although episodic migraine may occur at a lower frequency than chronic headache, both can be disabling at all times due to both headache experience and changes in behavior and function caused by concern about future headache episodes. Although research on the putative mechanisms of migraine is still developing, there are numerous treatment options available, many of which result in significant clinical improvement. Prophylactic and abortive medications can either prevent migraine onset or reduce episode duration, frequency or intensity, and NPIs (especially CBT) can significantly improve migraine with minimal side effects. Emerging treatments for migraine (e.g., CGRP mAb) offer great promise, though the research on these interventions is nascent.

Tension-Type Headache

Tension-type headache is one of the most common forms of headache with an estimated lifetime prevalence between 30% and 78% worldwide.[5] The International Classification of Headache Disorders—Third Edition differentiates TTH from migraine based on an absence of nausea or vomiting and an absence of photophobia and phonophobia. TTH is diagnosed if duration of headache episodes ranges between 30 min and 7 days and two of the following characteristics are present: the headache pain is bilateral, of a pressing or pulsing quality, mild or moderate intensity, and/or *not* aggravated by physical activity. TTHs can be further differentiated based on the frequency of the headache. TTH occurring less than 1 day per month is considered *infrequent episodic TTH*, one to 14 days a month is *frequent episodic*, and 15 or more days per month for more than 3 months is considered *chronic*. Notably, there is some debate about the distinction between chronic TTH and migraine without aura, making treatment for chronic TTH somewhat difficult.[34] When classifying TTH frequency, it is important to note that the headache episodes may change over time and repeated assessment of headache frequency is required to ensure appropriate classification (Table 2.3).

TTH is a deceptive form of headache which presents with similar clinical characteristics to muscular pain, but the mechanisms that drive TTH are not purely muscular and likely involve a host of factors including central pain sensitization, peripheral excitability, muscle hyperalgesia, changes in neurotransmitters, and genetics and psychiatric comorbidities.[35,36] Neurophysiological studies of TTH have identified roles for brainstem hyperexcitability and generalized abnormality of neural excitability beyond cranial nerves, though an overview of these studies warned that extant neurophysiological TTH studies are methodologically weak.[37] Attempts to experimentally induce TTH has shed some light on their underlying pathophysiology. Exposto and colleagues[38] used a tooth clenching task to induce TTH and found that changes in pericranial tenderness did not predict headache onset, as expected based on some theories of TTH origin. Pain modulation profiles (which use information from conditioned pain modulation and temporal summation of pain to predict pain and response to

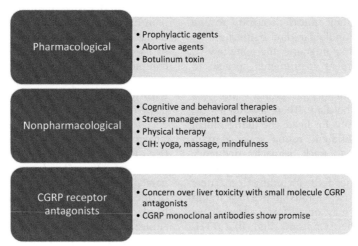

FIG. 2.2 Accepted migraine treatments.

TABLE 2.3
Diagnositic criteria for tension-type headache.

TTH Subtype	Frequency	Duration	Characteristics	Rule-Outs
Infrequent, episodic	10 episodes < 1 day/month	30 min to 7 days	Bilateral pressing or tightening mild to moderate	No nausea No vomiting Not worsened by activity
Frequent, episodic	10 episodes 1-14 days/month for > 3 months			
Chronic	Headache occurs ≥ 15 days/month	Hours to days unremitting		No more than one photo/phonophobia No moderate/severe nausea or vomiting

pain treatment[39]) also failed to predict TTH onset leading the authors to suggest that pain modulation may be an effect of TTH instead of a cause. Unfortunately, TTH often cooccurs with migraine making mechanistic studies of TTH very difficult.[40] Much more research is needed to further elucidate mechanisms specific to TTH.

TTH may be perpetuated and exacerbated through co-morbid conditions like insomnia and myofascial pain syndromes that add considerable complexity to assessment and treatment. Sleep problems are highly prevalent among individuals with TTH, particularly those who fit criteria for chronic TTH.[41] Jay and Barkin[42] offer a nice description of the various pathways through which sleep difficulties influence TTH, noting disturbance in stage 4 sleep (which may be beneficially addressed with low-dose tricyclic antidepressants) and increased pain accompanying poor sleep that could worsen the impact of TTH. TTH is also associated with myofascial pain syndromes, characterized by regional pain experience and cranial, temporomandibular, sternal/clavicular, and trapezius trigger points.[42] Myofascial pain may influence TTH through chronic muscle tension, posture changes, and temporomandibular joint dysfunction.[43]

TTH assessment: Unlike migraine, there are few (if any) headache assessment instruments specific to TTH. Due to the variable and episodic nature of most TTH, the most recommended assessment tool is a comprehensive headache diary. There are numerous, publicly available options for headache diaries, most of which include a numeric rating scale of pain intensity, mechanisms to track headache frequency and duration, and fields for recording circumstantial factors that may affect headache including sleep, stress levels, and medication use. Various studies have found that headache diaries may outperform retrospective self-report of headache symptoms and that TTH-sufferers, especially children, are likely to overreport

pain intensity using retrospective recall compared to prospective diary entries.[44] Some warn, however, that retrospective report of headache does provide valuable information about headache experience, and the best approach for TTH assessment is to combine headache diaries and interviews.[45] Despite their usefulness, there is concern that headache diaries may offer limited data about headache experience due to poor patient adherence to completing diary entries. One study found a high number of missing diary entries over a 30-day assessment period (15 mean missing entries) using a long-form paper diary and several recording or transcription errors in diary entries that affected data validity.[46] However, the investigators found fewer omissions and errors on brief electronic headache diaries, suggesting that transition to now ubiquitous e-diaries for headache could improve their validity and utility.

Scoring and using headache diary data can be difficult. Most chronic pain conditions are meaningfully assessed and easily summarized using measures of pain intensity (cf. [47]), self-reported disability,[48] functional quantification, and pain interference.[49] Because of its episodic presentation, however, headache is a complex phenomenon to measure. Regular headache diaries assess the quality, frequency, duration, and intensity of headaches, but there is little guidance on how to weigh these dimensions of headache experience to produce a summary of headache pain. Some suggest that headache dimensions can be multiplied (e.g., frequency * duration) resulting in a "headache index" (cf.[50]) or "headache ratio" (cf.[51]). Unfortunately, there are no extant studies supporting the use of these index varables and no data showing how headache index scores link to other meaningful clinical variables (e.g., psychiatric comorbidity). Most diaries will rely on either headache frequency or intensity without attempting to combine these metrics into a headache index.

Pharmacological treatment: Patients with TTH seek treatment at notably lower rates (16%) than migraineurs (56%;[52]), but when accounting for headache frequency (TTH is generally more frequent than migraine), TTH patients use pharmacological interventions at much higher rates.[40] The broad array of factors contributing to TTH allows for a similarly broad scope of pharmacological interventions, though analgesics and nonsteroidal anti-inflammatory drugs (NSAIDs) are the most recommended and studied treatments.[35] One meta-analysis of TTH analgesic studies found that NSAIDs and acetaminophen were significantly more effective for TTH management than placebo, and there were equivocal findings comparing NSAIDs to acetaminophen for acute TTH.[53] The investigators found no significant difference in efficacy across different NSAID drugs, though they did note differences in adverse event profiles that may guide selection of some compounds (e.g., aspirin use was associated with higher risk of gastrointestinal complaints compared to ibuprofen). Fumal and Schoenen[35] note that COX-2 inhibitors have shown some benefit for acute TTH management, though data comparing these compounds to NSAIDs are limited. Some suggest that adjuvant caffeine may increase the effectiveness of NSAIDs and simple analgesics.[54,55] Unfortunately, overreliance on analgesic medication is a significant concern for TTH patients. Schnider and colleagues[56] studied analgesic use in a cohort of 80 TTH patients and found very high levels of use resulting in "considerable risk" for medication overuse headache (MOH) (described in more detail below).

Most TTH pharmacotherapy targets acute treatment of episodic headache, but there is an evolving literature on the prophylactic use of certain compounds for patients with chronic TTH. Most available research supports amitriptyline as the best frontline prophylactic agent for chronic TTH.[57,58] The success of amitriptyline and other tricyclic antidepressants and mirtazapine (a tetracyclic antidepression) in preventing chronic TTH may be due to alterations in central pain processing (cf.[40]), though this mechanism is not strongly addressed in extant research. Recent studies of prophylactic pharmacotherapy for chronic TTH found that almost all patients taking a prophylactic agent are taking amitriptyline, and over 70% in one study found it effective,[59] though there are studies that found an insignificant change in TTH with amitriptyline (cf.[60]). Boz and colleagues[61] compared prophylactic amitriptyline to the selective serotonin reuptake inhibitor sertraline and found that both agents significantly reduced TTH symptoms. However, outcomes associated with amitriptyline were noticeably superior to sertraline, further cementing amitriptyline as the best frontline prophylactic agent.

Nonpharmacological treatment: Many of the nonpharmacological treatments recommended for migraine are also recommended, and strongly supported, for TTH. CBT can significantly improve TTH through the same stress management and cognitive restructuring mechanisms that are effective in migraine studies. Holroyd and Stensland[62] found that CBT interventions are just as effective as tricyclic medication for TTH, but found that CBT produced broader benefits than the medication that likely added to improved headache coping. Motoya and colleagues[63] explored cognitive mechanisms through which CBT might benefit TTH in a small pilot sample and found that TTH patients who complete CBT report fewer catastrophic/alarming thoughts about their pain and decreased pain-related activity avoidance, both of which are likely to significantly improve disability. As is the case for migraine, complementary and integrative health approaches are receiving increasing attention in the management of TTH. One recent study tested acupuncture and massage for TTH and found that both treatments resulted in significant decrease in the frequency and intensity of tension headaches.[64] Studies of chiropractic care for TTH offer some promising findings of decreased headache frequency[65] though the research on chiropractic for headache is underdeveloped and nascent, and more research is needed to reliably conclude that chiropractic care is truly beneficial for TTH (Fig. 2.3).

Conclusion: TTH is one of the most common and understudied forms of headache. Although mechanisms of TTH are still not well-understood, there is widespread agreement that these headaches are multifactorial, and patients are likely to benefit most from treatment plans that combine pharmacotherapies with effective nonpharmacological self-management strategies. Most patients with TTH will benefit from analgesic medications, and amitriptyline is often recommended as a first-line agent for prophylaxis of chronic TTH. TTH clinical characteristics (including frequency, duration, and intensity of episodes) can change over time, so repeated assessment with a brief pain diary is vital to good TTH treatment. Furthermore, TTH is vulnerable to exacerbation from comorbid conditions, so assessment of other pain conditions (especially myofascial pain), sleep, and mood disorders is necessary to ensure a comprehensive and effective treatment plan.

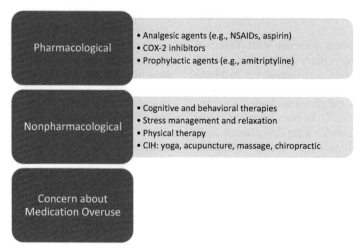

FIG. 2.3 Accepted tension-type headache treatments.

Trigeminal Autonomic Cephalgia

Trigeminal autonomic cephalgia (TACs) represent a relatively uncommon (affecting approximately 0.1% of the population) but clinically significant group of headaches (including cluster headaches, paroxysmal hemicranias, and hemicranias continua) that are regarded by some to be among the most painful and disabling headache presentations.[66] The ICHD-3[5] describes TACs as headaches with "prominent cranial parasympathetic autonomic features" often presenting as unilateral headache and putatively caused by activation of "a normal human trigeminal-parasympathetic reflex." Parasympathetic autonomic TAC features (including conjunctival injection and cranial autonomic symptoms) almost always occur ipsilateral to unilateral TAC headache. This is a clear distinction from other unilateral headache types with comorbid autonomic or aura symptoms (e.g., migraine) for which aura is rarely (if ever) identified as solely ipsilateral to the headache side.[66] There is some debate about the role of peripheral versus central nervous system mechanisms in TAC headache, though emerging evidence is starting to confirm that the central nervous system, especially the hypothalamus, may be particularly important in terminating TAC.[67] Fortunately, our understanding of therapeutic targets for TAC is rapidly expanding leading to novel treatments that show great promise.[69]

Several headache "subtypes" appear within the TAC category; prominent among them are cluster headaches and paroxysmal hemicranias. Cluster headache (which accounts for almost 90%) of TAC,[69] is defined by the ICHD-3 as severe or very severe sub-/ superorbital and/or temporal headache pain lasting between 15 min and 3 hours. Per the ICHD-3 diagnostic criteria, cluster headaches present as "bouts" of severely painful headaches with up to eight discrete headaches experienced in a single day. Cluster headache present with ipsilateral trigeminal symptoms like lacrimation, rhinorrhea, facial sweating, miosis/ ptosis, and/or restlessness or agitation. The ICHD-3 defines paroxysmal hemicranias, like cluster headache, as severe unilateral headache with cooccurring ipsilateral symptoms. Paroxysmal hemicranias diverge from cluster headache, however, through evidence of absolute arrest of headache with indomethacin (an NSAID) and headache duration between 2 and 30 min. Short-lasting unilateral neuralgiform headaches share all of the common characteristics of cluster headache and paroxysmal hemicranias, though these headaches present as single "stabbing" headaches or a series a "stabbing" pain episodes. Generally, cluster headaches present with longer episode duration (about 45–90 min) and lower frequency compared to other TACs; peripheral hemicrania headaches are of relative intermediate duration and frequency, and hemicrania continua are the most frequent.[66]

Treatment: In some cases, the front line of treatment for TAC is prevention through trigger avoidance.[68] For example, alcohol is a common trigger for cluster headache, so many cluster headache patients should be advised to avoid alcohol to prevent headache.[69] Some individuals with cluster headache (around 4% in one published study) and hemicrania continua reported worsening of headache symptoms with medication overuse, so education and behavior change around overuse of medication are recommended to prevent TAC headaches from worsening or transitioning into chronic, daily headaches.[70] TAC headaches tend to develop quickly, so abortive medications must be fast-acting to be useful. Cluster headache patients benefit most from abortive treatment with triptan medication (e.g., 6 mg of sumatriptan) or 15—20 min of exposure to pure oxygen. Agents like verapamil (a calcium channel blocker) are recommended as first-line preventative treatment for chronic cluster headache. As noted above, paroxysmal hemicrania diagnostically requires complete relief with indomethacin, thus indomethacin is considered a frontline treatment for these TAC headaches. For patients who are intolerant to indomethacin, cyclooxygenase 2 selective inhibitors may be beneficial.[66] Short-lasting unilateral neuralgiform headache is rare, so the literature-guiding treatment of these severely painful headaches is somewhat limited. Most neuralgiform headache will respond well to lamotrigine, though a few small trials have also found some support with topiramate.[66] Research on NPI for TAC is extraordinarily rare, and NPI is not often used to address these very brief headaches because of the extended time it takes to establish a meaningful dose of NPI versus the short duration of TAC headache.

Conclusion: TACs, though rare, are a significant concern because of the severe or very severe intensity of TAC symptoms. Because many TAC headaches are brief, there is limited research guiding the assessment and treatment of these headaches. Fortunately, many TAC headaches are characterized by strong response to medication, which will benefit most patients. As noted above, some behavior change (e.g., avoidance of alcohol) may help prevent TAC onset.

SECONDARY HEADACHE

Secondary headaches are differentiated from primary headaches due to onset attributable to another health condition. It is important to note that some primary headaches may be reclassified or coclassified as secondary headache if the course or presentation of the headache is altered by a comorbid medical condition. Thus, there is no defining clinical characteristic for secondary headache, and some secondary headaches may best be addressed through effective treatment of the causal condition and frontline therapies that suit the headache phenotype. For example, if migraine headache is worsened after head injury, treatment may start with therapeutic agents that are effective for chronic migraine. Headache that starts after

misuse/abuse or withdrawal of a substance can be treated through management of withdrawal and withdrawal symptoms. Because of the heterogeneity of these headaches, this chapter will not cover all possible secondary headaches. However, headache related to an injury to the head or neck (also called PTH) and headache related to medication overuse will both be discussed because of their high prevalence and associated disability.

Headache Related to Injury to Head or Neck (Posttraumatic Headache)

Posttraumatic headache is the most common and disabling symptom of traumatic brain injury (TBI), and federal agencies have dedicated significant resources to the diagnosis, management, and treatment of PTH.[71,72] The International Classification of Headache Disorders, Third Edition[5] defines PTH as persistent or acute headache attributed to traumatic injury to the head or the neck. Persistent PTH (lasting longer than 3 months) is highly prevalent among military veterans with TBI, and these headaches are increasingly recognized as the most disabling component of TBI.[73] Military veterans report significantly higher rates of PTH after a head injury (81%—97%) compared to civilians (6%—85%[71,74,75]; with a high rate of migraine-type symptoms and comorbid posttraumatic stress disorder (PTSD[76]). The exact mechanisms driving PTH remain a mystery, but growing evidence supports a significant role of posttraumatic stress disorder (PTSD) in headache chronicity and intensity[77] that may be stronger than that of more proximal headache causes like TBI.[73]

Treatment: Treatments for persistent PTH are slowly evolving and mounting evidence of predominant migraine characteristics in PTH have led some to explore existing migraine treatments for these debilitating headaches.[78] Chronic PTH can be highly disabling and a better understanding of this phenomenon is needed to identify treatments that can help patients overcome the impact of PTH on work absenteeism, decreased engagement with family, and decreased quality of life.[79] As of 2017, there were no FDA-approved medications that specifically treat PTH, and NPIs that are effective in primary headache have shown only modest benefits for patients with PTH and, in some cases, may actually increase disability due to paying more attention to headache symptoms during the treatment.[80] Fraser and colleagues identified some small studies of NPIs that appear promising, but the sample sizes were too small to draw firm conclusions about the efficacy of nonpharmacological treatments like cognitive-behavioral therapies and biofeedback-assisted relaxation. Pharmacological interventions currently under study include prophylactic and abortive agents for migraine and nonvasconstrictile agents like CGRP antagonists and 5-HT1F agonists, though side effect profiles of these agents may leave some patients unwilling to use them long-term,[71] and long-term medication use can actually worsen headache symptoms resulting in MOH. Because pharmacological agents are limited to headache symptoms and fail to address psychiatric comorbidities that contribute to headache chronicity and disability, contemporary research emphasizes comprehensive nonpharmacological strategies that can address both military PTH and comorbid trauma symptoms.[76,77]

Controversy about PTH definition: PTH is unique among headache disorders because PTH is classified by the mechanism of headache onset instead of the profile of headache symptoms. This results in PTH as a headache "type" without any defining clinical characteristics. PTH tends be more prevalent after a mild TBI (54%) compared to moderate or severe TBI (44%) and, unlike migraine, neither sex nor age appears to influence PTH presentation.[78] According to the ICHD-3 criteria, PTH is broadly classified in two ways: by chronicity and by mechanism of injury. PTH can be either acute (duration less than 3 months, 90% of which will abate without intervention) or chronic (duration greater than 3 months, few of which abate within a year). Distressingly, there is growing evidence showing that individuals who suffer mild TBI have a high likelihood of developing chronic PTH that is recalcitrant to frontline interventions for primary headache.[81] ICHD-3 criteria account for PTH caused by mild or severe trauma but make no distinction for onset mechanisms that may result in clinically complex or distinct phenotypes (e.g., headache caused by blast exposure[81]).

Even the most defining characteristic of PTH, onset or exacerbation of headache within 7 days of head or neck injury, is arbitrary and lacks clinical meaning.

Because PTH is likely to present with symptoms that replicate primary headaches (especially migraine), the diagnosing provider must rule out a primary headache process by identifying the development of a new (e.g., de novo) headache or the exacerbation of preexisting headache symptoms (defined by the ICHD-3 as a twofold or greater increase in the frequency or severity of a headache). Second, the diagnosing provider must identify a "close temporal relation" of the new or exacerbated headache to an injury to the head or neck. The ICHD-3 established a latency of 7 days between head injury and headache onset/exacerbation as a "somewhat arbitrary" onset latency criterion for PTH, chosen due to the close proximity of seven-day onset to the head injury event and a lack of available evidence to better define this criterion. There are some ongoing efforts to validate or change the 7-day headache onset criterion for PTH. Until more is known, there is a general consensus on using 7-day onset to establish PTH but allow up to 3 months headache onset latency based on clinical judgment and patient report.

Assessment: Most practitioners assess PTH using standard headache diaries and self-report measures of headache disability, which are particularly valuable for PTH because this headache is so disabling (similar measures are available for primary headaches as well). The 6-Item Headache Impact Test (HIT-6) is a gold standard, valid, and reliable assessment of headache-related disability.[82] In studies of migraine, HIT-6 scores demonstrated significant correlation with quality of life,[83] depression,[84] migraine disability assessment score,[85] and measures of PTSD.[86] As is the case for TTH and migraine, a headache diary is highly recommended as a way to track headache frequency and headache phenotype. Also, because PTH has no distinct clinical characteristics, a regular diagnostic interview assessing symptoms of both migraine and TTH may be necessary to note changes in clinical presentation that may indicate a new course of treatment (Table 2.4).

TABLE 2.4
Diagnostic criteria for posttraumatic headache (PTH).

PTH Subtype	Frequency	Duration	Characteristics	Rule-Outs
Acute PTH	Any	< 3 months	Any Pain	Not accounted for by primary headache
Persistent PTH	Any	> 3 months	Any Laterality Onset within 7 days of head injury	
• May be further specified as due to an injury to mild or moderate/severe head injury				

Daily Pain Self-Monitoring Form

Name:_____

Directions: Four times each day, please update the pain graph using the pain *intensity* scale below. Please indicate the type and amount of all medications you use each day using the symbols in the *medication* table below. For samples of filed out tables/scales, see examples given below.

I	[10]	EXTREMELY PAINFUL - My pain is so severe I can't do anything, I faint or black out
N	[9]	- My pain is so severe I can't concentrate on anything else, I have sweat flashes, and may feel panicky
T	[8]	VERY PAINFUL - My pain makes concentration difficult, but I can perform undemanding tasks
E	[7]	My pain makes it difficult to perform normal daily activities, with concentrated effort they can be performed
N	[6]	PAINFUL - I am in pain, but can continue what I am doing, performing slower and with a concentrated effort
S	[5]	My pain is to the point I must take medication
I	[4]	MILDLY PAINFUL - I can ignore my pain most of the time, or for several hours at a time.
T	[3]	My pain is similar to a nagging headache or getting a shot
Y	[2]	SLIGHTLY PAINFUL - I only notice my pain when I focus my attention on it, or it draws my attention to it.
	[1]	My pain is similar to a mild headache or sore muscle
	[0]	NO PAIN

PAIN INTENSITY SCALE

I [10]
N [9]
T [8]
E [7]
N [6]
S [5]
I [4]
T [3]
Y [2]
 [1]
 [0]
Med's

6   8   10   12   2   4   6   8   10   12
AM   PM

DAY: DATE: COMMENTS

I [10]
N [9]
T [8]
E [7]
N [6]
S [5]
I [4]
T [3]
Y [2]
 [1]
 [0]
Med's

6   8   10   12   2   4   6   8   10   12
AM   PM

DAY: DATE: COMMENTS

I [10]
N [9]
T [8]
E [7]
N [6]
S [5]
I [4]
T [3]
Y [2]
 [1]
 [0]
Med's

6   8   10   12   2   4   6   8   10   12
AM   PM

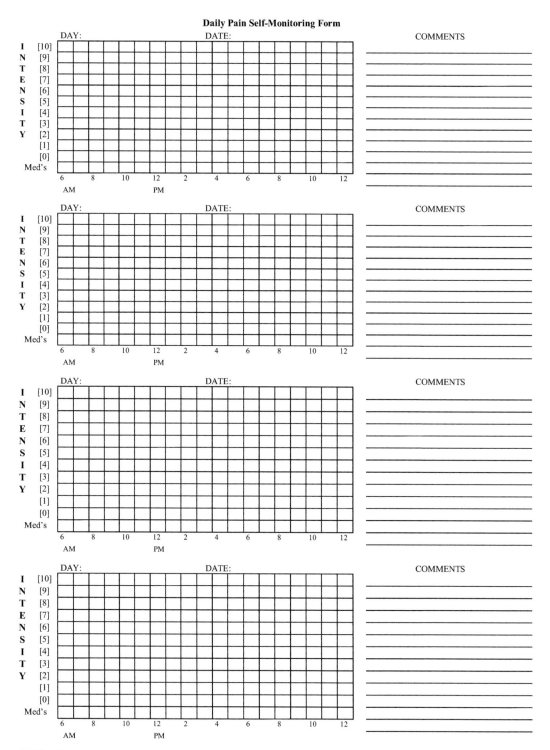

Daily Pain Self-Monitoring Form

Additional notes or comments:

Daily Pain Self-Monitoring Form

Treatment: Treatments designed to address both chronic musculoskeletal and headache pain target disability as a primary endpoint of care because disability is strongly correlated with multiple biopsychosocial domains and is a strong predictor of activity and work engagement. There is ample evidence supporting the contribution of pain characteristics (e.g., intensity, frequency, duration, quality) to disability, but there is surprisingly little research exploring the unique effects of common pain comorbidities on pain-related disability. Among military pain sufferers, for example, posttraumatic stress disorder (PTSD) adds significant complexity and intensity to pain experience often resulting in great levels of disability for patient with comorbid.[87] The unique nature of post-9/11 combat has led to a dramatic rise in the frequency with which veterans present with both pain and comorbid trauma symptoms. Trauma conditions (especially posttraumatic stress disorder, PTSD) that accompany pain can complicate the clinical phenotype and worsen pain symptoms and treatment response through a number of putative mechanisms.[87] Studies of chronic pain and PTSD comorbidity have found that veterans with PTSD report more severe pain, higher pain-related disability, higher interference of pain in daily activity, and lower perceptions of efficacy about controlling pain compared to veterans without PTSD.[88] High symptom severity is particularly troubling for veterans with comorbid headache and PTSD who are statistically less likely to seek mental health treatment to address PTSD compared to those with PTSD and no comorbid pain[89]. The relationship between PTSD and headache is notoriously complex, and individuals who develop PTSD have a twofold increased odds of developing headache after their trauma with odds of frequent headache increasing by 55% or more among individuals with more intrusive PTSD symptoms.[77] Indeed,

there is growing evidence showing that pain conditions (like PTH) are more likely to develop among individuals with prepain PTSD,[90] and PTSD is more likely to develop among individuals with persistent headache.[91]

Medication Overuse Headache

Medication overuse headache is a relatively new headache phenomenon, first identified as "drug-related headache" in the first edition of the International Classification of Headache Disorders (ICHD). The third edition of the ICHD (ICHD-3[5]) has established several criteria for MOH including chronic headache (15 headache days per month for 3 months) caused by overuse of headache medication for at least 3 months. Although MOH has been estimated to affect approximately 1%—2% of the world population (affecting more women than men), there is little guidance on effectively treating MOH.[92,93] Chen and Wang [92] appropriately note that the relationship between medication overuse and MOH is not clear, and that there are many headache patients with both migraine and TTH who may overuse medication and still never develop MOH. Thus, regular assessment of both medication use and headache symptoms (using a headache diary) is the best approach to capture concurrent medication overuse and consequent emergence of an MOH phenotype. Russel [93] explains that patients who are not compliant with a headache diary could be assessed for MOH using a modified "severity dependence scale questionnaire" that relies on brief numeric ratings to assess perception of control over medication use, anxiety related to missed medication dose, worry about use or overuse of medication, desire to stop using medication, and difficulty stopping headache medication. Risk factors for MOH are complex, and numerous factors can predict an increased likelihood of MOH in some patients. Hagen and colleagues[94] completed an 11-year trial of MOH and found over four times greater odds of developing MOH for headache sufferers who regularly used tranquilizer medication, had musculoskeletal or gastrointestinal complaints, or who reported high levels of anxiety or depression symptoms. As noted above, there are no accepted guidelines for managing MOH, though recent studies encourage prevention of medication overuse through strong patient assessment, surveillance of headache patients with multimorbidity that may increase MOH risk (e.g., chronic migraine, mental health disorder, circulatory conditions, endocrine conditions), providing education to patients about the risks of medication overuse, carefully monitored medication withdrawal (though this may only work for some patients), and NPIs (esp. biofeedback-assisted CBT) to help prevent relapse.[94–96]

CONCLUSION

Headache is complex and prevalent throughout the world. Despite very high representation in industrialized society, surprisingly little is known about the putative mechanisms that drive headache. Evolution in diagnostic criteria through the ICHD-3 has brought the medical system closer to effective treatments based on standardized typing and subtyping of headache, and research continues to broaden therapeutic targets by uncovering new mechanisms for headache onset and arrest. Most headaches can be addressed through thorough assessment and consideration of prophylactic and abortive treatments designed to minimized headache frequency and moderate disability after headache onset. In most cases, a headache diary (preferably in an electronic format) can help track, diagnose, and treat headache. NPIs are receiving increasing attention and provide effective treatment options with minimal side effect profiles.

REFERENCES

1. Stovner LJ, Nichols E, Steiner TJ, et al. Global, regional, and national burden of migraine and tension-type headache, 1990–2016: a systematic analysis for the Global Burden of Disease Study 2016. *Lancet Neurol.* 2018;17(11):954–976.
2. Burch RC, Buse DC, Lipton RB. Migraine: epidemiology, burden, and comorbidity. *Neurol Clin.* 2019;37(4):631–649.
3. Vetvik KG, MacGregor EA. Sex differences in the epidemiology, clinical features, and pathophysiology of migraine. *Lancet Neurol.* 2017;16(1):76–87.
4. Scher AI, Buse DC, Fanning KM, et al. Comorbid pain and migraine chronicity: the chronic migraine epidemiology and outcomes study. *Neurology.* 2017;89(5):461–468.
5. Headache Classification Committee of the International Headache Society (ICHD-3). The international classification of headache disorders, 3rd edition. *Cephalalgia.* 2018;38:1–211.
6. Hansen JM, Charles A. Differences in treatment response between migraine with aura and migraine without aura: lessons from clinical practice and RCTs. *J Headache Pain.* 2019;20(1):1.
7. Jackson JL, Cogbill E, Santana-Davila R, et al. A comparative effectiveness meta-analysis of drugs for the prophylaxis of migraine headache. *PloS One.* 2015;10(7).
8. Lipton RB, Stewart WF, Sawyer J, Edmeads JG. Clinical utility of an instrument assessing migraine disability: the Migraine Disability Assessment (MIDAS) questionnaire. headache. *J Head Face Pain.* 2001;41(9):854–861.
9. Ha H, Gonzalez A. Migraine headache prophylaxis. *Am Fam Physician.* 2019;99(1):17–24.
10. Sumelahti ML, Mattila K, Sillanmäki L, Sumanen M. Prescription patterns in preventive and abortive migraine medication. *Cephalalgia.* 2011;31(16):1659–1663.
11. Lucas S. Initial abortive treatments for migraine headache. *Curr Treat Options Neurol.* 2002;4(5):343–350.
12. Al-Quliti KW, Assaedi ES. New advances in prevention of migraine: review of current practice and recent advances. *Neurosciences.* 2016;21(3):207.
13. Bonafede M, Wilson K, Xue F. Long-term treatment patterns of prophylactic and acute migraine medications and incidence of opioid-related adverse events in patients with migraine. *Cephalalgia.* 2019;39(9):1086–1098.
14. Connelly M, Glynn EF, Hoffman MA, Bickel J. Rates and predictors of using opioids in the emergency department to treat migraine in adolescents and young adults. *Pediatr Emerg Care.* 2019. https://doi.org/10.1097/PEC.0000000000001851.
15. Jassar H, Nascimento TD, Kaciroti N, et al. Impact of chronic migraine attacks and their severity on the endogenous μ-opioid neurotransmission in the limbic system. *Neuroimage.* 2019;23:101905.
16. Dodson H, Bhula J, Eriksson S, Nguyen K. Migraine treatment in the emergency department: alternatives to opioids and their effectiveness in relieving migraines and reducing treatment times. *Cureus.* 2018;10(4).
17. Silberstein S, Mathew N, Saper J, Jenkins S, BOTOX Migraine Clinical Research Group. Botulinum toxin type A as a migraine preventive treatment. *Headache J Head Face Pain.* 2000;40(6):445–450.
18. Russo M, Manzoni GC, Taga A, et al. The use of onabotulinum toxin A (Botox®) in the treatment of chronic migraine at the Parma Headache Centre: a prospective observational study. *Neurol Sci.* 2016;37(7):1127–1131.
19. Moriarty M, Mallick-Searle T, Barch CA, Oas K. Monoclonal antibodies to CGRP or its receptor for migraine prevention. *J Nurse Pract.* 2019;15(10):717–724.

20. Goadsby PJ, Edvinsson L, Ekman R. Vasoactive peptide release in the extracerebral circulation of humans during migraine headache. *Ann Neurol*. 1990;28(2): 183−187.
21. Hansen JM, Hauge AW, Olesen J, Ashina M. Calcitonin gene-related peptide triggers migraine-like attacks in patients with migraine with aura. *Cephalalgia*. 2010;30(10): 1179−1186.
22. Bigal ME, Escandon R, Bronson M, et al. Safety and tolerability of LBR-101, a humanized monoclonal antibody that blocks the binding of CGRP to its receptor: results of the phase 1 program. *Cephalalgia*. 2014;34(7): 483−492.
23. Fang J, Xiaoli X, Wang R, Yuan Q, Pan L, Chen C. The treatment efficacy of galcanezumab for migraine: a meta-analysis of randomized controlled trials. *Clin Neurol Neurosurg*. 2019:105428.
24. Cousins S, Ridsdale L, Goldstein LH, Noble AJ, Moorey S, Seed P. A pilot study of cognitive behavioural therapy and relaxation for migraine headache: a randomised controlled trial. *J Neurol*. 2015;262(12):2764−2772.
25. Klan T, Liesering-Latta E, Gaul C, Martin PR, Witthöft M. An integrative cognitive behavioral therapy program for adults with migraine: a Feasibility study. *Headache J Head Face Pain*. 2019;59(5):741−755.
26. Ng QX, Venkatanarayanan N, Kumar L. A systematic review and meta-analysis of the efficacy of cognitive behavioral therapy for the management of pediatric migraine. *Headache J Head Face Pain*. 2017;57(3): 349−362.
27. Powers SW, Kashikar-Zuck SM, Allen JR, et al. Cognitive behavioral therapy plus amitriptyline for chronic migraine in children and adolescents: a randomized clinical trial. *J Am Med Assoc*. 2013;310(24):2622−2630.
28. Kroner JW, Hershey AD, Kashikar-Zuck SM, et al. Cognitive behavioral therapy plus amitriptyline for children and adolescents with chronic migraine reduces headache days to ≤ 4 per month. *Headache J Head Face Pain*. 2016 Apr; 56(4):711−716.
29. Kroon Van Diest AM, Powers SW. Cognitive behavioral therapy for pediatric headache and migraine: why to prescribe and what new research is critical for advancing integrated biobehavioral care. *Headache J Head Face Pain*. 2019 Feb;59(2):289−297.
30. Mullally WJ, Hall K, Goldstein R. Efficacy of biofeedback in the treatment of migraine and tension type headaches. *Pain Physician*. 2009;12(6):1005−1011.
31. Sharma N, Singhal S, Singh AP, Sharma CM. Effectiveness of integrated yoga therapy in treatment of chronic migraine: randomized controlled trial. *J Headache Pain*. 2013;14(1):1.
32. Bevilaqua-Grossi D, Gonçalves MC, Carvalho GF, et al. Additional effects of a physical therapy protocol on headache frequency, pressure pain threshold, and improvement perception in patients with migraine and associated neck pain: a randomized controlled trial. *Arch Phys Med Rehabil*. 2016;97(6):866−874.
33. Carvalho GF, Schwarz A, Szikszay TM, Adamczyk WM, Bevilaqua-Grossi D, Luedtke K. Physical therapy and migraine: musculoskeletal and balance dysfunctions and their relevance for clinical practice. *Braz J Phys Ther*. 2019. https://doi.org/10.1016/j.bjpt.2019.11.001.
34. Yu S, Han X. Update of chronic tension-type headache. *Curr Pain Headache Rep*. 2015;19(1):469.
35. Fumal A, Schoenen J. Tension-type headache: current research and clinical management. *Lancet Neurol*. 2008; 7(1):70−83.
36. de Tommaso M, Fernández-de-las-Penas C. Tension type headache. *Curr Rheumatol Rev*. 2016;12(2):127−139.
37. Rossi P, Vollono C, Valeriani M, Sandrini G. The contribution of clinical neurophysiology to the comprehension of the tension-type headache mechanisms. *Clin Neurophysiol*. 2011;122(6):1075−1085.
38. Exposto FG, Bendixen KH, Ernberg M, Bach FW, Svensson P. Characterization and predictive mechanisms of experimentally induced tension-type headache. *Cephalalgia*. 2019;39(10):1207−1218.
39. Yarnitsky D, Granot M, Granovsky Y. Pain modulation profile and pain therapy: between pro-and antinociception. *Pain*. 2014;155(4):663−665.
40. Jensen RH. Tension-type headache—the normal and most prevalent headache. *Headache J Head Face Pain*. 2018 Feb; 58(2):339−345.
41. Mathew NT, Glaze D, Frost J. Sleep apnea and other sleep abnormalities in primary headache disorders. In: *Migraine*. Karger Publishers; 1985:40−49.
42. Jay GW, Barkin RL. Primary headache disorders-part 2: tension-type headache and medication overuse headache. *Dis Mon*. 2017;63(12):342−367.
43. Fricton JR, Kroening R, Haley D, Siegert R. Myofascial pain syndrome of the head and neck: a review of clinical characteristics of 164 patients. *Oral Surg Oral Med Oral Pathol*. 1985;60(6):615−623.
44. Larsson B, Fichtel Å. Headache prevalence and characteristics among adolescents in the general population: a comparison between retrospect questionnaire and prospective paper diary data. *J Headache Pain*. 2014;15(1):80.
45. Krogh AB, Larsson B, Salvesen Ø, Linde M. Assessment of headache characteristics in a general adolescent population: a comparison between retrospective interviews and prospective diary recordings. *J Headache Pain*. 2016; 17(1):14.
46. Bandarian-Balooch S, Martin PR, McNally B, Brunelli A, Mackenzie S. Electronic-diary for recording headaches, triggers, and medication use: development and evaluation. *Headache J Head Face Pain*. 2017 Nov;57(10): 1551−1569.
47. McGeary DD, Mayer TG, Gatchel RJ. High pain ratings predict treatment failure in chronic occupational musculoskeletal disorders. *J Bone Jt Surg Am*. 2006;88(2):317−325.
48. Gatchel RJ, McGeary DD, Peterson A, et al. Preliminary findings of a randomized controlled trial of an interdisciplinary military pain program. *Mil Med*. 2009;174(3): 270−277.

49. Buckenmaier III CC, Galloway KT, Polomano RC, McDuffie M, Kwon N, Gallagher RM. Preliminary validation of the defense and veterans pain rating scale (DVPRS) in a military population. *Pain Med.* 2013; 14(1):110−123.

50. Mitsikostas DD, Thomas AM. Comorbidity of headache and depressive disorders. *Cephalalgia.* 1999;19(4):211−217.

51. Kudrow L. Lithium prophylaxis for chronic cluster headache. *Headache J Head Face Pain.* 1977;17(1):15−18.

52. Bendtsen L, Jensen R. Tension-type headache: the most common, but also the most neglected, headache disorder. *Curr Opin Neurol.* 2006;19(3):305−309.

53. Verhagen AP, Damen L, Berger MY, Passchier J, Merljin V, Koes BW. Is any one analgesic superior for episodic tension-type headache? This systematic review suggests good tolerance of any given agent may be the deciding factor. *J Fam Pract.* 2006;55(12):1064−1073.

54. Migliardi JR, Armellino JJ, Friedman M, Gillings DB, Beaver WT. Caffeine as an analgesic adjuvant in tension headache. *Clin Pharmacol Therapeut.* 1994;56(5):576−586.

55. Diamond S, Balm TK, Freitag FG. Ibuprofen plus caffeine in the treatment of tension-type headache. *Clin Pharmacol Therapeut.* 2000;68(3):312−319.

56. Schnider P, Aull S, Feucht M, et al. Use and abuse of analgesics in tension-type headache. *Cephalalgia.* 1994;14(2): 162−167.

57. Bendtsen L, Evers S, Linde M, Mitsikostas DD, Sandrini G, Schoenen J. EFNS guideline on the treatment of tension-type headache−Report of an EFNS task force. *Eur J Neurol.* 2010;17(11):1318−1325.

58. Bendtsen L, Jensen R, Olesen J. A non-selective (amitriptyline), but not a selective (citalopram), serotonin reuptake inhibitor is effective in the prophylactic treatment of chronic tension-type headache. *J Neurol Neurosurg Psychiatr.* 1996;61(3):285−290.

59. Palacios-Ceña M, Wang K, Castaldo M, et al. Variables associated with the use of prophylactic amitriptyline treatment in patients with tension-type headache. *Clin J Pain.* 2019;35(4):315−320.

60. Vernon H, Jansz G, Goldsmith CH, McDermaid C. A randomized, placebo-controlled clinical trial of chiropractic and medical prophylactic treatment of adults with tension-type headache: results from a stopped trial. *J Manipulative Physiol Therapeut.* 2009;32(5):344−351.

61. Boz C, Altunayoglu V, Velioglu S, Ozmenoglu M. Sertraline versus amitriptyline in the prophylactic therapy of non-depressed chronic tension-type headache patients. *J Headache Pain.* 2003;4(2):72−78.

62. Holroyd K, Stensland M. Separate and combined effects of CBT and drug therapy: psychosocial outcomes in the treatment of chronic tension-type headache. *J Pain.* 2005; 6(3):S4.

63. Motoya R, Oda K, Ito E, et al. Effectiveness of cognitive behavioral therapy based on the pain sustainment/exacerbation model in patients with tension-type headache: a pilot study. *Fukushima J Med Sci.* 2014;60(2):133−140.

64. Kamali F, Mohamadi M, Fakheri L, Mohammadnejad F. Dry needling versus friction massage to treat tension type headache: a randomized clinical trial. *J Bodyw Mov Ther.* 2019;23(1):89−93.

65. Vernon H, Borody C, Harris G, Muir B, Goldin J, Dinulos M. A randomized pragmatic clinical trial of chiropractic care for headaches with and without a self-acupressure pillow. *J Manipulative Physiol Therapeut.* 2015; 38(9):637−643.

66. Goadsby PJ. Trigeminal autonomic cephalalgias. *Continuum.* 2012;18(4):883−895.

67. Leone M, Bussone G. Pathophysiology of trigeminal autonomic cephalalgias. *Lancet Neurol.* 2009;8(8):755−764.

68. Wei DY, Jensen RH. Therapeutic approaches for the management of trigeminal autonomic cephalalgias. *Neurotherapeutics.* 2018;15(2):346−360.

69. Cohen AS, Matharu MS, Goadsby PJ. Trigeminal autonomic cephalalgias: current and future treatments: CME. *Headache J Head Face Pain.* 2007 Jun;47(6):969−980.

70. Goadsby PJ, Cittadini E, Burns B, Cohen AS. Trigeminal autonomic cephalalgias: diagnostic and therapeutic developments. *Curr Opin Neurol.* 2008;21(3):323−330.

71. Holtkamp MD, Grimes J, Ling G. Concussion in the military: an evidence-base review of mTBI in US military personnel focused on posttraumatic headache. *Curr Pain Headache Rep.* 2016;20(6):37.

72. Bourn LE, Sexton MB, Raggio GA, Porter KE, Rauch SA. Posttraumatic stress disorder and somatic complaints: contrasting Vietnam and OIF/OEF Veterans' experiences. *J Psychosom Res.* 2016;82:35−40.

73. Leung A, Shukla S, Fallah A, et al. Repetitive transcranial magnetic stimulation in managing mild traumatic brain injury-related headaches. *Neuromodulation: Technology at the Neural Interface.* 2016;19(2):133−141.

74. Lew HL, Lin PH, Fuh JL, Wang SJ, Clark DJ, Walker WC. Characteristics and treatment of headache after traumatic brain injury: a focused review. *Am J Phys Med Rehabil.* 2006;85(7):619−627.

75. Theeler BJ, Flynn FG, Erickson JC. Headaches after concussion in US soldiers returning from Iraq or Afghanistan. *Headache J Head Face Pain.* 2010 Sep;50(8):1262−1272.

76. Jaramillo CA, Eapen BC, McGeary CA, et al. A cohort study examining headaches among veterans of Iraq and Afghanistan wars: associations with traumatic brain injury, PTSD, and depression. *Headache J Head Face Pain.* 2016; 56(3):528−539.

77. Arcaya MC, Lowe SR, Asad AL, Subramanian SV, Waters MC, Rhodes J. Association of posttraumatic stress disorder symptoms with migraine and headache after a natural disaster. *Health Psychol.* 2017;36(5):411.

78. Lucas S. Posttraumatic headache: clinical characterization and management. *Curr Pain Headache Rep.* 2015; 19(10):48.

79. Theeler BJ, Erickson JC. Posttraumatic headache in military personnel and veterans of the Iraq and Afghanistan conflicts. *Curr Treat Options Neurol.* 2012;14(1):36−49.

80. Fraser F, Matsuzawa Y, Lee YS, Minen M. Behavioral treatments for post-traumatic headache. *Curr Pain Headache Rep.* 2017;21(5):22.

81. Kamins J, Charles A. Posttraumatic headache: basic mechanisms and therapeutic targets. *Headache J Head Face Pain.* 2018;58(6):811−826.

82. Kosinski M, Bayliss MS, Bjorner JB, et al. A six-item short-form survey for measuring headache impact: the HIT-6™. *Qual Life Res.* 2003;12(8):963−974.

83. Nachit-Ouinekh F, Dartigues JF, Henry P, et al. Use of the headache impact test (HIT-6) in general practice: relationship with quality of life and severity. *Eur J Neurol.* 2005; 12(3):189−193.

84. Sauro KM, Rose MS, Becker WJ, et al. HIT-6 and MIDAS as measures of headache disability in a headache referral population. *Headache J Head Face Pain.* 2010;50(3): 383−395.

85. Shin HE, Park JW, Kim YI, Lee KS. Headache Impact Test-6 (HIT-6) scores for migraine patients: their relation to disability as measured from a headache diary. *J Clin Neurol.* 2008;4(4):158−163.

86. Peterlin BL, Tietjen GE, Brandes JL, et al. Posttraumatic stress disorder in migraine. *Headache J Head Face Pain.* 2009;49(4):541−551.

87. McGeary D, Moore M, Vriend CA, Peterson AL, Gatchel RJ. The evaluation and treatment of comorbid pain and PTSD in a military setting: an overview. *J Clin Psychol Med Settings.* 2011;18(2):155.

88. Ang DC, Wu J, Sargent C, Bair MJ. Pain experience of Iraq and Afghanistan veterans with comorbid chronic pain and posttraumatic stress. *J Rehabil Res Dev.* 2014;51(4):559.

89. Outcalt SD, Hoen HM, Yu Z, Franks TM, Krebs EE. Does comorbid chronic pain affect posttraumatic stress disorder diagnosis and treatment? Outcomes of posttraumatic stress disorder screening in Department of Veterans Affairs primary care. *J Rehabil Res Dev.* 2016;53.

90. Cichowski SB, Rogers RG, Clark EA, Murata E, Murata A, Murata G. Military sexual trauma in female veterans is associated with chronic pain conditions. *Mil Med.* 2017; 182(9−10):e1895−e1899.

91. Theeler B, Lucas S, Riechers RG, Ruff RL. Post-traumatic headaches in civilians and military personnel: a comparative, clinical review. *Headache J Head Face Pain.* 2013; 53(6):881−900.

92. Chen PK, Wang SJ. Medication overuse and medication overuse headache: risk factors, comorbidities, associated burdens and nonpharmacologic and pharmacologic treatment approaches. *Curr Pain Headache Rep.* 2019;23(8):60.

93. Russell MB. Epidemiology and management of medication-overuse headache in the general population. *Neurol Sci.* 2019;40(1):23−26.

94. Hagen K, Linde M, Steiner TJ, Stovner LJ, Zwart JA. Risk factors for medication-overuse headache: an 11-year follow-up study. The Nord-Trøndelag Health Studies. *Pain.* 2012;153(1):56−61.

95. Kocasoy OE. Current approach to medication overuse headache. *Noro Psikiyatri Arsivi.* 2019;56(4):233.

96. D'Amico D, Sansone E, Grazzi L, et al. Multimorbidity in patients with chronic migraine and medication overuse headache. *Acta Neurol Scand.* 2018;138(6):515−522.

CHAPTER 3

Central Pain Syndromes

CHANEL DAVIDOFF, DO • ERIC LEUNG, MD

INTRODUCTION

Central pain (CP) is a term used to describe pain associated with an insult to the central nervous system (CNS). It is formally defined by the International Association for the Study of Pain (IASP) Taxonomy Taskforce as "pain caused by a lesion or disease of the central somatosensory system."[1] Clinically, it can be observed as neuropathic pain evolving or persisting in patients with neurologic complications as a result of an injury to the brain or spinal cord. There is a wide spectrum of CP-associated CNS injuries that exist resulting from vascular, infectious, demyelinating, neoplastic, or traumatic etiologies.[2] The most commonly studied conditions associated with CP are spinal cord injury (SCI) and stroke. Although these conditions are different entities, research suggests an overlap in the pathophysiologic mechanisms, as well as similarities in their clinical characteristics. Therefore, initial treatment modalities for CP have been similar in both populations.[3] CP has a number of clinical implications due to its medical complexity and potential to result in significant disability in those affected.

HISTORY AND TERMINOLOGY

The concept of "central arising pains" first appeared in published literature in the early 19th century by German neurologist Dr. L. Edinger.[4] Up until then, there have only been observational case reports describing pain arising from brain or cord origin.[5,6] This gave rise to a number of case studies describing pain, or "hyperesthesia" following damage in specific CNS locations (cortex, subcortex, internal capsule, thalamus, and brainstem) found through autopsy investigations. Furthermore, in the early 20th century, Dejerine and Roussy concluded that damage to the thalamus resulted in pain in association with other symptoms, and thus earning its name "thalamic syndrome."[5] Later, Head and Holmes published a seminal review identifying and quantifying sensory disturbances in CP, mainly as it related to thalamic injury.[7] Holmes also observed similar pains associated with spinal cord lesions in WWI solders. Although it was becoming increasingly known that CPs could arise from extrathalamic regions, the anatomical origin of CP remained a mystery. Later, a pivotal review by Cassinari and Pagni in the 1960s suggested that CP occurs as a result from lesion in the spinothalamic tract.[8]

Even with such discoveries, the terms "thalamic syndrome" and "central pain syndrome" remained interchangeable. With the rise of neuroimaging (CT scans and MRI) and functional neurophysiologic testing, evidence supported that neurological insults at any point within the CNS, from the spinal cord and up to the sensory cortex, could manifest with CP.[6] As a result, the term CP syndrome has been increasingly adapted to reflect this shift in thought.

CLINICAL CHARACTERISTICS

CP is often categorized as a type of neuropathic pain, presenting similarly to other types of neuropathies. Some common descriptors include burning, pins and needles, tingling, shooting, stabbing, electrical, squeezing, cramping, extreme cold, and itching, which can occur alone or in various combinations.

Pain intensity can vary between individuals, ranging from mild discomfort to agonizing pain. Studies have demonstrated that the degree of neurological deficit, nature of pain components, and comorbid mood disturbances may play a role in the severity of pain.[5] The degree of sensory deficits, specifically of pinprick and thermal sensations, has been shown to be correlated with pain severity. In a study of 157 patients with CP, deficits in pinprick and thermal sensations were more pronounced in areas of greatest pain, whereas tactile sensation, vibration, and two-point discrimination was uninfluenced in areas of pain.[9]

In addition, CP may present with different qualities of neuropathic pain and it is not uncommon for several qualities to present in the same person.[5,10] The characteristics of CP can be classified as steady, intermittent, or

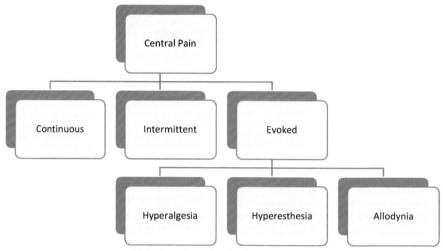

FIG. 3.1 Central pain characteristics.

evoked pain components (see Fig. 3.1). Intermittent pain tends to be spontaneous and more severe compared with steady pain. Evoked pain is often induced and can result in hyperesthesia (increased sensitivity to normal stimuli), allodynia (pain as a result of nonpainful stimuli), or hyperalgesia (increased pain as a result of normally painful stimuli). Often, patients experience a combination of intense, intermittent pain superimposed on dull, constant pain.[11,12] In general, the more components of pain present, the more intense the perceived pain. The severity of pain is usually higher in individuals with an incomplete sensory deficit compared with those with complete sensory deficits as they exhibit intense evoked pain in areas with mildly impaired sensory loss.[5]

Regardless of the characteristics and intensity, pain can become functionally limiting and have a negative impact on quality of life.[2,13] Functional impairment and pain was found to coexist with depression and sleeping difficulties 1 year after stroke.[14,15] Therefore, it is important to consider mood and sleep dysfunction when evaluating or treating CP, as difficulties with either may change the perception of pain intensity.

DIAGNOSIS

The diagnosis and classification of CP has been an ongoing discussion between researchers as well as clinicians. As a type of neuropathic pain, the presence of characteristic neuropathy often prompts investigation.

Neuropathic pain scales such as the Leeds Assessment of Neuropathic Symptoms and Signs (LANSS) pain scale[16], Neuropathic Pain Questionnaire[17], and the Douleur Neuropathique 4 (DN4)[18] were developed to aid in identifying the presence of neuropathic pain; however, these scales are limited in identifying CP. The Neuropathic Pain System Inventory (NPSI), which further characterizes neuropathic pain into subtypes, provides some insight into identifying CP; however, the NPSI is limited in sensitivity and specificity.[19] In general, these scales are not recommended to be used as diagnostic tools, but rather in conjunction with history and examination and review of ancillary testing if available.[20]

The grading system for neuropathic pain is a tool used to identify, with a level of certainty, that neuropathic pain is present. This was developed based on the definition outlined by the IASP "neuropathic pain caused by a lesion or disease of the somatosensory nervous system." The criteria require history and the distribution of pain to be consistent with sensory changes on physical exam and congruent with location of lesion confirmed on imaging.[13,20]

There are a number of limitations to consider when diagnosing CP. First, the presence of neuropathic pain does not delineate whether or not the lesion is localized to the central or peripheral nervous system (i.e., "burning" sensation can be found in both diabetic neuropathy and central post stroke pain [CPSP]). Second, CP may overlap with other pain entities, which can confound the diagnosis (i.e., a patient with CPSP may have concomitant lumbar radiculopathy affecting the same extremity). Further, there is high variability of clinical presentation that exists in patients with CP.

CP is often a multifactorial diagnosis, sharing overlapping features with other chronic pain conditions, further complicating evaluation and management.[21] This is commonly demonstrated in neurologically impaired patients with limited mobility, who are at risk for musculoskeletal complications as a result of their impairments. A cross-sectional study by de Oliveira et al. investigated the presence of myofascial pain (MP) in stroke patients diagnosed with CP syndrome.[22] It was found that the presence of MP cannot be excluded after stroke and may be present as a comorbid condition. Failure to consider other causes of pain could result in ineffective treatment.

As a result of the difficulty in evaluating and treating CP, the American Pain Society Pain Taxonomy (AAPT) provided evidence-based, multidimensional diagnostic criteria based on the classification of CP associated with SCI, stroke, and multiple sclerosis.[20] The proposed criteria includes 5 dimensions: 1) core diagnostic criteria, 2) common features, 3) common medical and psychiatric comorbidities, 4) neurobiological, psychosocial, functional consequences, and 5) putative neurobiological mechanisms, risk factors, and protective factors.

CENTRAL POST STROKE PAIN

Definition and Epidemiology

Chronic pain is a long-term complication of stroke. Data suggest that one-fifth to half of patients experience some pain following a stroke.[23,24] Pain can be further characterized as stroke-related pain and nonstroke-related pain where the latter tends to be explained by premorbid conditions such as arthritis or polyneuropathy. Stroke-related pain is categorized into subtypes that classically occur as a consequence of stroke. This includes CP, spasticity, complex regional pain syndrome, nociceptive/myofascial (i.e., shoulder) pain, and headaches.[3]

Central post stroke pain (CPSP) describes pain or sensory abnormalities following a stroke that corresponds to the area of cerebrovascular insult.[12] For example, an infarct in the left hemisphere of the brain resulting in right-sided hemiplegia may potentially result in pain in the hemiplegic limbs. The prevalence of CPSP has been highly variable in studies over the past two decades, ranging from 3% to 35%.[10,25,26] This can be partially explained by differences in study design and specific definition of post stroke pain.[23] In addition, CPSP is often underrecognized by clinicians, due to the lack of a specific pain scale or inquiry, and has been underreported by patients, which can add to the inconsistency in prevalence studies.[23] Risk factors for developing CPSP include young age, premorbid depression, tobacco use, and significant sensory and motor impairments.[24,27] Its

development is also strongly associated with the severity of stroke-related deficits, depression, and other pain conditions.[25] Screening and recognition of CPSP should include examination of functional and cognitive impairments as well as emotional well-being.

Onset and Description

The onset of CPSP occurs around 3−6 months; however, there has been reports of a latency period of up to 18 months.[28] The onset of pain has been suggested to be correlated with improvement in sensory and motor deficits. It can be sudden or gradual and may precede neurological recovery.[5,23,26] As mentioned earlier in the chapter, pain can be continuous, intermittent, and/or evoked. Continuous pain is most common to be present and is often dull in nature. Intermittent and evoked pain tends to be more severe.[5,23]

The heterogenous nature of reported symptoms can lead to challenges in recognizing CPSP. For this reason, more efforts have been made in identifying characteristics and patterns suggestive of CP as opposed to other pain syndromes.[26] Although pain descriptors, such as burning, tingling, or shooting, are not necessarily exclusive to CP, a distinguishing feature to consider is the area of pain distribution. If pain corresponds with the area of the central lesion, one can attribute these symptoms to be of central origin.

Diagnostic Criteria

The diagnostic criteria for CPSP set forth by the AAPT was created on the basis of neuropathic pain. There are six diagnostic criteria (see Fig. 3.2). The first requirement is a diagnostic test confirming recent or remote stroke. Second, pain must be present immediately after stroke or up to 1 year following the event, must be present for at least 3 months duration and distributed in the area affected by stroke. Third, there must be neuropathic features present such as allodynia or decreased sensation to stimuli. Lastly, there must be no other plausible diagnosis to explain the pain.[20]

Brain Localization

Classically, thalamic lesions have been shown to have the greatest association with pain after stroke, first described by Dejerine-Roussy as "thalamic pain syndrome."[29] However, subsequent studies have challenged this theory by demonstrating that only a minority of patients with post stroke pain was of thalamic origin.[30] It appears that a lesion anywhere along the neuroaxis responsible for transmitting and regulating pain correlates with the development of CPSP. Three areas have been relevant in the discussion

AAPT Diagnostic Criteria for Chronic CPSP	
1	Diagnostic Test Confirming stroke
2	Continuous or recurrent pain after stroke from immediately after onset for up to 1 year
3	Duration of pain for at least 3 months
4	Pain is distributed in area affected of stroke
5	Sensory changes in distribution of deficit At least 1 positive sign (i.e. allodynia) Or 1 negative sign (decreased sensations)
6	No other diagnosis to explain pain

FIG. 3.2 American pain society pain taxonomy diagnostic criteria for chronic central post stroke pain. (Adapted and modified from Widerström-Noga E, Loeser JD, Jensen TS, Finnerup NB. AAPT diagnostic criteria for central neuropathic pain. *J Pain*. 2017; 18(12):1417−1426. doi:10.1016/j.jpain.2017.06.003.)

of CPSP which include the spinothalamic tract, the medullary tract, and areas of the cerebral cortex.[12]

The spinothalamic tract is located at the anterolateral spinal cord, travels rostral, and synapses at the ventroposterior thalamus. This tract is generally responsible for both pain and temperature transmission. The medullary tract involves the trigeminothalamic pathway, which regulates similar nociception (i.e., pain and temperature) within the face. The medullary tract is implicated in brainstem strokes such as Lateral Medullary "Wallenberg" Syndrome, where about 25% of patients report ipsilateral facial pain.[31] Generally, infarcts within the cerebral cortex are rarely associated with the development of CPSP; however, lesions in cerebral structures involved in regulating and processing pain, such as the posterior insular cortex and medial operculum, have been shown to contribute to the development of CP.[32] These structures contribute to the pain due to their role as a receiving area for the spinothalamic tract and having close connections to the limbic and sensory cortices.[32]

Interestingly, right hemispheric infarcts are more likely to develop CPSP. This is suspected to be due to the right hemisphere playing a larger role in pain processing.[23,30] Other areas of the brain which are associated with the development of CPSP include the thalamus and brainstem generally seen in the setting of lacunar infarcts (small vessel strokes).[24]

Pathophysiology
The exact pathophysiology of CPSP is unknown; however, there are a few theories that have been proposed

on the basis of neuronal and biochemical pathways which include central disinhibition and sensitization.[33]

Studies by Head and Holmes in the early 1900s suggested the theory of central disinhibition observed with injury to the lateral thalamus. Pain was thought to be as a result of injury to the inhibitory, GABAnergic, pathways which communicate with the ventral-posterior lateral nuclei and medial thalamus, thus disinhibiting them from regulating pain control. This theory, later confirmed by SPECT studies, remains widely accepted as a mechanism of CPSP.[7,34]

Later, it was found that lesions along the spinothalamic-cortical pathway (responsible for pain and temperature sensation) can result in disinhibition and subsequent hyperactivity in the thalamus which lead to painful symptoms. This is further evident by multiple studies which have demonstrated impaired pinprick pain as well as temperature (especially cold) disturbances in the development of CP.[9,10] Moreover, disinhibition requires the integrity of the sensory tract to be somewhat maintained in order to explain the hyperactive component of this mechanism. Studies have shown that pain was more common in patients with partial lesions of the spinothalamic tract compared with complete involvement, further supporting this theory.[35]

Central sensitization is a sequela of chronic pain and is not to be confused with CP syndrome. Central sensitization is thought to occur from loss of inhibition or increased neuronal activity leading to overexcitability and hypersensitivity. It remains one of the mechanisms thought to drive chronic pain states. Its implication in

CPSP is suggested by studies in post stroke cohorts, which concludes that CP occurs as a result of spontaneous discharges from thalamic and cortical areas causing further neuronal hyperexcitability and central sensitization.[36] Central sensitization can be evaluated clinically by identifying hypersensitive areas and measuring thresholds in response to various stimuli.

Hyperexcitability on a cellular level can be explained by firing patterns of neurons, specifically in the thalamus. A review by Kumar et al. suggested two firing patterns: 1) bursting during hyperpolarization and 2) single-spike depolarization, both of which are modulated by neurotransmitters.[37] Regulation of firing patterns is determined by serotonergic, noradrenergic, and cholinergic input and plays a role in pain processing.[38] For instance, serotonin and noradrenaline was shown to increase GABAnergic transmission, which explains the benefit of using antidepressants in the treatment of CPSP (to be discussed later in the chapter). Biochemical pathways involving opioid receptors have also been investigated suggesting that decreased opioid receptor binding is a consequence of post stroke pain,[39] though clinical implications with opioids are limited and often discouraged in this population.[12]

SPINAL CORD INJURY CENTRAL PAIN
Definition and Epidemiology
CP in patients with SCI refers to neuropathic pain as a result of damage to the CNS, specifically the spinal cord and not the nerve roots. This pain is often classified as at-level neuropathic pain or below-level neuropathic pain according to the International Spinal Cord Injury Pain classification.[40] A significant number of patients with SCI experience pain with the prevalence estimated to be around 45% for both at-level and below-level neuropathic pain.[40-42] Pain interferes with rehabilitations, daily activities, and significantly affects the quality of life in individuals with SCI.

Spine Localization
In SCI, at-level CP is thought be the result of damage to the substance of the spinal cord. At-level CP is defined as neuropathic pain perceived in a segmental pattern within the dermatome or up to three dermatomes below the neurological level.[40] Thus, this type of pain is often referred to as "segmental" or "transitional zone pain." This is not to be confused with at-level peripheral neuropathic pain in the setting of SCI which can be secondary damage to the nerve roots at the level of injury. Pain is described as either spontaneous or stimulus evoked. Evoked pain typically has additional characteristics of allodynia, hyperalgesia, wind-up pain (abnormal temporal summation of pain), and aftersensations (persistent pain after painful stimulation has ceased).[43] Pain generally follows the dermatome of the neurological level of injury and can be present on one or both sides of the body.

Similar to at-level CP, below-level SCI neuropathic pain is considered to be a CP syndrome caused by spinal cord trauma. It has been previously referred to as "deafferentation central pain."[42] Below-level neuropathic pain is defined as neuropathic pain that is perceived more than three dermatomes below the neurological level.[40] It often has similar clinical characteristics as at-level CP with both spontaneous and stimulus-evoked neuropathic pain. However, unlike at-level CP, below-level CP is often described as being asymmetric, patch, and not characteristically dermatome. It may be perceived as coming from a particular body party (i.e., rectal, bladder, genitals).

Pathophysiology
The mechanisms of at- and below-level neuropathic pain are poorly understood and likely multifactorial in nature. It is often associated with neurochemical and excitotoxic changes. There is evidence of postinflammatory cytokines and excitatory amino acids (glutamate) briefly released in and around the site of SCI.[44,45] This is thought to contribute to pathologic changes in the spinal cord leading to increased sensitivity due to loss of normal neuronal input, removal of inhibitory influences, increased efficacy of alternative synapses and deafferentation, hyperexcitability of spinal and/or thalamic neurons, and further alterations in cellular activity of neurochemical and excitatory amino acids due to changes in ion channels and transport activity.[45]

There are also anatomical changes at the level of injury resulting in structural changes in the gray/white matter and subsequent structural reorganization. These changes alter the balance between spinal pathways (i.e., spinothalamic tract-dorsal column, spinothalamic-spinoreticulothalamic tract), which may contribute to development of CP.[43]

In addition to dysfunction of neurons, recent evidence indicates that alterations in the neuroimmune system also contribute to chronic pain, specifically to the microglia.[45] Microglia are thought to be principally phagocytes that are mobilized after injury, infection, disease, and seizures. When activated, glial cells produce proinflammatory cytokines, excitatory amino acids, and nitric acid which mediate pain following neural injury and produce neuronal hyperexcitability in the dorsal horn.[45] Dysfunction of the microglia is associated with neuropathic pain-related behaviors (i.e., allodynia and hyperalgesia) and is hypothesized to be responsible for the development of chronic CP.[45,46]

TREATMENT

Pharmacologic

There has been a variety of treatment options shown to be effective in managing CP disorders; however, supporting data are limited to only a few studies. Pharmacologic agents shown to be effective in treating CP include antidepressants, anticonvulsants, steroids, and opioid analgesia.

Neuropathic pain medications

Anticonvulsants and antidepressants are commonly prescribed as first-line therapy for CP disorders.[47] Pregabalin and gabapentin are anticonvulsants agents that have been a well-accepted choice for the treatment of neuropathic pain due to their relative affordability and tolerability.[12,43,44,47,48] While similar medications, pregabalin has been more frequently tested in CP disorders. Although the data on pain control have been marginal, large studies have demonstrated the efficacy of pregabalin for improved sleep and anxiety in patients with post stroke CP.[48]

Tricyclic antidepressants are also considered first-line agents for CP disorders. These medications are thought to produce analgesia through blocking reuptake of serotonin and norepinephrine transmitters. In a small (n = 15) double blinded-placebo controlled trial, amitriptyline was shown to produce significant reduction of pain and well tolerated in CPSP syndrome.[49] Still, this agent is known to have anticholinergic side effects as well as risk for developing cardiac arrhythmia.[48]

Second-line neuropathic medications include serotonin reuptake inhibitors (SSRIs) and serotonin norepinephrine reuptake inhibitors (SNRIs), which have been effective in treating various neuropathic pain states. However, there are limited studies about its efficacy in CP syndrome.[43,44,50] Other neuropathic agents, including carbamazepine and lamotrigine, have been studied in CP and are generally used as second-line agents due to higher incidence of side effects[49,51] (see Table 3.1).

Nonneuropathic pain medications

In central post stroke disorder, methylprednisolone was demonstrated to be a potential therapeutic option. In a retrospective study of stroke patients with CPSP, the group treated with a methylprednisolone steroid taper demonstrated a significant decrease in numerical rating scale pain score, as well as a marginal reduction of as needed pain medication.[52] The methylprednisolone taper in the study were reported to be a 6 day taper, starting at 24 mg, with subsequent reduction of dosing by 4 mg on each consecutive day.

Ketamine, an NMDA receptor antagonist, may also be therapeutic in management of CP disorders.[44] Animal studies have demonstrated an antinociceptive effect of ketamine in CP models. It is thought to "reset the CNS" due to its role in blocking the excitatory NMDA receptor; however, the evidence suggests that its mechanism may not be as simple.[53] Studies have suggested that ketamine has an effect at a cellular level on the HCN1 channel (on nociceptive neurons) and glial cells, which are implicated in chronic pain development.[54] Ketamine may also affect other systems involved in chronic pain transmission, including the cholinergic, aminergic, and opioid pathways. Ketamine has been studied in patients with SCI pain and were demonstrated to significantly reduce of VAS pain scores temporarily (up to 2 weeks).[53,55] These studies demonstrate promise of the use of ketamine as a potential therapeutic option in the treatment of CP disorders.

Opioid analgesics can be recommended for patients with intractable CP. Tramadol, morphine, and oxycodone have been studied in this population[44] with noted efficacy in pain control; however, side effects and risks of opioid abuse/complications can limit long-term use. Prescribers should follow the CDC and VA/DOD clinical practice guidelines which provide appropriate recommendations for prescribing monitoring and ensuring safety for patients on opioid pain management.[56,57]

Nonpharmacologic

Psychological and behavioral interventions play an important role in the management of CP disorders. CP is a complex stressor especially in patients with concomitant neurological deficits. There is significant evidence demonstrating the efficacy of these interventions in patients with multiple types of chronic pain disorders, including CP disorders.[42,58] Other nonpharmacologic techniques that have been employed included hypnosis, cognitive behavioral techniques, and biofeedback. These interventions focus on the physical, emotional, social, and occupational functioning aspects of pain and can be employed in conjunction to conventional medical treatment.

Other integrative therapies, such as acupuncture, transcutaneous electrical stimulation (TENS), have

TABLE 3.1
Pharmacologic Therapy for Central Pain Syndrome.

Drug Class	Agent	Mechanism	Effective Daily Dose	Side Effects/ *Precautions	Evidence
Anticonvulsant	Gabapentin (Neurontin)	Modulates voltage-gated Ca + channels in neural synapses	At least 1800 mg	Sedation, drowsiness, confusion, edema, tremors	**First-line agent** No RCTs performed for CPSP.
	Pregabalin (Lyrica)	Antagonist of voltage-gated Ca + channels	410 −460 mg	Similar to gabapentin	**First-line agent** Conflicting data for CPSP; however, improvement in sleep and anxiety. Favorable evidence for SCI pain.
	Lamotrigine	Neuronal membrane stabilizer via sodium channel blockade	200 −400 mg	Rash, Steven Johnsons syndrome (SJS), abdominal pain, diarrhea	Favorable evidence for CPSP and post SCI pain. Second-line agent. However effective dose is high. Must consider risks of adverse side effects.
	Carbamazepine	Sodium channel blocker and membrane stabilization	500 −760 mg	SJS, aplastic anemia, hepatic dysfunction, nausea, dizziness, hyponatremia *Monitor CBC and LFTs	Second-line treatment; however, efficacy for use is limited due to side effects.
Antidepressant	*SSRIs/SNRIs* Duloxetine	Analgesia through blocking reuptake of serotonin and norepinephrine (SNRI) neurotransmitters	60 mg	Sedation, fatigue, dizziness, nausea *Caution for serotonin syndrome * Withdrawal syndromes	Insufficient evidence for Duloxetine.
	Fluvoxamine		125 mg		Fluvoxamine effective in CPSP within 1 year
	Tricyclic antidepressant Amitriptyline	Adrenergically active antidepressant	75 mg	Sedation, dry mouth, orthostasis, constipation, urinary retention *Lowers seizure threshold *Risk of cardiac arrhythmias	**First-line agent** Evidence for CPSP; however, insufficient for post SCI pain.
NMDA antagonist	Ketamine	Blocking excitatory NMDA receptor	None established	Hypertension, hallucinations, respiratory depression *Cardiac precautions	Low level evidence; uncontrolled trials. Reserved for refractory pain as short-term measure.

Continued

TABLE 3.1
Pharmacologic Therapy for Central Pain Syndrome.—cont'd

Drug Class	Agent	Mechanism	Effective Daily Dose	Side Effects/ *Precautions	Evidence
Opioid	Tramadol Morphine Oxycodone	Presynaptic and postsynaptic inhibition of neurons in the CNS and PNS	None established	Sedation, dizziness, nausea, constipation, respiratory depression, confusion, urinary retention	Indicated for intractable pain; however, risks/side effects limit use. Morphine is ineffective in CPSP and side effects are frequent.
Steroid	Methylprednisolone		None established	Confusion, restlessness, nausea, abdominal pain, weight gain, hyperglycemia	Only retrospective studies. May be beneficial to CPSP patient with concurrent complex regional pain syndrome.
Cannabinoids	Tetrahydrocannabinol Cannabidiol		None established	Palpitations, hypotension, dry mouth, hallucinations, paranoia	Evidence is variable in RCTs.

Adapted and modified from Watson JC, Sandroni P. Central neuropathic pain syndromes. In: *Mayo Clinic Proceedings*; Vol. 91: Elsevier Ltd.; 2016: 372–385. doi:10.1016/j.mayocp.2016.01.017.

been employed to treat CP syndrome. Acupuncture has been used empirically for the treatment of SCI-related pain. There have been several small studies demonstrating a meaningful effect of acupuncture on neuropathic pain and CP in patients with SCI[59–61]; however, the methods and acupuncture technique employed vary from each study. Acupuncture techniques that were studied include electroacupuncture,[61] battle acupuncture,[59] as well as different schools of traditional acupuncture.[60,62] TENS is an integrative intervention where alternating current is delivered to electrodes positioned near painful areas. It activates large afferent fibers, which in turn activates descending inhibitory systems within the CNS.[63] Overall, the evidence in the utilization of TENS in CP disorders is limited; however, these studies do suggest that TENS may be of benefit in CP management.[64–66]

Cannabis has gained popularity as an alternative to pharmacologic therapy. There have been positive outcomes in the use of cannabinoid therapy in chronic neuropathic and oncologic pain.[67] Initial pilot studies demonstrated mixed results in the effect of cannabis for central spinal cord pain[44]; however, more studies are needed to determine dosing and efficacy. Adverse effects of medical cannabis include dizziness, dry mouth, nausea, fatigue, somnolence, euphoria, depression, vomiting, diarrhea, disorientation, asthenia, drowsiness, anxiety, confusion, balance disorders, hallucinations, dyspnea, paranoia, psychosis, weakness, falls, hypotension, palpitations, tachycardia, infections, urinary retention, and seizures. In patients with a preexisting CNS injury, these adverse effects place individuals at a significant increased risk of falls and injury secondary to motor incoordination and altered judgment.[67,68]

There are numerous ongoing studies on management for CP syndrome. Some nonpharmacologic interventions worth noting include vestibular caloric stimulation for CPSP syndrome and botulinum toxin for central neuropathic pain.

Vestibular caloric stimulation for CPSP was first reported by Ramachandran et al.[69] and later replicated with similar effect.[70,71] In these case series, vestibular caloric stimulation significantly reduced pain with a sustained benefit of at least 7 weeks for one patient.[69] The authors hypothesize that caloric stimulation activates the vestibular cortex in the posterior insular cortex which in turn inhibit the sensation of pain arising from the anterior cingulate. Botulinum toxin has been studied in the setting of neuropathic pain of the CNS, specifically in pain arising from SCI. Recent animal studies have also demonstrated that BTX-A has a significant effect on both peripheral and central-mediated neuropathic pain.[72,73] Jabbari et al. describe two patients with cervical spinal cord lesions (tumor and cord ischemia) who developed at-level neuropathic pain and failed oral medications.[74] He administered subcutaneous BTX-A injections to both of these patients with good results and persistent pain relief. Subsequent studies studying at-level CP in patients with SCI support his initial findings. While these interventions demonstrate promise, more studies are needed to determine efficacy and safety of the proposed treatments.

Interventional

There is limited evidence on interventional approaches to treat pain in persons with SCIs. Studies do not support the routine use of spinal cord stimulation in treating SCI-related CP[42,75]; however, there have been reports that it may be useful in incomplete SCI injuries.[41]

In CPSP syndrome, repetitive transcranial magnetic stimulation, deep brain stimulation (DBS), and motor cortex stimulation (MCS) have been studied as alternatives for treatment of refractory CP. Repetitive transcranial magnetic stimulation (rTMS) is a noninvasive procedure that involves a magnetic coil placed around the patient's head, which delivers impulses to the cortex.[12] A 2005 study examined a cohort of patients with poststroke pain and trigeminal neuralgia who underwent daily rTMS to the motor cortex for 5 days resulting in sustained relief at follow-up visit, 15 days following rTMS.[76] This is similar to MCS, which involves implanting electrodes over the motor cortex surgically. By stimulating hypothetical fourth-order neurons in the precentral gyrus (motor strip), nociceptive inputs from the cortex were thought to be inhibited, resulting in the reduction of pain.[77]

Another intervention for the management of CP is DBS. This involves implanting electrodes into deep structures of the brain, often thalamus or periventricular gray matter, to modulate sensory inputs and outputs by mechanisms that are not completely understood. However, positive results have been achieved in those with chronic pain. In a study of 15 patients with CPSP, 80% achieved pain relief, and 58% were able to wean off pain medications.[48,77,78]

While pharmacological management is considered to be first line in treatment, a multimodal approach with nonpharmacological interventions should be employed concurrently. The goal being to provide enough analgesia without compromising cognitive and physical recovery in the setting of known neurologic deficits.

CONCLUSION

CP syndrome is a condition that continues to be difficult to manage despite recent advances in the understanding of pathophysiology and treatment of the disorder. Challenges include, but are not limited to, difficulty in diagnosis due to its variable nature, as well as limited efficacious treatment. Early recognition and diagnosis of CP syndrome is imperative and remains an important step in initial management. It is best managed with a multimodal pain management program which includes pharmacologic and nonpharmacologic therapies. Evidence on interventional procedures is limited; however, studies in DBS in CP syndrome have shown some promising results.

CP remains an important topic in pain research as incomplete management of these patients can result in greater functional decline and dependence. It would be of interest to establish a means of identifying patients with higher risk of developing CP in order to optimize recovery. Further research into its pathophysiology may identify targets for management which would contribute to our understanding of the mechanism behind CP. Additionally, existing treatments need to be systematically studied further to determine efficacy and its psychosocial impact.

REFERENCES

1. IASP Terminology — IASP. https://www.iasp-pain.org/Education/Content.aspx?ItemNumber=1698. Accessed 12 October 2019.
2. Watson JC, Sandroni P. Central neuropathic pain syndromes. In: *Mayo Clinic Proceedings*. Vol. 91. Elsevier Ltd; 2016: 372−385. https://doi.org/10.1016/j.mayocp.2016.01.017.
3. Huang-Lionnet JH, Brummett C, Benzon H, et al. Central pain states. In: *Essentials of Pain Medicine*. 4th ed. Elsevier; 2018:251−260.
4. Edinger L. Giebt es central entstehendeSchmerzen? Dtsch Z Nervenheilkd. *J Neurol.* 1891;1(3−4):262−282. https://doi.org/10.1007/BF01796578.
5. Cavanero S, Bonicalzi V. *Central Pain Syndrome: Pathophysiology, Diagnosis, and Management.* Cambridge University Press; 2007.
6. Canavero S, Bonicalzi V. Central pain syndrome: elucidation of genesis and treatment. *Expert Rev Neurother.* 2007;7(11): 1485−1497. https://doi.org/10.1586/14737175.7.11.1485.
7. Head H, Holmes G. Sensory disturbances from central brain lesions. *Brain.* 1911;34(2−3):102−254. https://doi.org/10.1093/brain/34.2-3.102.
8. Cassinari VPC. *Central Pain: A Neurosurgical Survey.* Cambridge, MA: Harvard University Press; 1969.

9. Bowsher D. Central pain: clinical and physiological characteristics. *J Neurol Neurosurg Psychiatry.* 1996;61(1):62–69. https://doi.org/10.1136/jnnp.61.1.62.

10. Andersen G, Vestergaard K, Ingeman-Nielsen M, Jensen TS. Incidence of central post-stroke pain. *Pain.* 1995;61(2):187–193. https://doi.org/10.1016/0304-3959(94)00144-4.

11. Tasker RR, DeCarvalho GT, Dolan EJ. Intractable pain of spinal cord origin: clinical features and implications for surgery. *J Neurosurg.* 1992;77(3):373–378. https://doi.org/10.3171/jns.1992.77.3.0373.

12. Treister AK, Hatch MN, Cramer SC, Chang EY. Demystifying poststroke pain: from etiology to treatment. *PM R.* 2017;9(1):63–75. https://doi.org/10.1016/j.pmrj.2016.05.015.

13. Finnerup NB, Haroutounian S, Kamerman P, et al. Neuropathic pain: an updated grading system for research and clinical practice. *Pain.* 2016;157(8):1599–1606. https://doi.org/10.1097/j.pain.0000000000000492.

14. Appelros P. Prevalence and predictors of pain and fatigue after stroke: a population-based study. *Int J Rehabil Res.* 2006;29(4):329–333. https://doi.org/10.1097/MRR.0b013e328010c7b8.

15. Jönsson A-C, Lindgren I, Hallström B, Norrving B, Lindgren A. Prevalence and intensity of pain after stroke: a population based study focusing on patients' perspectives. *J Neurol Neurosurg Psychiatry.* 2006;77(5):590–595. https://doi.org/10.1136/jnnp.2005.079145.

16. Bennett M. The LANSS pain scale: the Leeds assessment of neuropathic symptoms and signs. *Pain.* 2001;92(1–2):147–157. https://doi.org/10.1016/S0304-3959(00)00482-6.

17. Krause SJ, Backonja M-M. Development of a neuropathic pain questionnaire. *Clin J Pain.* 2003;19(5):306–314. http://www.ncbi.nlm.nih.gov/pubmed/12966256.

18. Bouhassira D, Attal N, Alchaar H, et al. Comparison of pain syndromes associated with nervous or somatic lesions and development of a new neuropathic pain diagnostic questionnaire (DN4). *Pain.* 2005;114(1–2):29–36. https://doi.org/10.1016/j.pain.2004.12.010.

19. Bouhassira D, Attal N, Fermanian J, et al. Development and validation of the neuropathic pain symptom inventory. *Pain.* 2004;108(3):248–257. https://doi.org/10.1016/j.pain.2003.12.024.

20. Widerström-Noga E, Loeser JD, Jensen TS, Finnerup NB. AAPT diagnostic criteria for central neuropathic pain. *J Pain.* 2017;18(12):1417–1426. https://doi.org/10.1016/j.jpain.2017.06.003.

21. Maixner W, Fillingim RB, Williams DA, Smith SB, Slade GD. Overlapping chronic pain conditions: implications for diagnosis and classification. *J Pain.* 2016;17(9):T93–T107. https://doi.org/10.1016/j.jpain.2016.06.002.

22. de Oliveira RAA, de Andrade DC, Machado AGG, Teixeira MJ. Central poststroke pain: somatosensory abnormalities and the presence of associated myofascial pain syndrome. *BMC Neurol.* 2012;12:89. https://doi.org/10.1186/1471-2377-12-89.

23. Harrison RA, Field TS. Post stroke pain: identification, assessment, and therapy. *Cerebrovasc Dis.* 2015;39(3–4):190–201. https://doi.org/10.1159/000375397.

24. O'Donnell MJ, Diener HC, Sacco RL, Panju AA, Vinisko R, Yusuf S. Chronic pain syndromes after ischemic stroke: PRoFESS trial. *Stroke.* 2013;44(5):1238–1243. https://doi.org/10.1161/STROKEAHA.111.671008.

25. Lundström E, Smits A, Terént A, Borg J. Risk factors for stroke-related pain 1 year after first-ever stroke. *Eur J Neurol.* 2009;16(2):188–193. https://doi.org/10.1111/j.1468-1331.2008.02378.

26. Widar M, Samuelsson L, Karlsson-Tivenius S, Ahlström G. Long-term pain conditions after a stroke. *J Rehabil Med.* 2002;34(4):165–170. https://doi.org/10.1080/16501970213237.

27. Harno H, Haapaniemi E, Putaala J, et al. Central poststroke pain in young ischemic stroke survivors in the Helsinki Young Stroke Registry. *Neurology.* 2014;83(13):1147–1154. https://doi.org/10.1212/WNL.0000000000000818.

28. Klit H, Finnerup NB, Jensen TS. Central post-stroke pain: clinical characteristics, pathophysiology, and management. *Lancet Neurol.* 2009;8(9):857–868. https://doi.org/10.1016/S1474-4422(09)70176-0.

29. Jahngir MU, Qureshi AI. *Dejerine Roussy Syndrome;* 2019. http://www.ncbi.nlm.nih.gov/pubmed/30085589. Accessed October 12, 2019.

30. Leijon G, Boivie J, Johansson I. Central post-stroke pain — neurological symptoms and pain characteristics. *Pain.* 1989;36(1):13–25. https://doi.org/10.1016/0304-3959(89)90107-3.

31. MacGowan DJL, Janal MN, Clark WC, et al. Central poststroke pain and Wallenberg's lateral medullary infarction: frequency, character, and determinants in 63 patients. *Neurology.* 1997;49(1):120–125. https://doi.org/10.1212/WNL.49.1.120.

32. Garcia-Larrea L. *The Posterior Insular-Opercular Region and the Search of a Primary Cortex for Pain.* 2012.

33. Oh HS, Seo WS. A comprehensive review of central post-stroke pain. *Pain Manag Nurs.* 2015;16(5):804–818. https://doi.org/10.1016/j.pmn.2015.03.002.

34. Cesaro P, Mann MW, Moretti JL, et al. Central pain and thalamic hyperactivity: a single photon emission computerized tomographic study. *Pain.* 1991;47(3):329–336. https://doi.org/10.1016/0304-3959(91)90224-l.

35. Hong JH, Choi BY, Chang CH, et al. The prevalence of central poststroke pain according to the integrity of the spino-thalamo-cortical pathway. *Eur Neurol.* 2012;67(1):12–17. https://doi.org/10.1159/000333012.

36. Vestergaard K, Nielsen J, Andersen G, Ingeman-Nielsen M, Arendt-Nielsen L, Jensen TS. Sensory abnormalities in consecutive, unselected patients with central post-stroke pain. *Pain.* 1995;61(2):177–186. https://doi.org/10.1016/0304-3959(94)00140-A.

37. Kumar B, Kalita J, Kumar G, Misra UK. Central poststroke pain: a review of pathophysiology and treatment. *Anesth Analg.* 2009;108(5):1645–1657. https://doi.org/10.1213/ane.0b013e31819d644c.

38. McCormick DA, Wang Z. Serotonin and noradrenaline excite GABAergic neurones of the Guinea-pig and cat nucleus reticularis thalami. *J Physiol.* 1991;442(1):235–255. https://doi.org/10.1113/jphysiol.1991.sp018791.

39. Willoch F, Schindler F, Wester HJ, et al. Central poststroke pain and reduced opioid receptor binding within pain processing circuitries: a [11C]diprenorphine PET study. *Pain.* 2004;108(3):213–220. https://doi.org/10.1016/j.pain.2003.08.014.

40. Bryce TN, Biering-sørensen F, Finnerup NB, et al. International spinal cord injury pain classification: part I. Background and description. March 6–7, 2009. *Spinal Cord.* 2012;50(6):413–417.

41. Siddall PJ, Loeser JD. Pain following spinal cord injury. *Spinal Cord.* 2001;39(2):63–73.

42. Bryce TN, Ragnarsson KT. Pain after spinal cord injury. *Phys Med Rehabil Clin.* 2000;11(1):157–168.

43. Finnerup NB, Jensen TS. Spinal cord injury pain—mechanisms and treatment. *Eur J Neurol.* 2004;11(2):73–82.

44. Hagen EM, Rekand T. Management of neuropathic pain associated with spinal cord injury. *Pain Ther.* 2015;4(1):51–65.

45. Hulsebosch CE, Hains BC, Crown ED, Carlton SM. Mechanisms of chronic central neuropathic pain after spinal cord injury. *Brain Res Rev.* 2009;60(1):202–213.

46. Hains BC, Waxman SG. Activated microglia contribute to the maintenance of chronic pain after spinal cord injury. *J Neurosci.* 2006;26(16):4308–4317.

47. Kim JS, Bashford G, Murphy TK, Martin A, Dror V, Cheung R. Safety and efficacy of pregabalin in patients with central post-stroke pain. *Pain.* 2011;152(5):1018–1023. https://doi.org/10.1016/j.pain.2010.12.023.

48. Flaster M, Meresh E, Rao M, Biller J. Central poststroke pain: current diagnosis and treatment. *Top Stroke Rehabil.* 2013;20(2):116–123. https://doi.org/10.1310/tsr2002-116.

49. Leijon G, Boivie J. Central post-stroke pain — a controlled trial of amitriptyline and carbamazepine. *Pain.* 1989;36(1):27–36. https://doi.org/10.1016/0304-3959(89)90108-5.

50. Shimodozono M, Kawahira K, Kamishita T, Ogata A, Tohgo SI, Tanaka N. Reduction of central poststroke pain with the selective serotonin reuptake inhibitor fluvoxamine. *Int J Neurosci.* 2002;112(10):1173–1181. https://doi.org/10.1080/00207450290026139.

51. Vestergaard K, Andersen G, Gottrup H, Kristensen BT, Jensen TS. Lamotrigine for central poststroke pain: a randomized controlled trial. *Neurology.* 2001;56(2):184–190. https://doi.org/10.1212/WNL.56.2.184.

52. Pellicane AJ, Millis SR. Efficacy of methylprednisolone versus other pharmacologic interventions for the treatment of central post-stroke pain: a retrospective analysis. *J Pain Res.* 2013;6:557–563. https://doi.org/10.2147/JPR.S46530.

53. Cohen SP, Bhatia A, Buvanendran A, et al. Consensus guidelines on the use of intravenous ketamine infusions for chronic pain from the American Society of Regional Anesthesia and Pain Medicine, the American Academy of Pain Medicine, and the American Society of Anesthesiologists. *Reg Anesth Pain Med.* 2018;43(5):521–546.

54. Tajerian M, Leu D, Yang P, Huang TT, Kingery WS, Clark JD. Differential efficacy of ketamine in the acute versus chronic stages of complex regional pain syndrome in mice. *Anesthesiology.* 2015;123(6):1435–1447.

55. Amr YM. Multi-day low dose ketamine infusion as adjuvant to oral gabapentin in spinal cord injury related chronic pain: a prospective, randomized, double blind trial. *Pain Physician.* 2010;13(3):245–249.

56. Rosenberg JM, Bilka BM, Wilson SM, Spevak C. Opioid therapy for chronic pain: overview of the 2017 US Department of Veterans Affairs and US Department of Defense Clinical Practice Guideline. *Pain Med.* 2018;19(5):928–941.

57. Dowell D, Haegerich TM, Chou R. CDC guideline for prescribing opioids for chronic pain–United States, 2016. *J Am Med Assoc.* 2016;315(15):1624–1645.

58. Grzesiak RC. Cognitive and behavioral approaches to management of chronic pain. *N Y State J Med.* 1982;82(1):30–38.

59. Estores I, Chen K, Jackson B, Lao L, Gorman PH. Auricular acupuncture for spinal cord injury related neuropathic pain: a pilot controlled clinical trial. *J Spinal Cord Med.* 2017;40(4):432–438.

60. Rapson LM, Wells N, Pepper J, Majid N, Boon H. Acupuncture as a promising treatment for below-level central neuropathic pain: a retrospective study. *J Spinal Cord Med.* 2003;26(1):21–26.

61. Santos AB, Gozzani JL. Acupuncture as adjuvant therapy in thalamic syndrome: case report. *Rev Bras Anestesiol.* 2011;61(1):88–94.

62. Fan Q, Cavus O, Xiong L, Xia Y. Spinal cord injury: how could acupuncture help? *J Acupunct Meridian Stud.* 2018;11(4):124–132.

63. Vance CG, Dailey DL, Rakel BA, Sluka KA. Using TENS for pain control: the state of the evidence. *Pain Manag.* 2014;4(3):197–209.

64. Celik EC, Erhan B, Gunduz B, Lakse E. The effect of low-frequency TENS in the treatment of neuropathic pain in patients with spinal cord injury. *Spinal Cord.* 2013;51(4):334–337.

65. Sawant A, Dadurka K, Overend T, Kremenchutzky M. Systematic review of efficacy of TENS for management of central pain in people with multiple sclerosis. *Mult Scler Relat Disord.* 2015;4(3):219–227.

66. Leijon G, Boivie J. Central post-stroke pain–the effect of high and low frequency TENS. *Pain.* 1989;38(2):187–191.

67. Whiting PF, Wolff RF, Deshpande S, et al. Cannabinoids for medical use: asystematic review and meta-analysis. *J Am Med Assoc.* 2015;313(24):2456–2473.

68. Volkow ND, Baler RD, Compton WM, Weiss SR. Adverse health effects of marijuana use. *N Engl J Med.* 2014;370(23):2219–2227.

69. Ramachandran VS, Mcgeoch PD, Williams L, Arcilla G. Rapid relief of thalamic pain syndrome induced by vestibular caloric stimulation. *Neurocase.* 2007;13(3):185–188.

70. Mcgeoch PD, Williams LE, Lee RR, Ramachandran VS. Behavioural evidence for vestibular stimulation as a treatment for central post-stroke pain. *J Neurol Neurosurg Psychiatry.* 2008;79(11):1298–1301.

71. Spitoni GF, Pireddu G, Galati G, Sulpizio V, Paolucci S, Pizzamiglio L. Caloric vestibular stimulation reduces pain and Somatoparaphrenia in a severe chronic central post-stroke pain patient: a case study. *PloS One.* 2016;11(3):e0151213.

72. Park J, Chung ME. Botulinum toxin for central neuropathic pain. *Toxins.* 2018;10(6).

73. Chun A, Levy I, Yang A, et al. Treatment of at-level spinal cord injury pain with botulinum toxin A. *Spinal Cord Ser Cases*. 2019;5:77.

74. Jabbari B, Maher N, Difazio M. Botulinum toxin A improved burning pain and allodynia in two subjects with spinal cord pathology. *Pain Med*. 2003;4:10.

75. Cioni B, Meglio M, Pentimalli L, Visocchi M. Spinal cord stimulation in the treatment of paraplegic pain. *J Neurosurg*. 1995;82(1):35–39.

76. Khedr EM, Kotb H, Kamel NF, Ahmed MA, Sadek R, Rothwell JC. Longlasting antalgic effects of daily sessions of repetitive transcranial magnetic stimulation in central and peripheral neuropathic pain. *J Neurol Neurosurg Psychiatry*. 2005;76(6):833–838. https://doi.org/10.1136/jnnp.2004.055806.

77. Tsubokawa T, Katayama Y, Yamamoto T, Hirayama T, Koyama S. Chronic motor cortex stimulation in patients with thalamic pain. *J Neurosurg*. 1993;78(3):393–401. https://doi.org/10.3171/jns.1993.78.3.0393.

78. Owen SLF, Green AL, Stein JF, Aziz TZ. Deep brain stimulation for the alleviation of post-stroke neuropathic pain. *Pain*. 2006;120(1–2):202–206. https://doi.org/10.1016/j.pain.2005.09.03.

CHAPTER 4

Visceral Pain: Mechanisms, Syndromes, and Treatment

GAURAV SUNNY SHARMA, MD • KIRSTEN TILLISCH, MD

INTRODUCTION

Chronic visceral pain is a common medical condition that is experienced by more than 20% of the global population.[1] Visceral pain can be complex because of its vague constellation of symptoms and associated autonomic changes. Many patients avoid seeking medical treatment due to a lack of understanding, possible embarrassment, or even fear of judgment by friends, family, and providers. Persistent visceral symptoms and afferent transmission can lead to visceral hyperalgesia, with resulting structural and functional changes in the peripheral and central nervous systems. Chronic visceral pain can be debilitating and causes increased morbidity, decreased quality of life, and significant socioeconomic burden. Although there are organic causes that produce chronic and persistent symptoms such as inflammatory bowel disease (IBD), chronic pancreatitis, and malignancy, an absence of identifiable pathology is also common in disorders such as irritable bowel syndrome (IBS), functional dyspepsia, and interstitial cystitis (IC). This chapter reviews our current understanding of the physiology of visceral pain transmission, including peripheral and central processing mechanisms. We will discuss the clinical evaluation of and symptoms present in visceral pain conditions, as well as risk factors for developing symptoms. We will then highlight common visceral pain syndromes and discuss treatment modalities that may benefit patients.

PHYSIOLOGY OF VISCERAL PAIN

Visceral and somatic pain were once thought to share a single neurologic mechanism. Many previous studies have focused solely on mechanisms of somatic nociception, presumably due to increased complications in achieving adequate stimulation of visceral structures in research models.[2,3] While both are considered types of nociceptive pain and have some similarities, recent research has increased our understanding of the anatomic and physiologic basis of visceral pain signaling and its importance.

Peripheral Visceral Mechanisms

Embryologically, visceral organs arise from midline structures and thus receive dual innervation by primary afferents through autonomic parasympathetic and sympathetic nerves.[4] This is in contrast to cutaneous somatic tissue, which is innervated by afferent sensory fibers traveling along the spinal nerves to the dorsal horn of the spinal cord. Parasympathetic afferents are typically referenced by the nerve in which they travel, such as the vagal and pelvic afferents.[5] Vagal afferents provide innervation from the upper gastrointestinal system to the splenic flexure. Pelvic afferents provide innervation to the descending colon and remainder of the lower bowel. This is illustrated in Fig. 4.1. The sympathetic afferents are similar to spinal afferents, given their termination within the dorsal horn of the spinal cord, and are also named after the nerve in which they travel. Examples include the splanchnic spinal afferents projecting to the thoracolumbar segments and the pelvic spinal afferents projecting to the lumbosacral region.

Visceral sensory afferents are primarily composed of thinly myelinated A-delta nerve fibers and unmyelinated C nerve fibers. This is in contrast to cutaneous somatic mechanoreceptors, which are primarily A-beta nerve fibers and have specialized nerve endings including pacinian corpuscles, Meissner corpuscles, and Ruffini endings. Viscerosensory axons are polymodal and exhibit mechanosensitivity as well as chemosensitivity and thermosensitivity. Vagal afferents are thought to be a homogenous group responding primarily to low-intensity mechanical stimulation over a wide range.[4] This is thought to assist with the regulation of physiologic processes. Spinal afferents, in contrast,

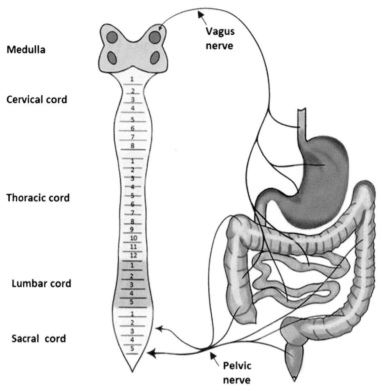

FIG. 4.1 Parasympathetic innervation of the gastrointestinal system. Vagal afferents provide innervation from the upper gastrointestinal system to the splenic flexure, whereas the pelvic afferents provide innervation to the descending colon.

have two physiologic classes of nociceptive receptors based on their responses. These include high-threshold receptors and low-threshold receptors. High-threshold receptors are activated by a mechanical stimulus intensity within the noxious range. These receptors innervate organs that produce conscious sensations of pain, including the heart, lungs, biliary system, small intestine, colon, ureter, bladder, and kidneys.[2,6] Low-threshold, or intensity-encoding, receptors are able to respond to a range of stimuli from innocuous to noxious and are able to encode the stimulus intensity based on the magnitude of their discharge.

Viscera are also innervated by a group of visceral afferents termed mechanically insensitive afferents, or silent afferents.[1] These silent afferents are suspected to be normally unresponsive to mechanical stimuli such as stretch and distention and instead are responsive to stimuli such as tissue injury and inflammation.[6] Silent afferents constitute approximately 25% of the afferents innervating the splanchnic and pelvic nociceptive pathways, but the exact mechanisms and

clinical importance of these receptors are still under investigation.[1] However, upon activation, they are believed to acquire mechanosensitivity and play a role in persistent visceral pain states.

Central Visceral Mechanisms

As discussed earlier, visceral sensation can be grouped into vagal afferents and spinal afferents. Vagal afferents project centrally to the inferior ganglion of the vagus nerve, or nodose ganglion, before terminating within the nucleus of the solitary tract. The solitary nucleus is located within the dorsal brainstem and assists with integration and regulation of autonomic function. Although vagal afferents are not specifically involved in the perception of pain, the nerve endings are sensitive to similar chemical mediators that affect spinal afferents, such as serotonin, prostaglandins, and capsaicin.[5] This may provide a mechanistic explanation for some of the autonomic symptoms, such as nausea and vomiting, that are frequently reported with visceral pain.

Spinal afferent pathways are known to be involved in the transmission of visceral pain. These afferents pass through the sympathetic ganglia and synapse along the dorsal horn of the spinal cord primarily in laminae I and V, but some also in laminae II and X.[6,7] Afferents then project rostrally along the dorsal column, spinothalamic, and spinoparabrachial pathways. The dorsal column and spinothalamic pathways are shown in Fig. 4.2. The dorsal column travels ipsilaterally within the spinal cord to the nucleus gracilis and nucleus cuneatus within the brainstem. Nociceptive input from there is transmitted to the ventral posterolateral

(VPL) nucleus of the thalamus. The spinothalamic tract projections are relayed from deeper within the dorsal horn and also synapse within the VPL nucleus of the thalamus. Third order neurons from the VPL travel to the primary and secondary somatosensory cortex. Nociceptive projections to these areas contribute to the sensory discriminative aspects of pain perception such as location, duration, and intensity.[8] The ventral postero-medial nuclei of the thalamus are the main target of the vagal afferents, as depicted in Fig. 4.3. Along with superficial dorsal horn projections from the spinopar-abrachial pathway, this nociceptive input is transmitted

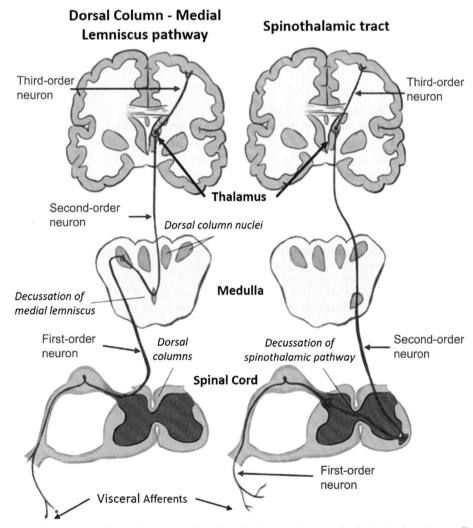

FIG. 4.2 Visceral pain afferent signals traveling along the dorsal column and spinothalamic pathways. Third-order neurons from the ventral posterolateral nucleus of the thalamus travel to the primary and secondary somatosensory cortices.

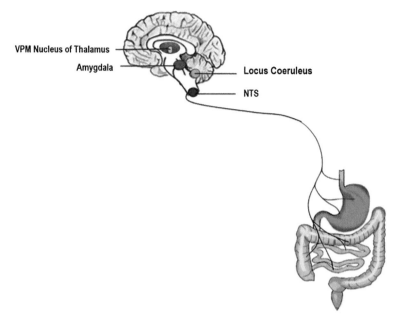

VPM Nucleus of Thalamus

Amygdala

Locus Coeruleus

NTS

FIG. 4.3 Vagal afferent pathways from the gastrointestinal tract to the nucleus tractus solitarius (NTS) and ventral posteromedial (VPM) nuclei of the thalamus that allow for processing of the affective aspects of pain.

to the limbic structures including the amygdala, insula, and anterior cingulate cortex to provide motivational and affective aspects of pain processing.[3,8]

Output traveling along descending pathways from the cortical and limbic areas in response to visceral pain input also plays a role in pain modulation, although these mechanisms are not well understood. The periaqueductal gray (PAG) and rostral ventromedial medulla (RVM) are the most studied structures involved. Nociceptive input is received in both the PAG and RVM, and in turn the PAG additionally projects to the RVM. The RVM acts as a supraspinal modulatory system providing facilitatory and inhibitory influences on spinal cord excitability.[3] Descending inhibitory projections to the dorsal horn of the spinal cord can assist in decreasing the intensity and emotional components of pain.[7]

The transmission and modulation of visceral afferents is only one aspect of the central mechanisms that may contribute to chronic visceral pain pathophysiology and symptom development. There is growing interest in the functional and structural alterations in brain regions and their association with various visceral pain conditions such as IBS, functional dyspepsia, and IC. This is often evaluated by the use of functional magnetic resonance imaging (fMRI) of the brain. Early fMRI studies identified pain-related brain regions that included the insular cortex, anterior cingulate cortex, primary sensory cortex, prefrontal cortex, and the thalamus.[9] These pain-related regions have been shown to have close connectivity with regions associated with emotional arousal, such as the amygdala. In a study comparing rectal distension in patients with IBS to healthy controls, the patients with IBS showed increased activation in regions associated with emotional arousal.[9] Healthy controls showed increased activation in the prefrontal cortex, possibly leading to suppression of arousal and to greater activation of descending inhibitory systems. Some of these brain regions are described as a salience network, which recognizes and interprets salient stimuli, modulating the organism's behavioral response to internal or external stimuli. In a review by Mayer et al.,[9] structural and functional changes in the salience network, sensorimotor network, and emotional arousal networks are the most commonly reported findings in visceral pain syndromes such as IBS. The use of neuroimaging studies has allowed for a greater understanding of the role of anticipation and context in visceral pain disorders, making it clear that the pain reported by patients is not solely related to peripheral input. Further studies are needed to understand these areas and identify possible central targets for treatment beyond our current options.

Viscerosomatic and Viscerovisceral Convergence

Both visceral and somatic afferent signals synapse on the dorsal horn of the spinal cord. Visceral afferents are thought to represent approximately 10% of all afferent signal inflow into the spinal cord, a relatively small number.[7] The convergence of afferent visceral and somatic signals into the supraspinal centers is thought to generate the symptoms of referred pain felt by many patients. Despite these neurons initially being activated by visceral nociceptors, central processing can create the perception that the input is arising from various somatic dermatomes, resulting in pain perception distant to the primary site. This is illustrated in Fig. 4.4. Sites of convergence may also be sources of nociceptive sensitization, although the exact mechanisms are not well understood.

Visceral pain conditions rarely occur in isolation and there is often significant symptom overlap. This is thought to occur as a result of viscerovisceral convergence, where pathology in one visceral organ can induce disease states in nearby organs.[1] As an example, both colonic and bladder afferents enter the spinal cord at similar levels resulting in possible cross-organ sensitization. This can explain why some studies have shown that patients with colitis can sometimes develop hypersensitivity of the bladder.[1]

Visceral Hyperalgesia

Visceral hyperalgesia and hypersensitivity are defined as an exaggerated response to a painful stimulus or a decreased pain threshold following nociceptor activation. This can often occur in chronic visceral pain states, making it difficult to identify the initial insult or

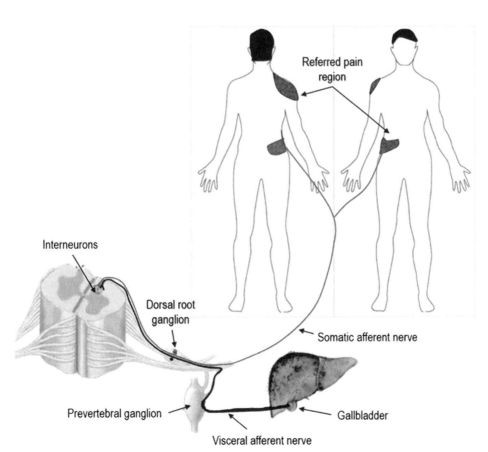

FIG. 4.4 Convergence of afferent visceral and somatic signals into the dorsal horn of the spinal cord. This viscerosomatic convergence can contribute to pain perception distant to the primary site. In this case, pain from the gallbladder can sometimes be felt in the abdominal region as well as the shoulder and scapular region.

pathology. Modulation in pain processing of visceral afferents can occur both peripherally and centrally resulting in hyperalgesia. Moshiree et al.[10] describe four potential mechanisms for visceral hypersensitivity. The first includes sensitization of primary afferent neurons innervating the viscera. The second is a result of spinal sensitization due to tonic impulse input from primary afferent neurons. The third potential mechanism involves descending facilitation from the brain to the spinal cord, and the final mechanism is a result of selective alteration in cortical processing of the afferent input.

Local ischemia, inflammation, and hypoxia can sensitize visceral afferent receptors in the periphery as mentioned previously with silent nociceptors. Degranulation of mast cells and secretion of inflammatory mediators causes an acute initial pain. This results in increased transmission and augmentation of the visceral afferents into the dorsal horn of the spinal cord. This persistent afferent stimulation can ultimately lead to sensitization, even after the initial insult has resolved.[3]

The mechanisms by which central sensitization contributes to visceral hyperalgesia have not been well studied in humans.[5] Centrally, positive feedback loops between spinal and supraspinal structures are thought to increase excitability and influence the development of visceral hyperalgesia. Additionally, psychologic stress and trauma can have significant effects on the perception of visceral pain.[1,5] Clearly, emotional states and a tendency to have heightened anticipation to threat can play a role in chronic persistent visceral pain.

CLINICAL FEATURES AND EVALUATION

The clinical presentation of patients with visceral pain poses a unique challenge for clinicians. On one hand, normal variations in visceral sensations are experienced throughout life. This may include the uneasiness felt in the stomach prior to a stressful event, sometimes referred to as "butterflies in the stomach." Bladder pain induced by stretching of a full bladder and abdominal pain due to constipation are normal responses to changes in visceral function. Acute-onset severe visceral pain can also be a normal signal indicating a medical emergency such as cholecystitis or myocardial infarction.[5] On the other hand, these normal visceral sensations can sometimes be altered or amplified into chronic visceral symptoms that cause significant morbidity without any identifiable cause.

Cervero and Laird[6] described five important clinical characteristics of visceral pain. The first is that pain is not evoked from all viscera. It has been noted that noxious stimuli such as cutting and burning are not perceived by all visceral organs, thus differentiating visceral sensations from somatic sensations.[4] The second is that pain is not always linked to visceral injury. The third characteristic is that visceral pain is often diffuse and poorly localized. The fourth characteristic states that pain is often referred to other locations. The final characteristic is that visceral pain is often accompanied by motor and autonomic reflexes. This can include nausea, vomiting, sweating, or changes in vital signs.

A common clinical condition to illustrate these visceral pain characteristics is pancreatitis resulting from inflammation of the pancreas. Patients often present with severe and generalized abdominal pain sometimes more localized to the upper quadrants. Symptoms can also radiate to the back or the shoulder. Autonomic symptoms such as nausea, vomiting, or increases in blood pressure and heart rate may also be present. An example of a condition that may not be due to a significant underlying pathology is severe gas pain. This too can present with vague abdominal symptoms and is a result of colonic stretching rather than true visceral injury. Stimuli that induce visceral pain can include distention, ischemia, and inflammation.[2] It is important to note that the severity of pain does not always correspond to the severity of the underlying condition. Malignancy or solid tumors such as those of the pancreas can sometimes go undetectable until the later stages, whereas more common conditions such as hunger pain or the urge to void can sometimes cause severe pain.

Visceral Referral Patterns

Visceral symptoms are most often experienced as a diffuse, generalized, and poorly defined pain within the abdominal region. However, pain from different visceral sources can refer to various somatic locations. Thought to be a response to viscerosomatic convergence, this can help explain some common pain referral patterns that are seen in visceral pain conditions.

Klineberg et al.[11] described examples of some visceral pain referral patterns that can be seen in patients presenting with back pain. For example, patients with aortic aneurysms can report mid-thoracic back pain that can be severe and described as tearing. Patients with gallbladder or liver pathology can have referred pain in the posterior scapular and shoulder region. This can be especially important in patients with spinal cord injury when there is sensation impairment below the level of injury and referred pain may be the only presenting symptom suggesting the underlying pathology. Ectopic pregnancy, kidney stones, and prostatitis may also present with referred pain to the back region. Pain and tenderness at McBurney point, located one-third the distance from the anterior superior iliac spine to the umbilicus, can suggest underlying appendicitis. Commonly referred pain patterns are shown in Fig. 4.5.

Risk Factors for Visceral Hyperalgesia

Symptoms of visceral hyperalgesia and hypersensitivity make the clinical evaluation and treatment of visceral pain disorders difficult. It is unclear exactly why patients' experience with these disorders can be highly variable, sometimes self-limiting and at other times causing significant pain and disability. Psychosocial factors are thought to influence the development of chronic visceral pain symptoms. Genetic factors and the body's stress response systems may also play a role.

Tillisch and Mayer[12] posit that an altered cognitive-emotional modulation of visceral afferent stimuli influences the clinical presentation of chronic visceral abdominal pain. In experimental fMRI studies, patients who have visceral pain with chronic pain, in contrast to healthy subjects, show activation of pain-related regions in the anticipation of pain, prior to pain delivery. This lends support to the notion that the perception of visceral pain is modulated by a psychologic state and helps explain why psychologic stressors and maladaptive coping strategies can thus pose a common risk factor for the development of chronic visceral pain. Clinically, patients with IBS, IBD, and IC have been seen to have symptoms that are exacerbated during periods of emotional distress.[1] Psychologic conditions such as depression, anxiety, and posttraumatic stress disorder, as well as chronic somatic pain syndromes, commonly overlap with chronic visceral pain and further reinforce the reporting of pain symptoms. Emotional trauma early in life, such as sexual abuse and maternal separation, can also be a risk factor for the development of chronic visceral pain in adulthood.[13] Clinical evaluation for potential psychologic comorbidities is essential in the diagnostic workup of chronic visceral pain symptoms, as these may be targets for potential treatment modalities.

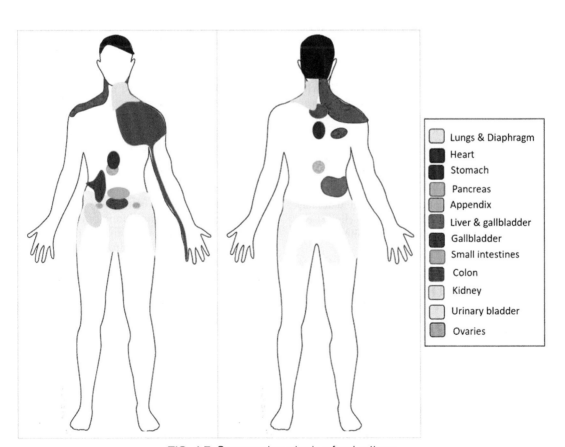

FIG. 4.5 Common visceral pain referral patterns.

Lungs & Diaphragm
Heart
Stomach
Pancreas
Appendix
Liver & gallbladder
Gallbladder
Small intestines
Colon
Kidney
Urinary bladder
Ovaries

Genetic disposition may play a role in the development of functional gastrointestinal disorders (FGIDs). This has been seen in twin and family studies associated with IBS, although no specific gene has been associated.[13] Organic causes of visceral pain, including IBD and celiac disease, are also known to have familial components. More recent research has sparked interest in possible epigenetic mechanisms that can alter gene expression without changing the underlying DNA sequence. These mechanisms include DNA methylation, histone modification, and microRNA activity. These environmental factors can play a role in the transfer of visceral pain characteristics and were seen in maternally separated rats exposed to stress.[8] It was noted that offspring cared for by maternally separated rats showed visceral hypersensitivity, whereas offspring cared for by conventionally raised rats did not show these symptoms in adulthood.

The autonomic nervous system and hypothalamic-pituitary-adrenal (HPA) axis both may be implicated in the development of chronic visceral pain in a response to stress. Autonomic dysfunction may be present in many conditions where chronic pain predominates, such as IBS, fibromyalgia, and chronic pelvic pain13. There appears to be a sex difference, with an altered autonomic nervous system responsiveness to a visceral stimulus being more prominent in men with IBS compared with women, as reported by Tillisch.[14] The HPA axis and specifically corticotropin-releasing factor (CRF) are influential in the body's stress response. CRF can be upregulated by intestinal inflammation as well as psychologic stressors and conditions, leading to enhanced visceral nociception. In rodent studies, CRF injections induced hyperalgesia to colorectal distention, while CRF receptor antagonism reduced visceral hyperalgesia.[1] Human studies to date have not been successful in achieving positive clinical outcomes with CRF receptor antagonists despite the strong preclinical models.[15]

Clinical Evaluation

A comprehensive clinical history and physical examination are essential in the evaluation of visceral pain syndromes. Psychosocial assessment is also very important, as the use of psychometric inventories and scales can help reveal underlying psychologic comorbidities and catastrophizing. Although functional disorders are not life threatening, they can have a significant impact on a patient's quality of life. FGIDs account for a large portion of chronic visceral abdominal pain; however, it is important not to overlook organic causes that could signal more serious or emergent conditions. Certain clues in the clinical history and physical examination can point toward organic disease such as weight loss, bloody or steatorrheic stools, jaundice, a history of malignancy, or a palpable abdominal mass.[16]

It is also important to be aware of factors that can aggravate and alleviate visceral pain symptoms to assist clinicians in the evaluation of patients. Food intake, for example, may worsen with reflux disease but does not often exacerbate IBS symptoms. Symptom relief after bowel movements may be associated with IBS. A history of recent life stressors such as bereavement, financial distress, and trauma is often associated with functional disorders, but can also be reported in IBD and gastroesophageal reflux disease.[16]

In the case of chronic visceral pain from suspected urogenital and pelvic disorders, symptoms may often involve more than one organ system. Additionally, there may be an association of psychologic comorbidities, such as anxiety, depression, and history of sexual abuse, with these disorders. Symptoms include private bodily functions such as sexual activity, voiding, and defecation. Thus it is important to establish good rapport with patients in order to create a strong physician-patient relationship. Essential components in the history may include cyclic patterns of pain, pain with intercourse, history of sexually transmitted diseases, prior abdominal or pelvic surgeries, and history of traumatic relationship or abuse. The physical examination should be performed in a methodical way minimizing discomfort to the patient. Utilization of a chaperone should be offered to patients during any sensitive physical examination.

CLINICAL SYNDROMES

A variety of clinical conditions can produce chronic visceral pain symptoms, spanning from organic pathology to functional syndromes. A few common visceral pain disorders are listed in Table 4.1. Visceral comorbidities often overlap with patients developing multiple conditions over time. For example, the incidence of IBS is two to three times higher in patients with IBD than that in the general population.[1,17] Patients with IC are also approximately 100 times more likely to have IBD symptoms than control patients.[1,18] Additionally, 20%−30% of patients with IC have IBS symptoms.[18] The overlap between these conditions makes it difficult for clinicians to identify the inciting pathology in order to help direct treatment. Here we will categorize different visceral pain syndromes and symptoms.

TABLE 4.1

Examples of Chronic Visceral Pain Disorders Grouped into Organic and Functional Syndromes.

CHRONIC VISCERAL PAIN DISORDERS	
Organic Syndromes	**Functional Syndromes**
Inflammatory bowel disease	Irritable bowel syndrome
Chronic pancreatitis	Functional abdominal pain syndrome
Cystitis	Interstitial cystitis/bladder pain syndrome
Malignancy	

Gastrointestinal Disorders

Visceral abdominal pain can have a multitude of causes spanning from acute to chronic. Chronic abdominal pain is one of the most frequent pain complaints with a prevalence of about 22.9 per 1000 individual-years.[16] Despite significant workup and diagnostic tests, the cause of symptoms often remains a mystery. Conditions that have been implicated in chronic visceral abdominal pain include IBD, chronic pancreatitis, IBS, functional abdominal pain syndrome, functional dyspepsia, and postsurgical abdominal adhesions.

IBD includes Crohn disease and ulcerative colitis and is an inflammatory disorder of the gastrointestinal tract that occurs as a result of an exaggerated immune response. Crohn disease can occur in any portion of the gastrointestinal tract, whereas ulcerative colitis is restricted to the colon region. Abdominal pain, diarrhea, and gastrointestinal bleeding, along with a chronic relapsing course, are the major clinical features of the syndrome. Diagnosis is usually achieved through colonoscopy or endoscopy with biopsy. IBD care results in significant economic cost in the United States, stated to be over $6 billion each year.[1] Exacerbations of Crohn disease can account for a large portion of this cost, as relapses can be more severe than ulcerative colitis. Complications can include strictures, fistulas, and perforation and these are also more commonly seen with Crohn disease. Goals of therapy with IBD primarily include symptom management and mucosal healing. Medications with immunosuppressive properties are usually the method of treatment, although colectomy is a treatment option for patients with ulcerative colitis. Despite continual improvements in medical therapy, chronic visceral pain often occurs in patients with IBD

because of refractory inflammation, scarring, postsurgical complications, or centrally medicated factors.

Chronic pancreatitis is another organic cause of visceral abdominal pain. Chronic or intermittent visceral symptoms can be present in up to 80%–90% of patients.[19] Although acute episodes may initially be self-limiting and resolve without any lasting injury, repeated insults can produce structural changes. Alcohol abuse is the primary cause in more than half the cases of chronic pancreatitis.[20] Other potential causes include smoking, previous trauma, ductal obstruction, hyperlipidemia, genetic factors, and α_1-antitrypsin deficiency.[20] Pain is often localized to the epigastric region and can radiate to the back. Symptoms can be aggravated by lying in a supine position and eating food and can sometimes be relieved with leaning forward. Elevated pancreatic enzyme levels are often present in acute episodes but are unreliable in chronic pancreatitis. Endoscopic ultrasonography and endoscopic retrograde cholangiopancreatography are used for diagnostic purposes. Imaging, such as computed tomography and MRI, can also assist with diagnosis, as it may show atrophy, dilation of the pancreatic duct, calcifications, or pseudocyst formation. Surgical diversion or resection may be a definitive treatment; however, treatment options more commonly center around symptom management and reduction of offending agents. Abstinence from alcohol can improve chronic visceral pain symptoms in up to 50% of patients.[20] Interventional procedures such as celiac plexus blocks have also been used to assist with symptoms and will be discussed later in this chapter.

FGIDs include a spectrum of conditions spanning from children to adults and are unique owing to their complexity of symptoms despite the absence of pathology. Because of the absence of organic disease, FGIDs are often diagnosed by symptom criteria. One of the well-known FGIDs is IBS, which affects more than 11% of the global population with a majority of patients, up to 65%, being women.[1] The Rome IV diagnostic criteria used for IBS state patients must have recurrent abdominal pain on average at least 1 day/week in the past 3 months associated with two of the following: symptoms related to defecation, symptoms associated with a change in frequency of stool, and symptoms associated with a change in the appearance of stool.[21] Symptoms must have been present for at least 6 months at the time of diagnosis. Symptoms can be highly variable and are sometimes exacerbated by stress, insomnia, or emotional distress. IBS is also further classified as constipation predominant or diarrhea predominant, with a mixed form also being present in some patients. Similar to other FGIDs, IBS is considered to be a disorder of the brain-gut axis. Altered gastrointestinal motility with high-amplitude propagating contractions has been described in the diarrhea-predominant subgroup but is not a universal feature.[16] In fact, the majority of patients with IBS have bowel habits with normal intestinal and colonic transit times by currently available measurement techniques. Altered intestinal microbial composition and a history of infectious gastroenteritis have been suspected to have contributions to the development of IBS and other FGIDs. Centrally, FGIDs may share certain features such as enhanced stress sensitivity associated with autonomic dysfunction and HPA axis dysfunction, as discussed earlier in this chapter. Coexistence of other psychiatric and chronic pain disorders and enhanced perception of visceral symptoms lead to altered modulation of visceral pain. Because of the complexity of symptoms associated with IBS and co-morbidity with psychologic and chronic pain conditions, the total direct and indirect costs of IBS in the United States is estimated at approximately $30 billion per year.[1] Current treatment strategies are suboptimal but include medications for the management of bowel habit and pain such as antidepressants, antispasmodic medications, or other targeted drugs, as well as dietary modifications, and psychologic interventions such as cognitive behavior therapy (CBT) or hypnotherapy.[20]

Pelvic and Urogenital Disorders

Pelvic and urogenital pain is most commonly seen in women, although it can affect men as well. Symptoms are complex and can lead to significantly decreased quality of life, decreased function, and loss of economic productivity. Symptoms can have varied causes including vascular, neurologic, musculoskeletal, and urologic. Because of the personal nature of these symptoms, patients may feel embarrassed and often underreport symptoms or do not seek medical care. In the United States, 14.7% of women between 18 and 50 years of age reported chronic pelvic pain.[16] Similar to FGIDs, chronic pelvic visceral pain symptoms may not have an obvious cause or diagnosis. Common acute and chronic conditions may include IC, endometriosis, adenomyosis, chronic pelvic pain, pudendal neuropathy, myofascial pelvic floor pain, dysmenorrhea, ectopic pregnancy, and pelvic congestion syndrome. Here we will focus on a few common causes of chronic visceral pelvic and urogenital pain.

IC and bladder pain syndrome (BPS) are the most common causes of urogenital and pelvic pain in both women and men. BPS is thought to be an early form of IC and serves as a descriptive diagnosis for a combination of complex urogenital and pelvic symptoms. There is no consensus on the cause and pathophysiology of this disorder. Cystoscopy may reveal the presence of mucosal ulcers, also known as Hunner ulcers. However, these findings on cystoscopy are not pathognomonic, and there is a subset of patients who may have normal cystoscopic findings.[22] These patients may be referred to as having BPS rather than IC, given the lack of inflammatory findings. Intravesical potassium sensitivity testing and urodynamic testing may also assist in supporting the diagnosis. For the purposes of this chapter, we will discuss IC and BPS together. IC/BPS is a female-predominant condition, with a female-to-male ratio of 10:1, and affects primarily young to middle-aged women.[19] Symptoms can progress rapidly and include pain, nocturia, frequency, and urgency. Pain may be localized to the lower abdomen, pelvis, or groin area. Symptoms can cause significant emotional and psychologic distress. It was reported that 25% of patients with IC/BPS also carried a diagnosis of depressive disorder and 19% carried a diagnosis of anxiety.[20] This can contribute to symptoms of visceral hyperalgesia, making treatment more difficult. In the United States, the costs associated with the treatment of IC/BPS are approximately $20–40 billion per year. There is no universally accepted treatment for IC/BPS and clinicians generally follow an approach from least invasive to most invasive treatments. Dietary modifications, stress management, and patient education are easy to implement. Unique treatment modalities used for IC/BPS include oral pentosan polysulfate and bladder hydrodistention. Pentosan polysulfate is believed to provide a protective coating to the damaged bladder wall, thus helping to improve pain as well as decrease urgency and frequency. Although some studies have seen improvement with pentosan polysulfate, others have had different results, including one that found cyclosporine to be more effective in reducing frequency.[20] Bladder hydrodistention and instillation with dimethyl sulfoxide, heparin, or lidocaine has shown some benefit in improving symptoms. Time itself has also shown to produce resolution of symptoms in some patients.

Endometriosis is the presence of endometrial glandular tissue in areas outside the uterus, such as the ovaries, fallopian tubes, bladder, or peritoneal cavity.[16,19] This results in a chronic inflammatory reaction. It is estimated to be present in approximately 1%–2% of the general female population.[20] The leading cause of endometriosis is thought to be a result of retrograde menstruation from the fallopian tubes into nearby structures causing the growth of endometrial tissue at these sites; however, this is not definitive, as retrograde menstruation has also been seen in women without endometriosis.[16] Variable symptoms are reported with endometriosis and some patients may even be asymptomatic. Thus a detailed history and physical examination is important to ensure that presenting symptoms are related to endometriosis. Pain is often described as cramping or stabbing, is usually cyclic in nature, and worsens with hormonal changes during menstruation. Associated symptoms may include dysmenorrhea, infertility, dyspareunia, urinary urgency, back pain, or thigh pain. On physical examination, a fixed retroverted uterus may be appreciated in addition to enlarged ovaries and rectovaginal nodules.[16] Surgical visualization via laparoscopy and histologic confirmation is the gold standard for diagnosis, but many clinicians may start empiric treatment based on a clinical diagnosis. Because of the hormonal sensitivity of the endometrial tissue, medical management often consists of hormonal treatments such as oral contraceptives or gonadotropin-releasing hormone (GnRH) agonists. These medications are often used to treat endometriosis-related pain symptoms, although symptoms often can recur if the medication is stopped. One study showed recurrence of symptoms 5.2 months after stopping a GnRH agonist.[16] More invasive treatments such as surgical management can sometimes be performed at the time of diagnostic laparoscopy if the lesions are small. Surgical excision has been shown to improve sexual function and reduce pain symptoms. Deep infiltrating endometrial lesions may carry a higher risk with surgery and these risks and benefits should be discussed with patients.

Chronic pelvic pain is a symptom that can be debilitating and can cause significant impairment of quality of life. In many patients, extensive diagnostic workup is unrevealing and no specific organic cause is appreciated. Often, the focus switches to symptomatic treatment management and patients are said to instead have a chronic pelvic and visceral pain syndrome. An exact definition of chronic pelvic pain syndrome has been difficult to establish, as in some cases there is no identifiable pathology and in other cases the pathology that is present may not be contributing to symptoms. A common definition used is pelvic pain in the same location that has lasted for at least 6 months.[23] A woman has a 5% risk of developing chronic pelvic pain, and this risk is multiplied in patients with a history of pelvic inflammatory disease.[23] Symptoms can be similar to other gynecologic and urologic conditions, highlighting the complexity of this syndrome. Patients may feel deep pain in the lower abdominal region radiating to the low back, buttocks, perineal area, or thighs. Other associated symptoms may include dyspareunia, changes in bowel or bladder habits, or a cyclic nature. Psychosocial factors such as depression, posttraumatic stress disorder, catastrophizing, or history of abuse may also be present. It is difficult to say if these psychologic comorbidities influenced the development of chronic pelvic pain or developed as a result of chronic pelvic pain. Thus a comprehensive history is essential in the initial patient evaluation. Additionally, a favorable patient rating of the initial consultation has been associated with better recovery.[16] It is important to allow patients to present their history, the effects pain has had on their life, and any thoughts they may have on the cause of the pain, as this itself may be therapeutic. Patients often desire to be taken seriously and reassured and this can lead to a more productive encounter. This condition is primarily prevalent in women but can also be present in men, in whom it is sometimes termed chronic prostatitis. Chronic pelvic pain is often poorly managed and difficult to treat. A pharmacologic trial of a GnRH agonist may be considered in women, especially if symptoms are cyclic. Diagnostic laparoscopy is often considered in refractory cases but the risks and benefits should be carefully evaluated. Medication classes utilized in other chronic pain syndromes, such as nonsteroidal antiinflammatory drugs, antidepressants, and anticonvulsants, have shown some benefit.[23]

TREATMENT MODALITIES

Chronic visceral pain and visceral hyperalgesia are complex clinical conditions that often require a multimodal treatment approach. Treatment is often directed at the underlying organic cause if it can be detected but, as discussed earlier in this chapter, this is often not the case. In patients without an identifiable cause, treatment goals often shift to symptomatic management to help patients improve their function and quality of life. Treatment regimens can consist of pharmacologic therapy, psychotherapy, integrative medicine, and interventional procedures.

Pharmacologic Therapy

Pharmacotherapy is divided into central- and peripheral-acting agents. Centrally acting medications are suspected to help reduce the mechanisms that modulate and interpret visceral afferent pain signals and the emotions associated with them.[16] They can also help treat coexisting psychologic disorders that often accompany chronic visceral pain. These medications include tricyclic antidepressants (TCAs), selective serotonin reuptake inhibitors (SSRIs), and serotonin and norepinephrine reuptake inhibitors, and they have been used in the treatment of chronic pain conditions for many years. A meta-analysis showed the superiority of both TCAs and SSRIs compared to placebo in patients with IBS with improvements in global assessment, symptom score, and abdominal pain.[24] In a study by Drossman et al.,[25] it was interestingly noted that a greater response was seen in patients without depression, suggesting the improvement in symptoms was not just due to treatment of the coexisting psychiatric condition. TCAs are generally started at low doses, as anticholinergic side effects can be a drawback with this medication. Anticonvulsive agents such as gabapentin and pregabalin have also shown some benefit in reducing chronic visceral pain symptoms.[4]

Peripherally acting antispasmodic medications are used in some FGIDs because they can help reduce stretch and contractions within the smooth muscle of the intestines thereby decreasing visceral afferent transmission. Medication classes can include anticholinergic agents and calcium channel blockers. Strong randomized controlled trials showing the benefits of these medications are limited; however, a meta-analysis did show that pinaverium bromide and trimebutine significantly reduced abdominal pain symptoms.[24] Peppermint oil has also been shown to have antispasmodic properties and can be beneficial in light of its favorable side effect profile.

Opioid medications are often requested by patients and have historically been a part of the treatment plan of patients with complex conditions and visceral hyperalgesia. Chronic opioid therapy with μ-agonists should be minimized, given the lack of long-term improvement and the known side effects of dependence, abuse, and opioid-induced hyperalgesia.[20] Patients with gastrointestinal disorders in particular may experience side effects of nausea, vomiting, and constipation, further exacerbating their overall symptoms. Peripheral visceral afferents express opioid κ receptors and thus κ-agonists have also been explored for their potential therapeutic effects. Central side effects of dysphoria and hallucinations may limit their use. Fedotozine was examined in chronic abdominal pain due to functional disorders over a short period and showed small improvements compared to placebo.[4] In 2015, eluxadoline was approved for use in diarrhea-predominant IBS. Further studies are indicated to explore the potential benefits and safety of these medications for visceral pain.

Psychotherapy

Psychologic and behavioral therapy is often used in patients with chronic visceral pain refractory to medications and in patients with psychologic comorbidities. However, consideration for earlier use of these interventions is warranted. As mentioned earlier, persistent visceral afferent activity can cause structural and functional changes in regions of the brain associated with pain processing and interpretation. A top-down treatment approach using psychologic interventions may provide significant benefits for patients. CBT is a commonly utilized treatment in functional visceral pain disorders. It aims to challenge and adjust cognitive thoughts and maladaptive behaviors such as avoidance and fear. Gut-directed CBT is well studied, and in a meta-analysis, it has been shown to reduce IBS-related symptoms versus placebo.[24] The difficulty is that CBT can be expensive and limited based on the availability of specialized therapists. Ljótsson et al.[26] describe an internet-based CBT program that has shown benefits specifically in patients with IBS. Lackner et al.[27] described a minimal contact CBT that performed as well as or better than traditional CBT. These types of minimal contact and patient-directed programs may help fill the need for trained therapists and conventional programs.

Hypnotherapy is another top-down intervention that has been shown to provide benefit to some patients. Specifically, gut-directed hypnotherapy in patients with IBS has shown improvements in pain symptoms and quality of life with a number needed to treat of two.[24] Studies in children and adults with functional dyspepsia have also shown benefits from hypnotherapy.[28] The exact mechanism underlying hypnotherapy is not fully understood, but possible theories include changes in brain responses to painful stimuli, decreased peripheral awareness, and reduction of central pain amplification.[16] Further studies of hypnotherapy across multiple visceral pain syndromes are needed, as are more studies evaluating uses of hypnotherapy in group settings or using online or minimal contact protocols to allow for increased availability.

Biofeedback is the process of gaining control over physiologic functions and has been well studied in chronic pain syndromes. Further research is needed to identify potential benefits in chronic visceral and abdominal pain syndromes.

Integrative Medicine Treatments

Integrative health modalities have become more incorporated in treatment regimens to advance patients' health and quality of life. These may include herbal therapies, acupuncture, tai chi, and meditation, among many others. There has been growing interest in the interaction between the gut microbiota and the regulation and processing of visceral afferents, as well as the gut-brain axis as a whole. Regarding patients with IBS, analysis has shown a shift in the diversity of bacterial species present in the bowel but consistent and clinically relevant changes in the microbiota across studies is still elusive.[29] The gut microbiome can be affected by various dietary, psychologic, infectious, and life stressors, thus modulating the responses to visceral pain.[29] To assist with this imbalance, prebiotics and probiotics have been utilized in an attempt to restore normal gut microbiota. *Lactobacillus salivarius* and *Bifidobacterium infantis* have both been shown to have some benefit in reducing IBS-related pain symptoms.[24] The magnitudes of these effects are small and further research is still needed to investigate which strains and in what combinations probiotics may be beneficial.

Acupuncture has also been utilized in the treatment of chronic visceral pain conditions. Acupuncture is thought to decrease pain through the activation of both endogenous opioid peptides and neurotransmitters, serotonin and norepinephrine, both peripherally and centrally.[30] Mindfulness-based stress reduction (MBSR) has been successful for symptomatic management in functional visceral disorders such as IBS in several clinical trials.[31] Because MBSR has also been shown to be beneficial for multiple types of chronic pain, depression, and anxiety, it is increasing in availability across health systems.[32] Integrative treatments have shown promise and additional well-controlled studies will assist in supporting their use in patients.

Interventional Treatments

Interventional procedures can be used both diagnostically and therapeutically for chronic visceral pain disorders, but they are of most benefit in those disorders with a clear anatomic cause. A transversus abdominis plane block is an abdominal field block performed with a local anesthetic agent between the internal oblique and transversus abdominis muscles. This will allow for analgesia to the lower and lateral abdominal wall, helping differentiate somatic from visceral pain. This can be used in the diagnostic workup of functional abdominal disorders when the underlying cause is not clear. Other somatic nerve blocks include a paravertebral nerve block, intercostal nerve block, and rectus abdominis sheath block.

Sympathetic nerve blocks can assist in the evaluation and treatment of visceral pain conditions. Spinal afferents innervate organs in the upper abdomen and travel to the celiac plexus and splanchnic nerves. Celiac plexus and splanchnic nerve blocks can be performed at this location.[4] A traditional dorsal approach under fluoroscopic guidance is used to deliver anesthetic medication at the target location. Neurolytic agents such as ethanol have also been used if longer-lasting treatment is desired, and recent research has also explored the use of radiofrequency nerve ablation treatments.[4] A superior hypogastric plexus block can be utilized to address the lower gastrointestinal tract and pelvic region. Sympathetic blocks have been used in visceral malignancy, chronic pancreatitis, and IC with some benefit; however, the risks and benefits should be discussed with patients and the long-term outcomes of these treatments may be limited.[4]

Spinal cord stimulation (SCS) has been utilized for many years to treat complex regional pain syndrome and postlaminectomy syndrome. There has been recent interest in the use of SCS in the treatment of chronic visceral pain syndromes refractory to multiple treatment modalities, but the evidence for this is limited. One case study utilized SCS for the treatment of chronic nonalcoholic pancreatitis.[33] The patient showed improvement in pain symptoms as well as decreased opioid use. Another study in 35 patients with chronic visceral abdominal pain showed SCS trial decreased pain at least 50% in 86% of the patients.[34] Of the 28 patients who received the implant, 19 were followed up for 1 year and showed maintenance of pain relief. Additional large studies and randomized controlled trials are needed to further validate the effectiveness and safety of SCS in these complex patients.

CONCLUSION

Chronic visceral pain is a complex clinical condition that can result in debility, decreased quality of life, and significant socioeconomic burden. Despite advancements in our understanding of the physiologic mechanisms of visceral pain and visceral hyperalgesia, patients continue to present a challenge for even experienced physicians. Central and peripheral mechanisms play a role in the development and treatment of chronic visceral pain symptoms. Psychologic stressors and emotional trauma are among the risk factors that exacerbate these conditions. A detailed clinical history and physical examination are essential to help identify organic causes amenable to treatment. A multimodal treatment approach directed at symptomatic management may utilize pharmacologic therapy, psychotherapy, integrative medicine, and interventional treatments. With a steady spotlight on understanding the physiology behind these symptoms and how this may contribute to future treatments, we can continue to improve the functional outcomes in these complex patients.

REFERENCES

1. Grundy L, Erickson A, Brierley S. Visceral pain. *Annu Rev Physiol.* 2019;81(1):261–284.
2. Al-Chaer E, Traub R. Biological basis of visceral pain: recent developments. *Pain.* 2002;96(3):221–225.
3. Sikandar S, Dickenson A. Visceral pain. *Curr Opin Support Palliat Care.* 2012;6(1):17–26.
4. Bielefeldt K, Gebhart G. Visceral pain. In: *Practical Management of Pain.* 2014, 441–448.e3.
5. Bulmer D, Roza C. Visceral pain. In: *The Oxford Handbook of the Neurobiology of Pain.* 2018.
6. Cervero F, Laird J. Visceral pain. *Lancet.* 1999;353(9170): 2145–2148.
7. Ness T, Gebhart G. Visceral pain: a review of experimental studies. *Pain.* 1990;41(2):167–234.
8. Tao Z, Traub R, Cao D. Epigenetic modulation of visceral pain. *EpigeneticsChronic Pain.* 2019:141–156.
9. Mayer E, Gupta A, Kilpatrick L, Hong J. Imaging brain mechanisms in chronic visceral pain. *Pain.* 2015;156: S50–S63.
10. Moshiree B, Zhou Q, Price D, Verne G. Central sensitisation in visceral pain disorders. *Gut.* 2006;55(7):905–908.
11. Klineberg E, Mazanec D, Orr D, Demicco R, Bell G, McLain R. Masquerade: medical causes of back pain. *Cleve Clin J Med.* 2007;74(12):905–913.
12. Tillisch K, Mayer E. Pain perception in irritable bowel syndrome. *CNS Spectr.* 2005;10(11):877–882.
13. Farmer A, Aziz Q. Gut pain & visceral hypersensitivity. *Br J Pain.* 2013;7(1):39–47.
14. Tillisch K. Sex specific alterations in autonomic function among patients with irritable bowel syndrome. *Gut.* 2005;54(10):1396–1401.
15. Coric V, Feldman H, Oren D, et al. Multicenter, randomized, double-blind, active comparator and placebo-controlled trial of a corticotropin-releasing factor receptor-1 antagonist in generalized anxiety disorder. *Depress Anxiety.* 2010;27(5):417–425.
16. Ballantyne J, Fishman S, Bonica J. *Bonica's Management of Pain.* 4th ed. Philadelphia: Lippincott Williams & Wilkins; 2010 Chapter 47, 61–65.
17. Ansari R, Attari F, Razjouyan H, et al. Ulcerative colitis and irritable bowel syndrome: relationships with quality of life. *Eur J Gastroenterol Hepatol.* 2008;20(1):46–50.
18. Alagiri M, Chottiner S, Ratner V, Slade D, Hanno P. Interstitial cystitis: unexplained associations with other chronic disease and pain syndromes. *Urology.* 1997;49(5):52–57.
19. Cheng J, Rosenquist R. *Fundamentals of Pain Medicine.* 1st ed. Cham, Switzerland: Springer International Publishing; 2018 Chapter 29–30.
20. Stannard C, Kalso E, Ballantyne J. *Evidence-Based Chronic Pain Management.* Singapore: Blackwell Publishing Ltd.; 2010 Chapter 15.
21. Schmulson M, Drossman D. What is new in Rome IV. *J Neurogastroenterol Motil.* 2017;23(2):151–163.
22. Wesselmann U. Interstitial cystitis: a chronic visceral pain syndrome. *Urology.* 2001;57(6):32–39.
23. Wesselmann U, Czakanski P. Pelvic pain: a chronic visceral pain syndrome. *Curr Pain Headache Rep.* 2001;5(1): 13–19.
24. Vanuytsel T, Tack J, Boeckxstaens G. Treatment of abdominal pain in irritable bowel syndrome. *J Gastroenterol.* 2014;49(8):1193–1205.
25. Drossman D, Toner B, Whitehead W, et al. Cognitive-behavioral therapy versus education and desipramine versus placebo for moderate to severe functional bowel disorders. *Gastroenterology.* 2003;125(1):19–31.
26. Ljótsson B, Hedman E, Andersson E, et al. Internet-delivered exposure-based treatment vs. Stress management for irritable bowel syndrome: a randomized trial. *Am J Gastroenterol.* 2011;106(8):1481–1491.
27. Lackner J, Keefer L, Jaccard J, et al. The Irritable Bowel Syndrome Outcome Study (IBSOS): rationale and design of a randomized, placebo-controlled trial with 12month follow up of self- versus clinician-administered CBT for moderate to severe irritable bowel syndrome. *Contemp Clin Trials.* 2012;33(6):1293–1310.
28. Palsson O. Hypnosis treatment of gastrointestinal disorders: a comprehensive review of the empirical evidence. *Am J Clin Hypn.* 2015;58(2):134–158.
29. Chichlowski M, Rudolph C. Visceral pain and gastrointestinal microbiome. *J Neurogastroenterol Motil.* 2015;21(2): 172–181.
30. Chen S, Wang S, Rong P, et al. Acupuncture for visceral pain: neural substrates and potential mechanisms. *Evid base Compl Alternative Med.* 2014;2014:1–12.
31. Garland E, Gaylord S, Palsson O, Faurot K, Douglas Mann J, Whitehead W. Therapeutic mechanisms of a mindfulness-based treatment for IBS: effects on visceral sensitivity, catastrophizing, and affective processing of pain sensations. *J Behav Med.* 2011;35(6):591–602.
32. Goyal M, Singh S, Sibinga E, et al. Meditation programs for psychological stress and well-being. *JAMA Intern Med.* 2014;174(3):357.
33. Kapural L, Rakic M. Spinal cord stimulation for chronic visceral pain secondary to chronic non-alcoholic pancreatitis. *J Clin Gastroenterol.* 2008;42(6):750–751.
34. Kapural L, Nagem H, Tlucek H, Sessler D. Spinal cord stimulation for chronic visceral abdominal pain. *Pain Med.* 2010;11(3):347–355.

CHAPTER 5

Neuropathic Pain

EDWARD K. PANG, DO • GABRIEL RUDD-BARNARD, MD

DEFINITIONS

There is a protective role in experiencing pain that warns of potential or actual tissue damage. Persistent pain, however, does not offer any such advantage. Chronic pain is a very disabling multifaceted disease that often requires multimodal treatments. Chronic pain can be classified broadly as nociceptive, neuropathic, or a mixture of the two. According to International Association for the Study of Pain (IASP), neuropathic pain is defined as pain caused by a lesion (an obvious trauma or abnormality in diagnostic testing) or disease (a known underlying cause such as stroke and diabetes mellitus) involving the somatosensory nervous system.[1] Neuropathic pain can be further subdivided into peripheral versus central depending on the location of the damage. This chapter focuses on neuropathic pain as a result of insult to the peripheral nerves.

Not all patients with peripheral neuropathy experience pain. In a large observational study of diabetic patients, the prevalence of painful diabetic neuropathy was 21%.[2] Whether neuropathy is affecting a single nerve, mononeuropathy, or multiple nerves, polyneuropathy, patients with neuropathy experience similar change in sensation. These changes include but are not limited to allodynia (pain after a commonly nonpainful stimulus), hyperalgesia (exaggerated pain after a commonly painful stimulus), paresthesia (abnormal nonpainful sensations that is not unpleasant), dysesthesia (abnormal painful sensation that is unpleasant), and hyperpathia (prolonged persistent painful sensation after repetitive stimulation). A type of neuropathy involving inflammation of the nerve is termed neuritis. This is often related to a viral or bacterial infection. A classic example is acute inflammatory demyelinating polyneuropathy (AIDP).

EPIDEMIOLOGY

Given the lack of validated clinical diagnostic tools to identify neuropathic pain, the incidence and prevalence of neuropathic pain has been challenging to estimate. The recent development of simple symptom-based screening tools has helped provide such information on the general population. One study demonstrated that the best estimate of prevalence of neuropathic pain ranges from 7% to 10%.[3] Neuropathic pain is also more frequently seen in women and in patients older than 50 years of age with the peak age between 50 and 64 years of age.[4]

MECHANISMS

Multiple mechanisms have been proposed for the development of neuropathic pain. Having a better understanding of the pathophysiology of neuropathic pain can in turn assist in finding better treatment options for patients. The pathological changes that cause neuropathic pain predominantly involve small sensory fibers, including unmyelinated C fibers and myelinated Aβ and Aδ fiber. After nerve injury, voltage-gated sodium channels accumulate around the injured site and along the length of the axon, which results in hyperexcitability and ectopic action potential discharges.[5] Sodium channel blockers and membrane stabilizers specifically target this mechanism to ease neuropathic pain. Transient receptor potential vanilloid type 1 (TRPV1) channels have been suggested to play a role in neuropathic pain. TRPV1 receptors are activated by heat (>42°C), low pH (pH < 6), and endogenous lipid molecules.[6] Nerve injury results in downregulation of TRPV1 receptors on the injured nerve and upregulation of uninjured C fibers resulting in spontaneous nerve activity, which in turn may be experienced as heat hyperalgesia along with burning pain.[7] Capsaicin is a naturally occurring vanilloid that activates TRPV1 receptors stimulating influx of cations that result in desensitization.[8]

Nerve injury can also induce sprouting of sympathetic fibers into the dorsal root ganglion (DRG), which presents as another mechanism for neuropathic pain and more specifically sympathetically mediated pain. After partial nerve injury, both damaged and undamaged axons begin expressing α-adrenoreceptors making them sensitive to various neurotransmitters from postganglionic sympathetic terminals. In both circumstances, the sympathetically mediated pain can theoretically be treated with sympathetic blocks or α1 antagonists.[5]

Changes in the central nervous system can occur after a peripheral nerve injury. Such change includes alteration of inhibitory control in the spinal cord. The disinhibition is orchestrated by multiple mechanisms. Opioid and gamma-aminobutyric acid (GABA) receptors have been found to be downregulated. The amount of GABA, an inhibitory transmitter, is reduced in the dorsal horn while the expression of cholecystokinin, an opiate receptor inhibitor, is upregulated. In addition, the death of inhibitory interneurons in lamina II is thought to be through an excitatory mechanism.[5] The culmination of these disinhibitory changes leads to spontaneous activation and an exaggerated painful response. As such, drugs targeting GABA receptors or drugs that mimic descending inhibition such as clonidine can have therapeutic value in treating neuropathic pain.

EVALUATION

Patients with neuropathic pain have distinctive symptoms that differ from patients with nociceptive pain. The patient can present with positive symptoms including paresthesia, dysesthesia, allodynia, hyperalgesia, and hyperpathia. Negative symptoms may also be present, such as reduced sensory perception to light touch, pinprick, vibration, or temperature. The most common symptoms a patient may describe are tingling, pins and needles, burning, and shooting sensations. Screening tools have been developed to identify patients with neuropathic pain in the form of questionnaires. These questionnaires focus on patient-reported verbal descriptors of their symptoms. Some of the most common scales are the Neuropathic Pain Questionnaire (NPQ), painDETECT, ID-Pain, and Douleur-Neuropathique 4 (DN4).[9] These screening tools are useful first-line instruments to identify patients with neuropathic pain; however, their efficacy of accurately identifying these patients is unknown.

Physical examination should include a thorough sensory examination including testing of light touch, vibration, pinprick, temperature, and temporal summation. Light touch can be assessed by application of cotton wool to skin, vibration by utilizing a tuning fork, pinprick by a sharp object such as body pin, temperature with cold and heat stimuli such as a metal object. Temporal summation can be tested with repetitive stimulation.[7] Peripheral neuropathy is often described as a stocking glove distribution of altered sensory perception during testing.

Diagnostic testing may be helpful in patients with suspected neuropathic pain. Electrodiagnostic testing (EDX) is one of the more common studies performed that involves two separate portions. The nerve conduction study measures electrical impulses by stimulating the nerves with electric current, whereas electromyography detects electrical activity of a muscle utilizing a fine needle. EDX may provide confirmation of neuropathy and differentiate whether the process is demyelinating or axonal as well as if the patient has mononeuropathy or polyneuropathy. However, EDX can be normal if the painful peripheral neuropathy (PPN) only involves small fibers as EDX only tests damage in large fibers.[10] Skin biopsy is an option to test for abnormality in small-fiber neuropathy; however, its utility is controversial and there is poor correlation between abnormal biopsy findings and pain.[11]

In addition, quantitative sensory testing (QST) is occasionally used to assess small and large fiber neuropathies as well as monitor somatosensory deficits and painful neuropathies.[2] QST is not meant to be used in isolation to determine neuropathic pain, but to provide complementary information.[13] It is also important to note that the treatment of neuropathic pain does not change with these confirmatory testing. Laboratory testing is another important tool to help identify potentially treatable causes of pain such as diabetes mellitus and other causes of peripheral polyneuropathy including metabolic, toxic, genetic, or infectious/inflammatory etiologies.

The IASP has developed a grading system intended to determine the likelihood that the patient's pain is neuropathic. "Possible" neuropathic pain is defined as symptoms consistent with neuropathic pain features as well as the pain distribution are anatomically consistent with the suspected lesion. "Probable" neuropathic pain requires additional clinical evidence on physical examination such as sensory changes. "Definite" neuropathic pain involves further objective diagnostic confirmatory tests, such as an electrodiagnostic study or advanced imaging study.[14]

PAINFUL NEUROPATHIES

Again, this section will focus on neuropathies whose symptoms are peripheral. The etiology of neuropathies with painful peripheral symptoms can further be categorized as injury/acquired, genetic, autoimmune/infectious, or as a result of systemic disease (i.e., diabetes mellitus). PPNs vary widely in their origin; therefore, a thorough medical history and physical exam should guide further diagnostic evaluation and treatment considerations. Reviewing all PPNs is outside the scope of this text, and therefore the focus will be on clinically relevant topics and special cases.

Injury/Acquired Painful Peripheral Neuropathies

Acquired peripheral neuropathies can be caused by injury or through iatrogenesis. They often become chronic, lasting longer than the inciting injury. Treatment is tailored to the specific injury and often requires a multimodal approach.

Complex regional pain syndrome

Complex regional pain syndrome (CRPS) is a potentially devastating painful condition that typically occurs following trauma such as wrist or ankle fracture or surgical procedure. CRPS has an approximate overall diagnosis rate of 0.07%, is more common in females, and peaks between ages 45–55.[15] It is important to identify CRPS early to improve outcomes and reduce disability.

Currently, CRPS is diagnosed clinically by criteria accepted by the IASP called the Budapest Criteria. It has been validated to have a sensitivity of 99% and a specificity of 68%.[16,17] The clinical criteria consist of four categories, both in patient-reported symptoms and signs examined by a physician as outlined by Harden et al. in Table 5.1. The first category is sensory. The hallmark of CRPS is allodynia, which is defined as pain to a nonpainful stimulus. Patients with CRPS may report that the affected extremity is subject to severe pain with nonnoxious stimuli, such as wind, clothing, bedsheets, or shoes.

The second category is vasomotor. This consists of skin temperature changes, skin color changes, or asymmetry in these findings. Sudomotor change is the third category and consists of edema, changes in sweating, or sweating asymmetry. The last category is motor or trophic changes. This could be weakness, dystonia, tremor, decreased range of motion, or hair, nail, or skin changes. The patient must exhibit a symptom in each of the four categories and at least two signs in separate categories at the time of diagnosis. Importantly a final criterion is that no other condition or disease can better explain the signs and symptoms exhibited by the patient.

Prompt treatment is important as CRPS can spread to different limbs and centrally as it affects the spinal cord and brain. Treatment should be guided by a pain specialist who has experience in treating this disorder to prevent disability and further impairment. Treatment is typically based upon symptom severity and may include a host of treatments. Neuropathic medications such as anticonvulsants and antidepressants, sympathetic nerve blocks, physical therapy, psychological therapy, spinal cord stimulation (SCS), DRG stimulation, ketamine infusions, and intrathecal drug pumps are all treatment modalities used in CRPS.[16]

Chemotherapy-induced peripheral neuropathies

Chemotherapy-induced peripheral neuropathy (CIPN) is a common problem occurring in approximately 30%–40% of those treated with neurotoxic chemotherapy. Traditional chemotherapeutic agents causing

---

TABLE 5.1
Budapest Clinical Diagnostic Criteria for CRPS.

Appendix II Budapest Clinical Diagnostic Criteria for CPRS

(1) Continuing pain, which is disproportionate to any inciting event
(2) Must report at least one symptom in *three of the four* following categories:
  - *Sensory:*repots of hyperesthesia and/or allodynia
  - *Vasomotor:*reports of temperature asymmetry and/or skin color changes and/or skin color asymmetry
  - *Sudomotor/edema:*reports of edema and/or sweating changes and/or sweating asymmetry
  - *Motor/trophic:*reports of decreased range of motion and/or motor dysfunction (weakness, tremor, dystonia) and/or trophic changes (hair, nail, skin)
(3) Must display at least one sign at time of evaluation in *two or more* the following categories:
  - *Sensory:*evidence of hyperalgesia (to pinprick) and/or allodynia (to light touch and/or deep somatic pressure and/or joint movement)
  - *Vasomotor:*evidence of temperature asymmetry and/or skin color changes and/or asymmetry
  - *Sudomotor/edema:*evidence of edema and/or sweating changes and/or sweating asymmetry
  - *Motor/trophic:*evidence of decreased range of motion and/or motor dysfunction(weakness, tremor, dystonia) and/or trophic changes (hair, nail, skin)
(4) There is no other diagnosis that better explains the signs and symptoms

CIPN are the platinum, taxanes, and vinca alkaloid medications. These drug classes cause CIPN by direct neuronal toxicity. Factors affecting the development of CIPN include route of medication delivery and dosing.[18]

The platinum-based chemotherapies, such as cisplatin, are believed to exert their CIPN producing action by attacking the DRG sensory neurons. They also have a unique characteristic of "coasting" wherein despite cessation of the drug, symptoms continue to worsen for months. Taxanes cause an axonopathy of sensory neurons that is both length and dose dependent. Vinca alkaloids also cause a length-dependent sensory neuropathy but may affect motor neurons as well. They are common in the treatment of hematological malignancies.[19]

Prevention of CIPN is difficult and there are currently no specific treatments except symptom management. Despite their lifesaving effects, these medications can lead to significant adverse effects. Multiple studies have investigated the treatment of CIPN with neuropathic pain medications with duloxetine showing some benefit.[19]

Nutritional deficiencies causing peripheral neuropathy

Nutritional deficiencies can lead to PPNs. Pain is typically not the only symptom but can be the most concerning for patients. Thiamine deficiency (vitamin B1) is common in chronic alcoholics, dialysis patients, and patients on specific diets that avoid thiamine. Thiamine deficiency leads to beriberi, which is a clinical syndrome consisting of cardiovascular effects and heart failure along with PPN. Thiamine deficiency caused by chronic alcoholism can cause a similar syndrome, Wernicke-Korsakoff.[20]

Vitamin B12 deficiency can also lead to a PPN. Vitamin B12 is absorbed in the gastrointestinal tract. Diseases, such as chronic gastritis or pernicious anemia, that affect absorption can lead to deficiency of vitamin B12. This leads to altered metabolism of homocysteine causing a peripheral neuropathy. The mainstay of treatment is B12 replacement therapy.[21]

Genetic Painful Peripheral Neuropathies
Charcot-Marie-Tooth disease

Charcot-Marie-Tooth disease (CMT) is the most commonly inherited PPN with a prevalence between 1 in 1213 and 1 in 2500. It is a group of differentially inherited diseases (CMT1-4 and CMT1X) that can cause a PPN. Most are inherited in an autosomal dominant pattern, but CMT4 is autosomal recessive and CMT1X

follows X-linked inheritance. This means that the majority of CMTs will have a 50% chance of transmission to future generations by the affected parent.[22] Clinical manifestations beyond PPN include distal symmetric leg weakness, decreased or absent reflexes, and significant foot deformities (pescavus and equinus protonation).

Hereditary sensory and autonomic neuropathies

The hereditary and sensory autonomic neuropathies (HSAN) are another group of genetically acquired diseases. They primarily affect the myelinated and unmyelinated sensory nerves. HSAN I is the most common pattern of inheritance and is autosomal dominant. The typical clinical presentation includes sensory loss and neuropathic pain. Onset of HSAN I commonly occurs in the early twenties. HSAN II—III are inherited in an autosomal recessive pattern and along with HSAN IV and V do not typically cause painful neuropathy. In fact, they often cause a degree of insensitivity to pain with type IV causing a profound lack of pain sensation with onset in infancy.[22]

Painful channelopathies

Channelopathies are a group of disorders resulting in an identified genetic mutation affecting pain receptors. The two most commonly affected receptors are voltage-gated sodium ion channels (Na1.7, Na1.8, and Na1.9) caused by mutations in the SCN genes (*SCN9A*, *SCN10A*, and *SCN11A*) and TRP channels.[23] Conditions resulting from these genetic alterations include inherited erythromelalgia, paroxysmal extreme pain disorder, small-fiber neuropathy, and familial episodic pain syndromes. Onset of these conditions varies but can occur as early as birth or later in adulthood. There are no genetic treatments currently available for these conditions, so treatment focuses on symptom management with strategies described later in this chapter. Interestingly, genetic mutations in the *SCN9A* and *SCN11A* can also cause insensitivity to pain.[23,24]

Autoimmune/Infectious Painful Peripheral Neuropathies
Postherpetic neuralgia

Postherpetic neuralgia (PHN) is the persistence of dermatomal pain 90 days after acute herpes zoster manifestation. It is the most common sequelae of herpes zoster infection. Herpes zoster is caused by reactivation of the varicella zoster virus that causes chicken pox. There is an annual incidence of one million cases in the

United States, and the condition affects roughly 20% of patients with herpes zoster. The pain may be described as burning and electric-like and is caused by damage to the nerve and secondary inflammation caused by the replicating virus. The American Academy of Neurology suggests initial treatment should focus on neuropathic pain medications and lidocaine patch 5%, which is FDA approved for PHN. The varicella zoster vaccine is suggested in patients over 60 years old and may prevent herpes zoster infection and presumably PHN. Interventional procedures for treatment-resistant cases can include nerve blocks at the nerve innervating the affected dermatome and neuromodulation.[25−28]

HIV/AIDS-associated peripheral neuropathy

HIV-associated peripheral neuropathy is the most common neurological complication of HIV/AIDS.[29] The most prevalent clinical manifestation is a distal symmetric polyneuropathy that can be burning in nature. Symptoms are not believed to be correlated with lower CD4 counts or higher viral load, but may be related to longer lifespans in HIV/AIDS- affected patients and increase in comorbid diseases with age.[29] The specific pathophysiology of HIV-associated peripheral neuropathy is unknown, but it is not believed to occur through direct damage of neurons from the virus itself. Studies have shown limited efficacy for most oral medications traditionally used for PPNs. Treatments that have shown improvement compared with placebo include capsaicin 8% and smoked cannabis.[30,31]

AIDP/CIDP

AIDP and chronic inflammatory demyelinating polyneuropathy (CIDP) are autoimmune disorders. PPN can be part of a patient's symptomatology, but the hallmark of these diseases is significant muscle weakness resulting from axonal damage.[32] AIDP is thought to be initiated most frequently by infections of campylobacter jejuni leading to anti-ganglioside antibodies and complement attacking the nodes of Ranvier at nerves.[32]

AIDP, also called Guillain-Barre syndrome (GBS) after the clinician who first described it, is the most common cause of adult onset acute flaccid paralysis in the United States, but can also cause painful neuropathy.[32] Approximately one-third of patients diagnosed with AIDP complain of pain during the initial presentation.[33] The yearly incidence of GBS is one per 100,000. Pain is common in GBS with approximately 89% of patients affected.[34] Suggested mechanisms leading to pain in GBS are inflammation and compression of the nerve roots. Aside from treating the underlying

cause of GBS, pain arising from GBS is typically treated with neuropathic pain medications, specifically gabapentin and carbamazepine. Epidural steroids have also shown efficacy.[34]

CIDP is rare and affects approximately 40,000 people in the United States.[35] Of those, 13%−17% have symptoms of severe pain. CIDP is characterized by relapsing and remitting symptoms, unlike AIDP. Although, individuals who initially present with AIDP may be later diagnosed with CIDP if their symptoms reoccur.[35] The most commonly used diagnostic criteria are published by the European Federation of Neurological Societies (EFNS).[36] Initial treatment of CIDP consists of immunoglobulin, corticosteroids, and/or plasma exchange.[35]

Painful Peripheral Neuropathies Resulting from Systemic Diseases

Diabetic painful peripheral neuropathy

Diabetic PPN is the most common peripheral painful neuropathy with a known etiology. Recent studies suggest a prevalence of approximately 18% of type 2 diabetics is affected.[37] According to the World Health Organization, diabetes occurs in 8.5% of the worldwide population over the age of 18 and continues to increase.[38] Although the exact mechanism of hyperglycemic-induced PPN is yet to be elucidated, both nerve injury and neurovascular alterations are likely to blame. Axonal atrophy, degeneration or regeneration, altered peripheral vascular flow, and peripheral sensitization all lead to neuropathic pain experienced by these patients.[39] Typical pain is in the classic "stocking and glove" distribution although it can vary and be manifested as radiculopathy, mononeuritis multiplex, and mononeuropathies. The quality of pain is usually described in terms of burning, electric, and stabbing sensations.[40]

Treatment of diabetic PPN is multimodal. Hyperglycemic control is pivotal in preventing neuropathy in type 1 diabetics but plays a much smaller roll in reducing PPN in type 2 diabetics.[40] Numerous studies have been performed and show level A evidence for first-line medications gabapentin, tricyclic antidepressants (TCAs), and duloxetine including the European Federation of Neurological Society guidelines.

TREATMENT OF PAINFUL PERIPHERAL NEUROPATHIES

Treatment of PPNs should follow a multimodal approach maximizing efficacy and reducing side effects. Ideally, less invasive techniques are preferred, but treatment should be tailored to each individual's symptoms. General treatment considerations include medications (enteral, parenteral, and topical), modalities, interventional techniques, and psychological intervention.

Medications

Oral medications are often first-line treatment for neuropathic pain conditions with common ones being outlined in Table 5.2. Recommendations for treatment by the European Federation of Neurological Societies Task Force (EFNS) were developed by reviewing the Cochrane Database and Medline for class 1 and 2 randomized control trials. These guidelines continue to recommend TCAs, gabapentin, and pregabalin as first-line, tramadol as second-line, and stronger opioids as third-line treatments.[41] This may vary among specific neuropathic conditions (i.e., HIV-induced neuropathy or trigeminal neuralgia) and many investigational studies have reviewed the use of these medications.

Anticonvulsants

Gabapentin and pregabalin are in the drug family of gabapentinoids and exert their effects at voltage-gated calcium channels whereby reducing channel function and the release of excitatory neurotransmitters, which in turn increase the function of inhibitory $GABA_A$ receptors.[42,43] They both have shown significant clinical efficacy in treating many neuropathic pain conditions.[44,45] The number needed to treat (NNT) for gabapentin and pregabalin is roughly 7 and 8–9,

respectively.[46] Their adverse effect profiles are similar and include drowsiness, ataxia, mental confusion, and respiratory depression.[47] Advantages of pregabalin are its twice per day dosing and the ability to reach a therapeutic level more quickly as dosing of 150 mg/day (often a starting dose) shows efficacy where 1200 mg/day of gabapentin is the lowest dose found to provide benefit in clinical studies.

Carbamazepine and oxcarbazepine deserve special mention as they are first-line drugs for the treatment of trigeminal neuralgia. In the anticonvulsant family, they both block sodium channels. Carbamazepine is quite effective in most patients with trigeminal neuralgia with an NNT of 1.7.[48] Due to cardiac, renal, and liver effects, baseline labs and EKG should be performed prior to initiation of either carbamazepine or oxcarbazepine and periodically monitored.[49] Both drugs are contraindicated in patients with atrioventricular block. Common side effects of both medications are dizziness, nausea, sedation, vomiting, diplopia, memory issues, elevated liver enzymes, and hyponatremia. Severe side effects are hepatotoxicity, Stevens-Johnson syndrome, aplastic anemia, and drug-induced systemic lupus erythematosus.[50] Because of these side effects, initial and periodic liver and renal function lab monitoring should be obtained. Starting doses of carbamazepine are 100–200 mg twice per day and can be increased daily by 100 mg. Starting doses for oxcarbazepine is 150 mg twice per day and increased by 300 mg every 3 days.[50–53]

Other anticonvulsants that have been studied for treatment of pain include lamotrigine, topiramate, lacosamide, valproic acid, and levetiracetam. Treatment trials for these medications have not shown great efficacy and they remain third-line agents.

Antidepressants

TCAs are a drug class that includes nortriptyline and amitriptyline, among others. They show clinically significant pain improvement in PPNs, but their use is often limited by undesirable adverse effects. They were originally developed as antidepressants and their mechanism of action is believed to occur by inhibiting the reuptake of serotonin and norepinephrine.[54–56] The NNT for the most well-studied TCA, amitriptyline, is approximately 5.[46] Significant anticholinergic adverse effects, interactions with cytochrome P450 enzymes, and cardiotoxicity causing prolonged QT intervals and arrhythmias can occur with TCAs. There is a target dosing of 75 mg/day and higher dosing can increase side effects.[55] Elderly populations should typically avoid TCAs due to potential adverse effects.

TABLE 5.2
Medications for Painful Peripheral Neuropathy.[120]

Chemical Modulator	Pharmacologic Option
Alpha 2 agonists	Clonidine
AMPA (Na + channel) antagonist	Gabapentin, carbamazepine, valproic acid, phenytoin
$GABA_B$ agonists	Baclofen
Glutamate antagonist	Gabapentin
NE reuptake inhibitors	TCAs
NMDA Ca^{2+} channel antagonist	Ketamine, amantadine, dextromethorphan, haloperidol
Non-NMDA Ca^{2+} channel blocker	Nifedipine

Other antidepressants increasingly used to treat neuropathic pain are serotonin-norepinephrine reuptake inhibitors (SNRIs) duloxetine and venlafaxine.[57−61] Their mechanisms of action are similar to TCAs blocking the reuptake of serotonin and norepinephrine but have significantly lower affinity for other receptors leading to less cholinergic side effects. Duloxetine appears to bind receptors with higher affinity than venlafaxine and has a higher bioavailability due to venlafaxine's first pass liver metabolism.[62] Most common side effects of SNRIs in descending order are somnolence, nausea, constipation, decreased appetite, and dry mouth. These occurred in a frequency greater than 3% of participants studied during the first 2 weeks of dose escalation (20 mg/day week one, 40 mg/day week two, then 60 mg/day weeks 3−14). Following week two of dose escalation, all side effects significantly decreased.[63]

Mirtazapine acts antagonistically at the 5HT-2, 5HT-3, and k-opioid receptors.[56] It has been studied in fibromyalgia and postamputation neuropathic pain.[64,65] No efficacy was found for the treatment of fibromyalgia as it was equivalent to placebo treatment. A case series suggested that mirtazapine may provide some benefit in phantom limb pain, but the study was small and lacked control groups. A recent study showed improvement in diabetes-induced hyperalgesia in rats treated with mirtazapine, but further clinical investigation is necessary.[66]

Cannabinoids

With increased availability and legalization of cannabis, its use in treating pain has grown. Cannabidiol is a ligand of the cannabinoid receptors, mainly the CB1 receptor, which is present in both the peripheral and central nervous system pain pathways. Numerous publications, including several randomized controlled trials, have investigated the reduction in pain from use of cannabinoids.[67−72] Neuropathic pain treated with smoked cannabis, specifically HIV-associated neuropathy, has shown the greatest treatment benefit compared with placebo.[30,73,74] Ongoing research into the treatment of neuropathic pain conditions with cannabis will hopefully elucidate the efficacy and risks to best guide future treatment decisions. Of note, cannabis is still considered a Schedule I medication.

Topical medications

Topical medications are commonly used for neuropathic pain including lidocaine, capsaicin, menthol products, and compounded topical medications. Capsaicin cream, at 0.025%, 0.075%, or 8% topical patch, has shown efficacy.[75−77] This is a paradoxical effect given capsaicin, when initially applied, causes pain. Capsaicin functions as a highly selective agonist at the transient receptor potential vanilloid-1 (TRPV1).[31] Capsaicin-induced desensitization is not completely understood, but possible mechanisms include the depletion of neuropeptides (substance P) in nerves expressing TRPV1 after repeated administration or high dose exposure. The TRPV1 receptors enter into a refractory state.[78] Topical cream forms should be applied three times per day continuously for efficacy. The 8% topical patch is applied once every 3 months to the area of pain and often with topical lidocaine to reduce the immediate burning effects. Efficacy has been shown specifically in painful diabetic neuropathy and PHN.[75]

Lidocaine topicals are either administered in a spreadable cream/ointment or as a patch. Lidocaine is a local anesthetic, which blocks voltage-gated sodium channels stabilizing nerve membranes and inhibiting pain signals from transduction.[79,80] Systemic absorption is limited when placed on intact skin. Lidocaine patches are FDA approved for PHN and are applied for 12 h followed by a 12-hour patch-free time period. Given its minimal adverse effect profile and demonstrated efficacy, it is considered first-line therapy in PHN.[81]

Compounded topical medications come in many forms and are created on an individual basis. Common medications included for neuropathic pain are gabapentin, ketamine, lidocaine, and clonidine. A recent randomized controlled trial enrolling 399 patients showed that compounded topical medications provided no benefit beyond placebo.[82] Furthermore, these medications are typically not covered by health insurance and are generally expensive. This suggests other treatment modalities should be considered.

Topical cannabidiol (CBD) oils are becoming widespread despite lack of clinical studies. One group found significant improvement in pain with four-week application of 250mg/3oz CBD oil for lower extremity neuropathy. This was a small study population of 29 patients, 15 randomized to the treatment group and 14 to placebo. Symptoms were evaluated using the neuropathic pain scale and performed on a biweekly basis.[83] Further investigation is needed to better understand true treatment benefit.

Infusion Medications

Intravenous infusion of medications including ketamine, lidocaine, and others has long been used to treat neuropathic pain. Ketamine is the most commonly used and is a dissociative anesthetic that acts mainly as an NMDA-antagonist.[84] At higher doses, ketamine can also act at opioid receptors (mu > kappa > sigma). It has effect on mu opioid receptor by also acting at dopamine receptors.[83] Ketamine is a chemical derivative of phencyclidine (PCP), which is now most commonly seen as a drug of abuse. Ketamine has been used since 1964, approved by the FDA in 1970, and was widely used during the Vietnam War given its anesthetic effects while preserving hemodynamic and respiratory stability. In addition to its analgesic effects, ketamine has hypnotic and amnestic properties that make it unique. Treatment of CRPS with ketamine infusions has frequently been studied.[85–92] Original studies showed clinical benefit in the treatment of CRPS using doses at 100 mg over 4 hours for 10 consecutive days.[85] Currently, protocols for infusion for chronic neuropathic pain varies and optimal dosing is not known. Most study follow-up periods were 9–12 weeks and it is believed the efficacy for statistically significant pain reduction is congruent with that time frame.

When performing ketamine infusion therapy for chronic pain, expected side effects, adverse effects, and contraindications need to be considered. During infusions, patients often experience a degree of dissociation and/or hallucinations and therefore most protocols pretreat with midazolam at the time of induction and during infusion as needed. Nausea is also a very common adverse effect and use of ondansetron or another antiemetic is recommended. As with all levels of anesthesia, continuous hemodynamic monitoring should be performed. This includes monitoring blood pressure, heart rate, respirations, electrocardiogram, and pulse oximetry. Unlike other common anesthetics, ketamine often increases blood pressure and patients are pretreated with clonidine prior to infusion. Nystagmus during infusion is a common cause of blurry vision and desists shortly following completion of treatment. Cystitis and hepatic toxicity are serious side effects and typically occur most commonly in ketamine abusers.[93]

Lidocaine infusions have also been used to treat chronic neuropathic pain. It is believed lidocaine infusion therapy works by blocking both peripheral and centrally located sodium channels.[94] Multiple studies have demonstrated varying effects of lidocaine infusions in the treatment of neuropathic pain conditions including trigeminal neuralgia, CRPS, and PHN. A recent metaanalysis of IV lidocaine infusion suggested pain relief in the immediate postprocedural period, but that it is short-lived.[94] Studies comparing different doses of 1 mg/kg versus 3 mg/kg versus 5 mg/kg infused over 30 min suggest that doses less than 5 mg/kg are equivalent to placebo. Common side effects of lidocaine infusion are lightheadedness, somnolence, perioral paresthesia, nausea, headache, dysarthria, dry mouth, and a metallic taste.[94]

Therapeutic Modalities

Electrotherapeutic and physical agent modalities are commonly used in the treatment of painful conditions. Defined as physical agents used for therapeutic benefit, they are typically adjunctive to other treatments and include heat, cold, water, sound, electricity, and electromagnetic waves.[95] They are utilized as a component of multimodal treatment in neuropathic pain disorders.[96] Transcutaneous electrical nerve stimulation (TENS) is one of the most common modalities used to treat neuropathic pain with metaanalyses suggesting efficacy.[97,98] A 2017 Cochrane review comparing TENS to sham TENS in patients with neuropathic pain showed an effect size in a visual analog pain score favoring TENS of −1.58 (95% confidence interval (CI) −2.08 to −1.09, $P < .00001$). Although this met the investigators prespecified criteria for minimally important difference, because of low quality available research, the authors were unable to confidently comment on the effectiveness of TENS and stated that the actual effectiveness is likely different than what was obtained through their analysis.[99] TENS is believed to provide pain reduction by stimulation of large afferent nerve fibers inhibiting small nociceptive C and A-delta fibers as explained in Wall and Melzack's Gate Control Theory.[100] It is placed at the site of neuropathic pain and generally considered a temporary treatment as the effect diminishes once stimulation ceases.

Heat and cold modalities are generally avoided in neuropathic pain conditions as cooccurring decreased sensation is common and can lead to undesired skin injury. Where these modalities may provide benefit are in desensitization of hypersensitive neuropathic pain. For example, in patients with allodynia/hypersensitivity with CRPS or neuropathic pain of an extremity (e.g.,erythromelalgia), contrast baths can be suggested. Contrast bath desensitization is performed by using two buckets of water, one warm and the other cool. Care should be taken to avoid excessively hot or cold water to prevent burns. The affected limb(s) should be placed in one bucket for approximately 2 minutes until acclimatized then switched to the other bucket and repeated three times per day. There is limited evidence for these treatments in neuropathic pain, mostly anecdotal.

Virtual reality is an innovative, noninvasive, treatment modality with limited side effects that has recently been employed in many painful conditions. Virtual reality is part of a larger treatment group utilizing visual feedback to modulate painful responses. Predecessors to this technology would be mirror box therapy, which is commonly used in neuropathic pain conditions. The mechanisms believed to be affecting neural substrates in visual feedback therapy are mirror neurons located in the anterior cingulate gyrus.[101,102]

Neuropathic pain conditions studied with visual feedback treatment modalities include CRPS, phantom limb pain, and post spinal cord injury (SCI) neuropathic pain. Earlier studies by McCabe et al. in 2003 demonstrated both pain reduction and objective limb temperature changes with visual feedback (mirror box therapy).[103] Virtual reality has some advantages over previous visual feedback treatments including the ability to treat bilateral symptoms, enhanced virtual environments, and ability for customization, although this comes with considerable financial cost. Recent systematic review for neuropathic pain in SCI patients suggested statistical benefit, but unclear clinical improvement in neuropathic pain. The relief was also short-lived.[104] Visual feedback treatments as an adjunct to other treatments may be of clinical benefit and given limited adverse effects and their noninvasive nature is reasonable to consider as part of multimodal treatment in neuropathic pain.[105–107]

Interventional Procedures

Interventional procedures are often used in the treatment of neuropathic pain. Sympathetic blockade and neuromodulation are two interventional treatments that have been used for decades to help manage painful symptoms associated with peripheral neuropathy.

Sympathetic ganglion injections

In some pain conditions, most commonly seen in CRPS, the sympathetic nervous system malfunctions. Chronic stimulation of the somatosympathetic reflexes in the intermediolateral column of the spinal cord can lead to sympathetically mediated pain. Blockade of either the stellate or lumbar sympathetic ganglion can provide pain relief in the upper or lower extremity, respectively. The stellate ganglion is located in the posterior chest from the seventh cervical vertebrae to the first thoracic vertebrae. It measures approximately 2.5 cm in length, 1 cm in width, and 0.5 cm in thickness. Significant structures are in close proximity including the carotid artery, vertebral artery, and vagus nerve. Injection of local anesthetic into these structures can lead to hoarseness and seizures.[108] Although originally performed without image guidance, current standard of care uses ultrasound or fluoroscopic guidance

to enhance safety and efficacy. Lumbar sympathetic blocks are performed for sympathetically mediated pain in the lower extremity. The ganglion lies anterior to the lumbar 2–3 vertebrae. This block is performed with fluoroscopic guidance to ensure proper placement. In addition to sympathetic blocks at these two locations, neurolysis with phenol or alcohol, radiofrequency ablation, and injection with botulinum toxin have all been studied.[109]

Neuromodulation

Neuromodulation with electrical stimulation is an advanced technique used in the treatment of neuropathic pain. It has been thoroughly studied in CRPS and peripheral painful neuropathies. Two forms most commonly used are SCS of the dorsal columns of the spinal cord and DRG stimulation. These involve implanted devices consisting of metal leads and an implantable pulse generator (i.e., battery) that provides the required energy to the leads so they can affect nerve tissue. Many different waveforms have been used to deliver energy to the spinal cord or DRG, but currently optimal waveforms are unclear. A recent systematic review of placebo or sham control trials using SCS leads to a decrease in pain intensity compared with placebo.[110] Individual studies in patients with diabetic peripheral neuropathy and CRPS also show efficacy.[111–114] DRG stimulation for neuropathic pain has also been studied and now is a frequently utilized treatment modality.[115–117] DRG has been approved for use since 2011 in Europe and more recently in 2016 by the FDA in the United States. The intervention places electrical leads in proximity to the dorsal root ganglion of spinal nerves instead of over the spinal cord. Recent clinical trials have suggested that DRG stimulation in CRPS provides better pain relief and longer-term efficacy.[118,119]

REFERENCES

1. Vaegter HB, Andersen PG, Madsen MF, Handberg G, Enggaard TP. Prevalence of neuropathic pain according to the IASP grading system in patients with chronic non-malignant pain. *Pain Med.* 2014;15(1):120–127.
2. Abbott CA, Malik RA, van Ross ER, Kulkarni J, Boulton AJ. Prevalence and characteristics of painful diabetic neuropathy in a large community-based diabetic population in the U.K. *Diabetes Care.* 2011;34(10): 2220–2224.
3. van Hecke O, Austin SK, Khan RA, Smith BH, Torrance N. Neuropathic pain in the general population: a systematic review of epidemiological studies. *Pain.* 2014;155(4): 654–662.

4. Bouhassira D, Lanteri-Minet M, Attal N, Laurent B, Touboul C. Prevalence of chronic pain with neuropathic characteristics in the general population. *Pain*. 2008; 136(3):380−387.

5. Woolf CJ, Mannion RJ. Neuropathic pain: aetiology, symptoms, mechanisms, and management. *Lancet*. 1999;353(9168):1959−1964.

6. Gunthorpe MJ, Chizh BA. Clinical development of TRPV1 antagonists: targeting a pivotal point in the pain pathway. *Drug Discov Today*. 2009;14(1−2):56−67.

7. Baron R, Binder A, Wasner G. Neuropathic pain: diagnosis, pathophysiological mechanisms, and treatment. *Lancet Neurol*. 2010;9(8):807−819.

8. Palazzo E, Rossi F, Maione S. Role of TRPV1 receptors in descending modulation of pain. *Mol Cell Endocrinol*. 2008;286(1−2 Suppl 1):S79−83.

9. Jones 3rd RC, Backonja MM. Review of neuropathic pain screening and assessment tools. *Curr Pain Headache Rep*. 2013;17(9):363.

10. Mendell JR, Sahenk Z. Clinical practice. Painful sensory neuropathy. *N Engl J Med*. 2003;348(13):1243−1255.

11. Truini A, Biasiotta A, Di Stefano G, et al. Does the epidermal nerve fibre density measured by skin biopsy in patients with peripheral neuropathies correlate with neuropathic pain? *Pain*. 2014;155(4):828−832.

12. Deleted in review.

13. Backonja MM, Attal N, Baron R, et al. Value of quantitative sensory testing in neurological and pain disorders: NeuPSIG consensus. *Pain*. 2013;154(9):1807−1819.

14. Finnerup NB, Haroutounian S, Kamerman P, et al. Neuropathic pain: an updated grading system for research and clinical practice. *Pain*. 2016;157(8): 1599−1606.

15. Elsharydah A, Loo NH, Minhajuddin A, Kandil ES. Complex regional pain syndrome type 1 predictors - epidemiological perspective from a national database analysis. *J Clin Anesth*. 2017;39:34−37.

16. Harden RN, Oaklander AL, Burton AW, et al. Complex regional pain syndrome: practical diagnostic and treatment guidelines, 4th edition. *Pain Med*. 2013;14(2): 180−229.

17. Harden RN, Bruehl S, Perez RS, et al. Validation of proposed diagnostic criteria (the "Budapest criteria") for complex regional pain syndrome. *Pain*. 2010;150(2): 268−274.

18. Staff NP, Grisold A, Grisold W, Windebank AJ. Chemotherapy-induced peripheral neuropathy: a current review. *Ann Neurol*. 2017;81(6):772−781.

19. Kim PY, Johnson CE. Chemotherapy-induced peripheral neuropathy: a review of recent findings. *Curr Opin Anaesthesiol*. 2017;30(5):570−576.

20. Wiley KD, Gupta M. *Vitamin B1 Thiamine Deficiency (Beriberi)*. Treasure Island (FL): StatPearls Publishing StatPearls Publishing LLC.; 2019.

21. Yang GT, Zhao HY, Kong Y, Sun NN, Dong AQ. Correlation between serum vitamin B12 level and peripheral neuropathy in atrophic gastritis. *World J Gastroenterol*. 2018;24(12):1343−1352.

22. Ramchandren S. Charcot-marie-tooth disease and other genetic polyneuropathies. *Continuum*. 2017;23(5): 1360−1377. Peripheral Nerve and Motor Neuron Disorders.

23. Bennett DL, Woods CG. Painful and painless channelopathies. *Lancet Neurol*. 2014;13(6):587−599.

24. Waxman SG. Painful Na-channelopathies: an expanding universe. *Trends Mol Med*. 2013;19(7):406−409.

25. Lin CS, Lin YC, Lao HC, Chen CC. Interventional treatments for postherpeticneuralgia: asystematic review. *Pain Physician*. 2019;22(3):209−228.

26. Saguil A, Kane S, Mercado M, Lauters R. Herpes zoster and postherpeticneuralgia: prevention and management. *Am Fam Physician*. 2017;96(10):656−663.

27. Hadley GR, Gayle JA, Ripoll J, et al. Post-herpetic neuralgia: a review. *Curr Pain Headache Rep*. 2016;20(3):17.

28. Jones J. Postherpetic neuralgia. *J Pain Palliat Care Pharmacother*. 2015;29(2):180−181.

29. Kaku M, Simpson DM. HIV neuropathy. *Curr Opin HIV AIDS*. 2014;9(6):521−526.

30. Amaniti A, Sardeli C, Fyntanidou V, et al. Pharmacologic and non-pharmacologic interventions for HIV-neuropathy pain. A systematic review and a meta-analysis. *Medicina*. 2019;55(12).

31. Blair HA. Capsaicin 8% dermal patch: areview in peripheral neuropathic pain. *Drugs*. 2018;78(14):1489−1500.

32. Goodfellow JA, Willison HJ. Guillain-Barre syndrome: a century of progress. *Nat Rev Neurol*. 2016;12(12): 723−731.

33. Yao S, Chen H, Zhang Q, et al. Pain during the acute phase of Guillain-Barre syndrome. *Medicine*. 2018; 97(34):e11595.

34. Liu J, Wang LN, McNicol ED. Pharmacological treatment for pain in Guillain-Barre syndrome. *Cochrane Database Syst Rev*. 2015;(4):Cd009950.

35. Ryan M, Ryan SJ. Chronic inflammatory demyelinating polyneuropathy: considerations for diagnosis, management, and population health. *Am J Manag Care*. 2018; 24(17 Suppl):S371−s379.

36. Rajabally YA, Simpson BS, Beri S, Bankart J, Gosalakkal JA. Epidemiologic variability of chronic inflammatory demyelinating polyneuropathy with different diagnostic criteria: study of a UK population. *Muscle Nerve*. 2009;39(4):432−438.

37. Gylfadottir SS, Christensen DH, Nicolaisen SK, et al. Diabetic polyneuropathy and pain, prevalence, and patient characteristics: a cross-sectional questionnaire study of 5,514 patients with recently diagnosed type 2 diabetes. *Pain*. 2020;161(3):574−583.

38. Emerging Risk Factors C, Sarwar N, Gao P, et al. Diabetes mellitus, fasting blood glucose concentration, and risk of vascular disease: a collaborative meta-analysis of 102 prospective studies. *Lancet*. 2010;375(9733):2215−2222.

39. Sloan G, Shillo P, Selvarajah D, et al. A new look at painful diabetic neuropathy. *Diabetes Res Clin Pract*. 2018;144: 177−191.

40. Callaghan BC, Cheng HT, Stables CL, Smith AL, Feldman EL. Diabetic neuropathy: clinical manifestations

and current treatments. *Lancet Neurol.* 2012;11(6):521−534.

41. Attal N, Cruccu G, Baron R, et al. EFNS guidelines on the pharmacological treatment of neuropathic pain: 2010 revision. *Eur J Neurol.* 2010;17(9):1113−e1188.

42. Yu J, Wang DS, Bonin RP, et al. Gabapentin increases expression of delta subunit-containing GABAA receptors. *Ebiomedicine.* 2019;42:203−213.

43. Kremer M, Salvat E, Muller A, Yalcin I, Barrot M. Antidepressants and gabapentinoids in neuropathic pain: mechanistic insights. *Neuroscience.* 2016;338:183−206.

44. Wiffen PJ, Derry S, Bell RF, et al. Gabapentin for chronic neuropathic pain in adults. *Cochrane Database Syst Rev.* 2017;6:Cd007938.

45. Moore A, Derry S, Wiffen P. Gabapentin for chronic neuropathic pain. *J Am Med Assoc.* 2018;319(8):818−819.

46. Finnerup NB, Haroutounian S, Baron R, et al. Neuropathic pain clinical trials: factors associated with decreases in estimated drug efficacy. *Pain.* 2018;159(11):2339−2346.

47. Quintero GC. Review about gabapentin misuse, interactions, contraindications and side effects. *J Exp Pharmacol.* 2017;9:13−21.

48. Wiffen PJ, Derry S, Moore RA, McQuay HJ. Carbamazepine for acute and chronic pain in adults. *Cochrane Database Syst Rev.* 2011;(1):CD005451.

49. Asconape JJ. Use of antiepileptic drugs in hepatic and renal disease. *Handb Clin Neurol.* 2014;119:417−432.

50. Al-Quliti KW. Update on neuropathic pain treatment for trigeminal neuralgia. The pharmacological and surgical options. *Neurosciences.* 2015;20(2):107−114.

51. Spina A, Mortini P, Alemanno F, Houdayer E, Iannaccone S. Trigeminal neuralgia: toward a multimodal approach. *World Neurosurg.* 2017;103:220−230.

52. Maarbjerg S, Di Stefano G, Bendtsen L, Cruccu G. Trigeminal neuralgia - diagnosis and treatment. *Cephalalgia.* 2017;37(7):648−657.

53. Haanpaa M, Attal N, Backonja M, et al. NeuPSIG guidelines on neuropathic pain assessment. *Pain.* 2011;152(1):14−27.

54. Pereira VS, Hiroaki-Sato VA. A brief history of antidepressant drug development: from tricyclics to beyond ketamine. *Actaneuropsychiatrica.* 2018;30(6):307−322.

55. Gillman PK. Tricyclic antidepressant pharmacology and therapeutic drug interactions updated. *Br J Pharmacol.* 2007;151(6):737−748.

56. Feighner JP. Mechanism of action of antidepressant medications. *J Clin Psychiatr.* 1999;60(Suppl 4):4−11. discussion 12-13.

57. Aiyer R, Barkin RL, Bhatia A. Treatment of neuropathic pain with venlafaxine: asystematic review. *Pain Med.* 2017;18(10):1999−2012.

58. Fornasari D. Pharmacotherapy for neuropathic pain: areview. *Pain Ther.* 2017;6(Suppl 1):25−33.

59. Gallagher HC, Gallagher RM, Butler M, Buggy DJ, Henman MC. Venlafaxine for neuropathic pain in adults. *Cochrane Database Syst Rev.* 2015;(8):Cd011091.

60. Minami K, Tamano R, Kasai E, et al. Effects of duloxetine on pain and walking distance in neuropathic pain models via modulation of the spinal monoamine system. *Eur J Pain.* 2018;22(2):355−369.

61. Obata H. Analgesic mechanisms of antidepressants for neuropathic pain. *Int J Mol Sci.* 2017;18(11).

62. Bymaster FP, Dreshfield-Ahmad LJ, Threlkeld PG, et al. Comparative affinity of duloxetine and venlafaxine for serotonin and norepinephrine transporters in vitro and in vivo, human serotonin receptor subtypes, and other neuronal receptors. *Neuropsychopharmacology.* 2001;25(6):871−880.

63. Konno S, Oda N, Ochiai T, Alev L. Randomized, doubleblind, placebo-controlled phase III trial of duloxetine monotherapy in Japanese patients with chronic low back pain. *Spine.* 2016;41(22):1709−1717.

64. Welsch P, Bernardy K, Derry S, Moore RA, Hauser W. Mirtazapine for fibromyalgia in adults. *Cochrane Database Syst Rev.* 2018;8:Cd012708.

65. Kuiken TA, Schechtman L, Harden RN. Phantom limb pain treatment with mirtazapine: a case series. *Pain Pract.* 2005;5(4):356−360.

66. Bektur E, Sahin E, Ceyhan E, et al. Beneficial effect of mirtazapine on diabetes-induced hyperalgesia: involvement of TRPV1 and ASIC1 channels in the spinal cord and dorsal root ganglion. *Neurol Res.* 2019;41(6):544−553.

67. Wilsey B, Marcotte TD, Deutsch R, Zhao H, Prasad H, Phan A. An exploratoryhuman laboratory experiment evaluating vaporized cannabis in the treatment of neuropathic pain from spinal cord injury and disease. *J Pain.* 2016;17(9):982−1000.

68. Weizman L, Dayan L, Brill S, et al. Cannabis analgesia in chronic neuropathic pain is associated with altered brain connectivity. *Neurology.* 2018;91(14):e1285−e1294.

69. Mucke M, Phillips T, Radbruch L, Petzke F, Hauser W. Cannabis-based medicines for chronic neuropathic pain in adults. *Cochrane Database Syst Rev.* 2018;3:Cd012182.

70. Lee G, Grovey B, Furnish T, Wallace M. Medical cannabis for neuropathic pain. *Curr Pain Headache Rep.* 2018;22(1):8.

71. Donvito G, Nass SR, Wilkerson JL, et al. The endogenous cannabinoid system: abudding source of targets for treating inflammatory and neuropathic pain. *Neuropsychopharmacology.* 2018;43(1):52−79.

72. Aviram J, Samuelly-Leichtag G. Efficacy of cannabisbased medicines for pain management: asystematic review and meta-analysis of randomized controlled trials. *Pain Physician.* 2017;20(6):E755−e796.

73. Stavros K, Simpson DM. Understanding the etiology and management of HIV-associated peripheral neuropathy. *Curr HIV/AIDS Rep.* 2014;11(3):195−201.

74. Abrams DI, Jay CA, Shade SB, et al. Cannabis in painful HIV-associated sensory neuropathy: a randomized placebo-controlled trial. *Neurology.* 2007;68(7):515−521.

75. Tenreiro Pinto J, Pereira FC, Loureiro MC, Gama R, Fernandes HL. Efficacy analysis of capsaicin 8% patch

in neuropathic peripheral pain treatment. *Pharmacology*. 2018;101(5−6):290−297.

76. Mankowski C, Poole CD, Ernault E, et al. Effectiveness of the capsaicin 8% patch in the management of peripheral neuropathic pain in European clinical practice: the ASCEND study. *BMC Neurol*. 2017;17(1):80.

77. Finnerup NB, Attal N, Haroutounian S, et al. Pharmacotherapy for neuropathic pain in adults: a systematic review and meta-analysis. *Lancet Neurol*. 2015;14(2):162−173.

78. Fattori V, Hohmann MS, Rossaneis AC, Pinho-Ribeiro FA, Verri WA. Capsaicin: current understanding of its mechanisms and therapy of pain and other preclinical and clinical uses. *Molecules*. 2016;21(7).

79. Pickering G, Martin E, Tiberghien F, Delorme C, Mick G. Localized neuropathic pain: an expert consensus on local treatments. *Drug Des Dev Ther*. 2017;11:2709−2718.

80. Knezevic NN, Tverdohleb T, Nikibin F, Knezevic I, Candido KD. Management of chronic neuropathic pain with single and compounded topical analgesics. *Pain Manag*. 2017;7(6):537−558.

81. Davies PS, Galer BS. Review of lidocaine patch 5% studies in the treatment of postherpetic neuralgia. *Drugs*. 2004;64(9):937−947.

82. Brutcher RE, Kurihara C, Bicket MC, et al. Compounded topical pain creams to treat localizedchronic pain: arandomized controlled trial. *Ann Intern Med*. 2019;170(5):309−318.

83. Xu DH, Cullen BD, Tang M, Fang Y. The effectiveness of topical cannabidioloil in symptomatic relief of peripheral neuropathy of the lower extremities. *Curr Pharmaceut Biotechnol*. 2019.

84. Connolly SB, Prager JP, Harden RN. A systematic review of ketamine for complex regional pain syndrome. *Pain Med*. 2015;16(5):943−969.

85. Schwartzman RJ, Alexander GM, Grothusen JR, Paylor T, Reichenberger E, Perreault M. Outpatient intravenous ketamine for the treatment of complex regional pain syndrome: a double-blind placebo controlled study. *Pain*. 2009;147(1−3):107−115.

86. Schwartzman RJ, Alexander GM, Grothusen JR. The use of ketamine in complex regional pain syndrome: possible mechanisms. *Expert Rev Neurother*. 2011;11(5):719−734.

87. Kiefer RT, Rohr P, Ploppa A, et al. A pilot open-label study of the efficacy of subanesthetic isomeric S(+)-ketamine in refractory CRPS patients. *Pain Med*. 2008;9(1):44−54.

88. Kiefer RT, Rohr P, Ploppa A, et al. Efficacy of ketamine in anesthetic dosage for the treatment of refractory complex regional pain syndrome: an open-label phase II study. *Pain Med*. 2008;9(8):1173−1201.

89. Kiefer RT, Rohr P, Ploppa A, Altemeyer KH, Schwartzman RJ. Complete recovery from intractable complex regional pain syndrome, CRPS-type I, following anesthetic ketamine and midazolam. *Pain Pract*. 2007;7(2):147−150.

90. Goldberg ME, Torjman MC, Schwartzman RJ, Mager DE, Wainer IW. Enantioselective pharmacokinetics of (R)- and (S)-ketamine after a 5-day infusion in patients with complex regional pain syndrome. *Chirality*. 2011;23(2):138−143.

91. Goldberg ME, Torjman MC, Schwartzman RJ, Mager DE, Wainer IW. Pharmacodynamic profiles of ketamine (R)- and (S)- with 5-day inpatient infusion for the treatment of complex regional pain syndrome. *Pain Physician*. 2010;13(4):379−387.

92. Goldberg ME, Domsky R, Scaringe D, et al. Multi-day low dose ketamine infusion for the treatment of complex regional pain syndrome. *Pain Physician*. 2005;8(2):175−179.

93. Cohen SP, Bhatia A, Buvanendran A, et al. Consensus guidelines on the use of intravenous ketamine infusions for chronic pain from the American Society of Regional Anesthesia and Pain Medicine, the American Academy of Pain Medicine, and the American Society of Anesthesiologists. *Reg Anesth Pain Med*. 2018;43(5):521−546.

94. Zhu B, Zhou X, Zhou Q, Wang H, Wang S, Luo K. Intravenous lidocaine to relieve neuropathic pain: asystematic review and meta-analysis. *Front Neurol*. 2019;10:954.

95. Braddom R, ed. *Physical Medicine and Rehabilitation*. 4th ed. Elsevier; 2011.

96. Akyuz G, Kenis O. Physical therapy modalities and rehabilitation techniques in the management of neuropathic pain. *Am J Phys Med Rehabil*. 2014;93(3):253−259.

97. Jin DM, Xu Y, Geng DF, Yan TB. Effect of transcutaneous electrical nerve stimulation on symptomatic diabetic peripheral neuropathy: a meta-analysis of randomized controlled trials. *Diabetes Res Clin Pract*. 2010;89(1):10−15.

98. Johnson MI, Bjordal JM. Transcutaneous electrical nerve stimulation for the management of painful conditions: focus on neuropathic pain. *Expert Revi Neurother*. 2011;11(5):735−753.

99. Gibson W, Wand BM, O'Connell NE. Transcutaneous electrical nerve stimulation (TENS) for neuropathic pain in adults. *Cochrane Database Syst Rev*. 2017;9:Cd011976.

100. Johnson M. Transcutaneous electrical nerve stimulation: mechanisms, clinical application and evidence. *Rev Pain*. 2007;1(1):7−11.

101. Ramachandran VS, Altschuler EL. The use of visual feedback, in particular mirror visual feedback, in restoring brain function. *Brain*. 2009;132(7):1693−1710.

102. Fogassi L, Gallese V, di Pellegrino G, et al. Space coding by premotor cortex. *Exp Brain Res*. 1992;89(3):686−690.

103. McCabe CS, Haigh RC, Ring EF, Halligan PW, Wall PD, Blake DR. A controlled pilot study of the utility of mirror visual feedback in the treatment of complex regional pain syndrome (type 1). *Rheumatology*. 2003;42(1):97−101.

104. Chi B, Chau B, Yeo E, Ta P. Virtual reality for spinal cord injury-associated neuropathic pain: systematic review. *Ann Phys Rehabil Med*. 2019;62(1):49−57.

105. Mouraux D, Brassinne E, Sobczak S, et al. 3D augmented reality mirror visual feedback therapy applied to the treatment of persistent, unilateral upper extremity

neuropathic pain: a preliminary study. *J Man Manip Ther.* 2017;25(3):137−143.

106. Mendez-Rebolledo G, Gatica-Rojas V, Torres-Cueco R, Albornoz-Verdugo M, Guzman-Munoz E. Update on the effects of graded motor imagery and mirror therapy on complex regional pain syndrome type 1: a systematic review. *J Back Musculoskelet Rehabil.* 2017;30(3): 441−449.

107. Breivik H, Allen SM, Stubhaug A. Mirror-therapy: an important tool in the management of complex regional pain syndrome (CRPS). *Scand J Pain.* 2013;4(4):190−197.

108. Narouze S. Ultrasound-guided stellate ganglion block: safety and efficacy. *Curr Pain Headache Rep.* 2014;18(6): 424.

109. Gunduz OH, Kenis-Coskun O. Ganglion blocks as a treatment of pain: current perspectives. *J Pain Res.* 2017; 10:2815−2826.

110. Duarte RV, Nevitt S, McNicol E, et al. Systematic review and meta-analysis of placebo/sham controlled randomised trials of spinal cord stimulation for neuropathic pain. *Pain.* 2020;161(1):24−35.

111. Duarte RV, Andronis L, Lenders MW, de Vos CC. Quality of life increases in patients with painful diabetic neuropathy following treatment with spinal cord stimulation. *Qual Life Res.* 2016;25(7):1771−1777.

112. Slangen R, Schaper NC, Faber CG, et al. Spinal cord stimulation and pain relief in painful diabetic peripheral neuropathy: a prospective two-center randomized controlled trial. *Diabetes Care.* 2014;37(11):3016−3024.

113. de Vos CC, Meier K, Zaalberg PB, et al. Spinal cord stimulation in patients with painful diabetic neuropathy: a

114. de Vos CC, Bom MJ, Vanneste S, Lenders MW, de Ridder D. Burst spinal cord stimulation evaluated in patients with failed back surgery syndrome and painful diabetic neuropathy. *Neuromodulation.* 2014;17(2):152−159.

115. Koetsier E, Franken G, Debets J, et al. Mechanism of dorsal root ganglion stimulation for pain relief in painful diabetic polyneuropathy is not dependent on GABA release in the dorsal horn of the spinal cord. *CNS Neurosci Therapeut.* 2020;26(1):136−143.

116. Huygen F, Kallewaard JW, Nijhuis H, et al. Effectiveness and safety of dorsal root ganglion stimulation for the treatment of chronic pain: a pooled analysis. *Neuromodulation.* 2020;23(2):213−221.

117. Harrison C, Epton S, Bojanic S, Green AL, FitzGerald JJ. The efficacy and safety of dorsal root ganglion stimulation as a treatment for neuropathic pain: a literature review. *Neuromodulation.* 2018;21(3):225−233.

118. Levy RM, Mekhail N, Kramer J, et al. Therapy habituation at 12 months: spinal cord stimulation versus dorsal root ganglion stimulation for complex regional pain syndrome type I and II. *J Pain.* 2019.

119. Deer TR, Levy RM, Kramer J, et al. Dorsal root ganglion stimulation yielded higher treatment success rate for complex regional pain syndrome and causalgia at 3 and 12 months: a randomized comparative trial. *Pain.* 2017; 158(4):669−681.

120. Wright DV. Non-narcotic options for pain relief with chronic neuropathic conditions. *J Nurse Pract.* 2008; 4(4):263−270.

multicentre randomized clinical trial. *Pain.* 2014; 155(11):2426−2431.

CHAPTER 6

Musculoskeletal Pain

BRETT GERSTMAN, MD • KATHY CHOU, DO • LINDSAY BURKE, MD

INTRODUCTION

Musculoskeletal (MSK) pain disorders are the second most common cause of disability worldwide and have increased by 45% from 1990 to 2010.[1] This number is expected to continue to rise with an increasingly obese, sedentary, and aging population. In the United States, approximately 8%−10% of both emergency room and primary care visits are related to complaints of MSK pain.[2,3]

The term "musculoskeletal pain disorders" is a broad term that encompasses numerous pain disorders. In order to simplify our discussion, MSK pain disorders are organized into five subcategories: disorders of the (1) bone, (2) joint/bursae, (3) muscle/tendon/ligament, (4) nerve, and (5) systemic processes. This chapter will focus on the most common syndromes in each category (Table 6.1). Explanations of their pathophysiology, diagnostic approaches, and treatment strategies can be applied to less common disease processes that are not discussed in this chapter.

VERTEBRAL COMPRESSION FRACTURES

Vertebral compression fracture is defined as the loss of height of a vertebral body due to the failure of the structural osseous component of the vertebrae. This pathology has a variety of potential causes including osteoporosis, infection, malignancy, and trauma.[4] Individuals who smoke are postmenopausal, and those with a history of chronic or high-dose steroid use are at an increased risk of developing vertebral compression fractures.[5] Approximately 30%−50% of patients on long-term steroid therapy have atraumatic fractures.[6] Evidence suggests that genetics may also place individuals at increased risk. Specifically, vitamin D receptor polymorphisms, among others, lead to decreased bone mineral density thus increasing the risk of a compression fracture.[7−9]

Trabecular bone is the primary load bearing element in bone. When an axial load on the bone exceeds the vertebral body's strength, a compression fracture occurs. Reduction in bone density also results in loss of trabecular bone strength. This is most commonly seen in osteoporosis. The risk of developing future compression fractures in the setting of osteoporosis increases after the initial fracture, with up to 19% of patients developing an additional fracture within 1 year.[10−12] This increased risk is largely due to the altered force vectors that are created by the initial fracture. Compression fractures may also be caused by malignancy or in association with kyphosis or deconditioning.

Many patients with compression fractures are asymptomatic.[13,14] Patients who seek medical attention with an acute compression fracture commonly complain of severe localized pain and limited mobility. Pain with palpation and percussion over the injured spinous process and paravertebral structures may be observed on physical exam. Typically, pain is most

TABLE 6.1
Chapter Organization of Common Musculoskeletal Pain Disorders.

Bone	Joint/Bursae	Muscle/Tendon/Ligament	Nerve	Systemic Process
Vertebral compression fractures	Degenerative joint disease	Muscular sprain/strain	Radiculopathy	Fibromyalgia
	Bursitis	Tendinopathy	Entrapment neuropathies	
	Adhesive capsulitis			

intense at the fracture level and is exacerbated by movement and alleviated with bedrest.[15]

Suspected acute vertebral body compression fracture can be confirmed by plain radiographs of the spine (Fig. 6.1). Most often, compression fractures occur in the lower thoracic and upper lumbar spine and involve the anterior aspect of the vertebral body, resulting in anterior wedging.[15] Magnetic resonance imaging (MRI) can also be employed to determine the etiology of fractures as well as establish their age[16] (Fig. 6.2). The bone marrow signal on MRI can help determine the acuity of the fracture. Acute compression fractures will have a high signal intensity on T2-weighted scans and low signal on T1-weighted scans. Compression fracture due to osteoporosis may be indistinguishable from those due to metastasis on plain radiographs.[17] Distinguishing the etiology of the fracture impacts management significantly.

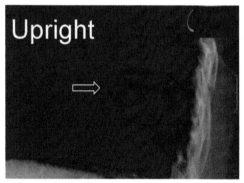

FIG. 6.1 Lateral X-ray of thoracic spine with T11 compression fracture (*arrow*).

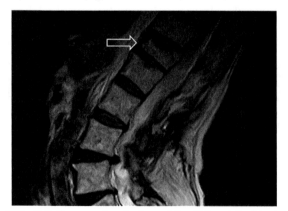

FIG. 6.2 Compression fracture of the T11 vertebral body (*arrow*) on sagittal T1-weighted magnetic resonance imaging.

The majority of patients can be managed conservatively with pain control and physical therapy.[18] First-line agents for symptom management include oral analgesics such as acetaminophen and ibuprofen. Opioids or a two to four-week course of calcitonin may be used as alternative options if pain persists.[19–22] Physical activity should be resumed as soon as possible as inactivity may worsen deconditioning. Physical therapy aimed at strengthening the core and improving gait may help patients return to their previous function.[23] Weight-bearing exercises can be used to combat the decrease in bone density seen in osteoporosis.[24] Care must be taken to instruct patients to restrict flexion-based activity as this maneuver loads the anterior vertebral body and thus places them at increased risk for worsening or additional fracture.[15] Bracing, such as thoracic lumbar sacral orthosis, can be considered—however, the efficacy remains inconclusive.[25] Intercostal nerve blocks may also be used for pain management. Lastly, vertebroplasty or kyphoplasty can be used in patients who fail conservative treatment.[26] A surgical consult should be obtained if an unstable fracture is identified on radiographic imaging.

DEGENERATIVE JOINT DISEASE

Degenerative joint disease (DJD), often called osteoarthritis, is one of the most common causes of disability due to pain and dysfunction of the joint. It most often involves the knees, hips, spine, and small hand joints and is characterized by deterioration of joint structures and remodeling of subchondral bone.[27,28]

DJD is commonly thought of as a progressive "wear and tear" process but the pathophysiology is multifaceted (Fig. 6.3). While the exact pathway leading to the disease varies between individuals, commonly the same pathological findings are observed in articular cartilage, bone, synovium, and surrounding soft tissues. Excess shear forces placed on the joint can lead to repetitive trauma and inflammation. This inflammation then leads to the production of proteolytic enzymes which degrade the extracellular matrix and ultimately compounds to lead to accelerated chondrocyte death and injure the articular cartilage of the joint and synovium.[29] Over time, this process leads to loss of joint space, eburnation of the subchondral bone, and hypertrophic repair of cartilage. Risk factors for the disease include age, joint injury, genetics, repetitive joint trauma or stress, neuromuscular weakness, obesity, occupation, biomechanics, and anatomical factors, as well as gender.[30]

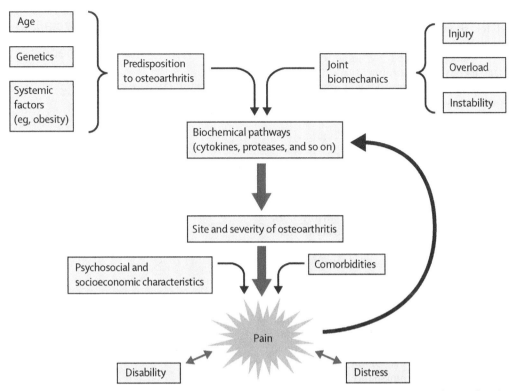

FIG. 6.3 Schematic representation of relations between environmental and endogenous risk factors for joint damage, osteoarthritis, joint pain, and their consequences. (From Dieppe PA, Lohmander LS. Pathogenesis and management of pain in osteoarthritis. *Lancet*. 2005;365:965–73; with permission.)

Typically, patients presenting with symptoms of DJD are older than 45 years, complain of activity-related joint pain, and may have morning joint stiffness lasting less than 30 min.[31] The quality of the pain varies, ranging from aching joint pain to less localized radiating pain. Joint locking and instability may also be observed.[28] On exam, patients may present with pain on range of motion (ROM) and swelling of the affected joint. In hip DJD, pain may radiate to the groin, anterior thigh, and knee.[27]

A comprehensive history and physical exam is essential to the diagnosis of DJD. Plain radiographs can be utilized to confirm the diagnosis and rule out other conditions. In the earliest stages of the disease, X-ray findings may be benign. As the underlying process advances, subchondral bony sclerosis, formation of osteophytes, and joint space narrowing are commonly seen. In the knee, narrowing tends to be seen at the medial joint space, whereas in the hip the superior lateral joint space is narrowed.[15] Additional laboratory testing may be appropriate in younger patients, those with atypical symptoms, or those with constitutional symptoms. Inflammatory markers are typically normal in DJD and may exclude other diagnoses.[32] If the diagnosis is unclear, imaging modalities such as MRI can be used to identify the disease at earlier stages before radiographic evidence is present. The use of MRI occurs most often when evaluating knee pathology to assess for pathology in other structures which may be contributing to patient presentation.[33]

Goals of treatment include pain relief and improvement of joint dysfunction. Nonpharmacologic treatment is first line of treatment and includes patient counseling focused on encouraging patients to exercise and strengthen local muscles.[34,35] Weight loss is essential if the patient is overweight or obese.[31] Physical therapy can be utilized to improve function and reduce pain in patients with mild to moderate symptoms. First-line pharmacological management includes the use of acetaminophen and/or topical nonsteroidal antiinflammatory drugs (NSAIDs). If further pain control is necessary, substitution with oral NSAIDs or COX-2 inhibitors may be used.[31] Tramadol can also be considered for initial management of hand, knee, or hip

DJD.[36] Intraarticular corticosteroid injections may be beneficial for short-term relief of symptoms.[37] The role of hyaluronic acid or platelet-rich plasma remains unclear.[38–40] Surgical referral for joint replacement can be made if conservative treatment fails or if quality of life is significantly impaired. Opioid analgesics are not indicated in the management of chronic osteoarthritic pain.[41]

TROCHANTERIC PAIN SYNDROME

Trochanteric bursitis is one of the most common causes of lateral hip pain in adults. The condition results from gluteus medius or minimus insertional tendinopathy along the greater trochanter and often involves the regional bursae.[42] Recently, the term "greater trochanteric pain syndrome" has gained wider use as the bursae are not always the source of pain. Risk factors for the disease include female gender, obesity, and hip and knee arthritis.[43]

Bursae are designed to reduce friction as soft tissues move over bony prominences. In the hip, a proximal bursa exists between the iliotibial band and the greater trochanter (Fig. 6.4). It may become inflamed as a result of trauma but often abnormal biomechanics lead to gradual inflammation. An imbalance in strength of the hip muscles may also contribute to development. The medial aspect of the greater trochanter serves as the insertion point of the short external rotators of the hip. These muscles along with the abductors work to maintain pelvic stability while walking. An imbalance or weakness of these muscles may contribute to development of greater trochanteric pain syndrome.[44]

Patients with trochanteric pain syndrome complain of lateral gluteal pain especially while lying on their affected side and will have difficulty tolerating weight bearing on the affected side. On examination, maximal tenderness occurs over the posterior corner of the trochanter[43,45] and commonly extends along the length of the iliotibial band. Motor testing often reveals weakness in hip abduction and external rotation. Tensor fascia lata inflexibility is also commonly seen.[46] There are no established criteria for diagnosing trochanteric pain syndrome. There is commonly no cardinal sign of inflammations such as erythema, edema, or rubor along the lateral buttock.[42] Concurrent intraarticular hip and lumbar spine pathology should be ruled out prior to making the diagnosis of primary trochanteric pain syndrome. Findings on plain radiography are highly variable and thus are not recommended.

There are no established treatment protocols for trochanteric bursitis.[47] Initial management may include

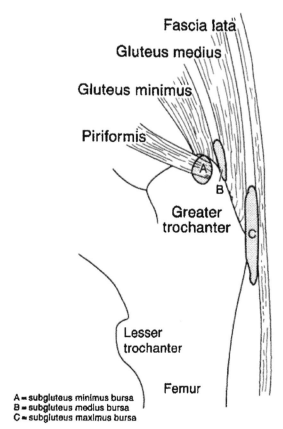

A = subgluteus minimus bursa
B = subgluteus medius bursa
C = subgluteus maximus bursa

FIG. 6.4 Peritrochanteric anatomy. (From Reid D. The management of greater trochanteric pain syndrome: A systemic literature review. *J Orthoped.* 2016;13:15–28; with permission.)

oral NSAIDs. If more immediate relief is required, local glucocorticoid injections may be considered.[48,49] Physical therapy or home exercises focused on isometric loading of the gluteus medius, minimus, and quadriceps should be a mainstay of treatment as it will both improve patient symptoms and treat the underlying cause of their symptoms. Additional conservative therapies include platelet-rich plasma injection, shock wave therapy, and weight reduction.[42] It is estimated that over 90% of cases will resolve with conservative therapy.[50] Trochanteric bursitis may also be self-limiting in many patients.[42] If symptom relief is not obtained after several months, investigation of a tear of the gluteus medius tendon should be performed using MRI. Refractory cases may also be managed with bursectomy, iliotibial band lengthening techniques, or gluteal tendon repair.[42,51]

Adhesive Capsulitis

Adhesive capsulitis (AC), often called frozen shoulder, has been defined as a condition characterized by the progressive development of global limitation of active and passive shoulder motion without radiographic findings other than osteopenia.[52]

AC can be primary or secondary to various conditions such as diabetes mellitus, thyroid pathology, or following trauma or surgery.[52–55] This condition commonly presents unilaterally, more often in women, and affecting the nondominant shoulder. The exact pathophysiology of the condition is unclear. A commonly cited hypothesis is that inflammation occurs in the joint capsule and leads to the development of adhesions and fibrosis in the synovial lining of the joint.[56] This leads to loss of joint volume due to thickening and contracture of the joint capsule and surrounding tissues. There is considerable debate as to whether the underlying pathology is predominantly inflammatory or fibrosing in nature.[57] The thickened glenohumeral joint capsule can form adhesions to itself and/or to the anatomic neck of the humerus. The joint volume is subsequently decreased as there is minimal synovial fluid present.[58]

Patients with frozen shoulder complain of severe shoulder pain and progressively worsening limited mobility. AC is described as progressive, and patients may present at any of the three distinct phases of the disease.[59] During the initial or freezing stage, the patient will complain of diffuse shoulder pain that is worse at night. Physical exam reveals limited active and passive ROM in two or more planes of motion. Often external rotation and abduction are most greatly affected. Loss of external rotation ROM more than internal rotation can be helpful in differentiating AC from rotator cuff pathology.[60] The initial/freezing phase can last anywhere from 3 to 9 months.[61] During the subsequent "frozen stage," which can last 4–12 months, pain does not necessarily worsen but limited use of the limb can lead to deconditioning.[61,62] ROM improves and pain improves during the final thawing phase which lasts 12–24 months[61,63] (Fig. 6.5).

The diagnosis of AC is based on an appropriate history and physical examination. Plain radiographs may be utilized to rule out other conditions such as osteoarthritis. MRI or ultrasound may also be used to rule out other pathologies and can be especially helpful in diagnostically challenging clinical situations. These include patients with concomitant osteoarthritis or rotator cuff pathology. An injection of anesthetic into the subacromial space can be employed to help differentiate AC from subacromial pathology. Symptoms will not improve in patients with AC but should improve in patients with subacromial impingement/rotator cuff dysfunction.

There is little high-level evidence supporting any specific treatment for AC. Rest and shoulder mobility exercises are recommended. Adequate pain control can usually be achieved with activity modification and acetaminophen or NSAIDs early in the disease course. Physical therapy should be initiated as mobility improves. An intraarticular injection of a combination of anesthetic and glucocorticoid can be considered in patient with severe symptoms for short-term relief.[64] Surgical referral for manipulation under anesthesia or arthroscopy and capsular release may be warranted if patients fail to find relief from conservative measures.[52] Future treatments in the development stage are aimed at targeting inflammatory cytokines in early disease and decreasing fibrosis and capsular remodeling in later stages.[65]

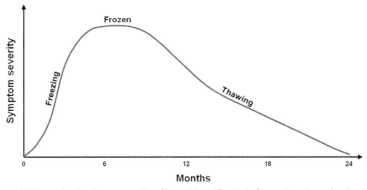

FIG. 6.5 Natural history of adhesive capsulitis. (From Hsu JE, et.al. Current review of adhesive capsulitis. *J Shoulder Elbow Surg.* 2011;20:502–514; with permission.)

MUSCLE STRAIN

Ninety percent of all muscle injuries are either contusions or sprains.[66] Contusions are caused by blunt extrinsic compressive trauma to the muscle, while strains are caused by intrinsic muscle tearing. Strains most commonly affect muscles spanning two joints, such as the semitendinosus or gastrocnemius.[67]

Excessive tensile forces and tearing of the myofibers at the myotendinous junction commonly leads to disruption of intramuscular vessels and necrosis. This muscle trauma results in release of adenosine triphosphate and protons which activate nociceptors (unmyelinated C or thinly myelinated Aδ nerves) in the muscle belly. Subsequently nociceptors transmit to the central nervous system where the depolarization is perceived as pain. Skeletal muscle healing occurs with regeneration of the myofibers and remodeling of scar tissue.[67]

Patients who sustain a muscle strain typically develop immediate sharp pain in the muscle and exhibit a decrease in ROM acutely. The pain develops into a cramping or pressure-like sensation throughout the muscle. On physical exam, point tenderness is noted along the injured muscle with possible concurrent warmth or edema in the area. ROM is expected to be decreased within the muscle and joint movement it contributes to. Muscle injury is a clinical diagnosis based on patient's history and physical exam, with findings described above. Imaging with ultrasound and/or MRI can be helpful in identifying small hematomas or muscular tears, but are not recommended unless a patient fails to exhibit expected symptomatic improvement with conservative care.[68]

There is limited research on the treatment of "muscle strain" due to the high variability in presentation and severity. The current treatment regimen is based on the underlying pathophysiology and expert recommendations. Immediate treatment should utilize the RICE protocol-rest, ice, compression, and elevation, which targets the initial bleeding and inflammation after injury.[66] Temporary immobility prevents further damage to the muscle and vasculature, reduces excessive scar formation, and minimizes risk of rerupture. Cryotherapy with ice packs or cold compresses decrease pain and intramuscular blood flow. Compression and elevation minimize edema and bleeding, which interfere with healing and regeneration.[67] NSAIDS are recommended for the acute phase and have been shown to reduce strength loss and soreness after injury.[69]

No specific duration for relative immobility has been formally recommended. Studies have demonstrated scar tissue approximating the ruptured muscle fibers achieves sufficient tensile strength for muscle contraction by day 10.[70] It is essential that patients return to graduated activity within the limits of pain. Early mobilization induces vasculature regrowth, aligns myofibers for faster recovery of preinjury strength, and prevents extensive scarring.[68,71] A graduated exercise program should be initiated after rest. The injured muscle should be progressed through isometric, isotonic, and finally dynamic training. Surgery is reserved for severe injuries, including complete thickness muscle tear or tears with significant loss of function. In full thickness muscle strains, injury recovery time can range from 4 to 6 weeks.[68]

TENDINOPATHY

Tendinopathy is a degenerative overuse tendon injury and describes both tendinitis and tendinosis.[72] Upper extremity tendinopathies frequently involve the biceps, supraspinatus, and medial and lateral elbow tendons. Lower extremity tendinopathies more commonly affect the gluteal, patellar, and Achilles tendons.

Tendinopathies occur with high stress, repeated strains, compression, or shearing forces. Injured tendons exhibit changes in tenocytes, extracellular matrix, and increased inflammation.[73] Biopsies of painful tendon have demonstrated disorganized collagen fibers, increased vascularity, and changes in cellularity and extracellular matrix.[74–76] Pain from tendon injuries is multifactorial in nature. Studies have shown that local elevations in substance P, prostaglandins,[77] glutamate,[78] and neovascularization with new innervation[76,79,80] may all contribute to stimulating nociceptors.

Patients with tendon-related pain present with localized tendon pain typically at the enthesis. Local swelling and warmth is commonly seen. Pain is exacerbated with tendon loading, short duration-high force movements, and focal pressure applied to the area.

Ultrasound with color doppler is a highly sensitive tool to visualize neovascularization, tendon thickening, and hypoechoic intratendinous which are changes suggestive of tendinopathy[81,82] (Fig. 6.6). MRI is a more specific imaging modality compared with ultrasound and is superior in evaluating degenerative changes.[83,84]

NSAIDs can provide acute pain relief and have been proven to improve the biomechanical properties of injured tendons in animal studies.[85,86] NSAID use should be limited to the acute period after injury as it may impair enthesis healing with prolonged

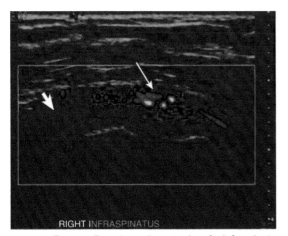

FIG. 6.6 Power Doppler ultrasound of infraspinatus tendinopathy showing hypoechogenicity with loss of fibrillary pattern and marked neovascularization. (From LaMartina II J, Ma B, LansdownD. Imaging for rotator cuff pathology. In: Provencher M (ed). *Disorders of the Rotator Cuff and Biceps Tendon*: Elsevier; 2020; with permission.)

use.[87–89] Similarly, local corticosteroid injections can provide short-term pain relief particularly in upper extremity tendinopathies but there are conflicting studies.[90–93] Eccentric strengthening exercises may improve pain, function, and strength, by stimulating mechanotransduction for healing,[94] but has not been proven superior or inferior to other isometric or isotonic exercises for pain relief.[95–97] Exercise is most beneficial when used in conjunction with other physical therapy modalities such as ice, heat, or ultrasound.[98,99] There is limited evidence for iontophoresis, phonophoresis, or deep friction massage.[100] Refractory tendinopathy can be treated surgically with tendon debridement, repair, or augmentation.

Several novel treatments are being investigated for tendinopathies. Transdermal and topical nitric oxide has been shown in randomized, double-blind, placebo-controlled trials to improve pain in some chronic tendinopathies.[101–103] Extracorporeal shock wave therapy (EWST) applies low-energy shock waves to stimulate tenocyte proliferation for repair. EWST is approved by US Food and Drug Administration for lateral epicondylitis and may be promising for other tendinopathies.[98,104,105] Sclerotherapy ablates neovascularization and potential pain-generating adjacent nerve fibers and has been shown to reduce pain in several small studies.[106,107] Regenerative therapies including plasma-rich plasma have shown promise

for pain relief and functional improvement.[108,109] Gene therapy for altering the inappropriate remodeling pathways in tendinopathy and tissue engineering is currently limited to animal studies.

RADICULOPATHY

Radiculopathy is dysfunction of a spinal nerve root, caused by mechanical compression and/or chemical irritation.[110,111] Degenerative changes of the spine and intervertebral disc protrusions are the most common causes for both cervical and lumbar radiculopathy.[112–115]

The pathophysiology of pain in radiculopathy is dependent on the underlying etiology. Nerve compression upregulates pain pathways.[116] In radiculopathy caused by herniated discs, proinflammatory cytokines are released by the discs which may stimulate nociceptive fibers causing sensitization and pain.[117–119] In facet injury, spinal hyperexcitability may cause and perpetuate pain.[120,121]

Radicular pain is commonly described as radiating electric or shooting pain in a dermatomal distribution (Fig. 6.7). In clinical practice, pain characterization is highly variable and can be dull or aching in character with a nondermatomal distribution. If related to mechanical nerve root compression from a disc herniation, symptoms may be exacerbated by coughing or Valsalva. Corresponding sensory, motor, or reflex changes should be noted on neurologic testing. Neurodynamic tests can also aid in diagnosis. The slump test is more sensitive (84%) than the straight leg test, but the straight leg test is more specific (89%) for lumbar radiculopathy secondary to herniated lumbar disc.[122] The Spurling's maneuver is 89%–100% specific for cervical radiculopathy.[123–125]

The diagnosis of radiculopathy can be made clinically with a comprehensive history and physical exam. MRI can be utilized to confirm the specific causes of the underlying nerve root dysfunction (Fig. 6.8). One obvious drawback to MRI is its high false-positive rate for discogenic radiculopathy.[126] Electrodiagnostic testing, nerve conduction studies/electromyography (NCS/EMG), is also helpful in confirming the underlying diagnosis and excluding concurrent diagnoses such as peripheral neuropathy, mononeuropathy, or plexopathy.[127]

Most cervical and lumbar radiculopathies resolve spontaneously.[113,128] 50% of patients with a lumbar radiculopathy will obtain symptom resolution by 2 weeks and 90% of patients will obtain symptom resolution within 12 weeks.[129] NSAIDs are the mainstay

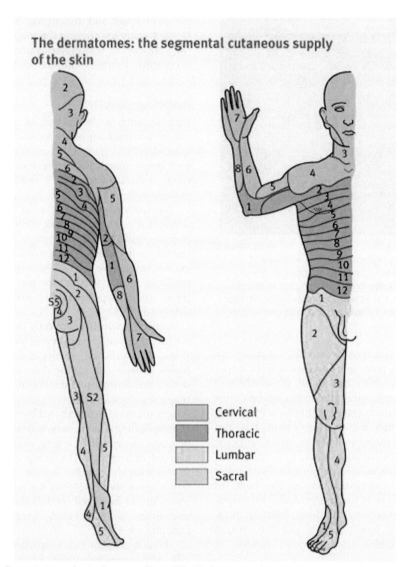

FIG. 6.7 Dermatomes of spinal nerves. (From Ellis H. Anatomy of the spinal nerves and dermatomes. *Anes Intensive Care Med.* 2009;10:536–537; with permission.)

treatment for radicular pain. For an acute inflammatory episode due to herniated disc, oral corticosteroids can be effective in improving function, but may not improve pain.[130] Common adjunctive therapy include opioids for severe pain, short courses of muscle relaxants for concurrent spasms, anticonvulsants (gabapentin, pregabalin), tricyclic antidepressants, or serotonin and norepinephrine reuptake inhibitors (SNRIs) for neuropathic pain relief.[131,132] With adequate pain control, physical therapy should be utilized for both

cervical and lumbar radiculopathies. Traction and spinal manipulation are controversial manual therapies, but may provide relief in select patients.[94,133,134]

Epidural steroid injections can provide both short- and long-term symptomatic relief[135–138] but responses vary based on the underlying etiology. Patients with symptoms of a cervical radiculopathy due to a disc herniation obtain more relief from an epidural steroid injection compared with those with radicular pain due to underlying spinal stenosis.[137] Operative management is

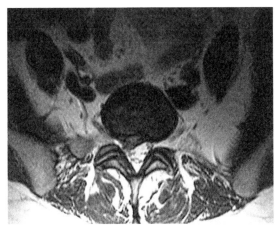

FIG. 6.8 Right-sided paracentral L5 herniated disc on axial MRI.

commonly reserved for patients with at least 6 weeks of persistent symptoms and failed nonsurgical treatments. Surgery is indicated on a more accelerated timeline in the setting of progressive weakness, bowel or bladder incontinence[139] (Fig. 6.9).

ENTRAPMENT NEUROPATHY

Entrapment neuropathies, also known as compression neuropathies, are highly prevalent and can cause significant pain and functional deficits. Median neuropathy at the wrist (carpal tunnel syndrome) is the most prevalent entrapment injury.[140] Ulnar neuropathy at the

elbow and fibular neuropathy at the fibular head are also common.

The course of a peripheral nerve can be narrowed or compressed by surrounding soft tissue or bony structures. Compression obstructs intraneural vasculature causing venous congestion and in severe cases arterial ischemia. Subsequent inflammation and edema lead to further breakdown of the blood-nerve barrier and the development of degenerative fibrosis and demyelination.[141–143] Demyelination results in partial or complete block of action potentials. Continuous or prolonged compression can result in chronic hypoxia with subsequent axonal degeneration.[144]

Entrapment neuropathies have highly variable presentations depending on the severity of the underlying nerve injury and location of the compression. In the setting of a compressive injury, patients may report intermittent paresthesia and pain in the sensory distribution of the peripheral nerve followed by persistent paresthesias. As compression worsens, weakness in corresponding innervated muscles can occur. In chronic and severe cases, atrophy of distally innervated muscles is seen as well. Common syndromes will be discussed below:

Carpal tunnel syndrome is an entrapment neuropathy of the distal median nerve as it passes through the volar wrist. Patients first report paresthesia in volar thumb, first and second digits, or possibly the entire hand. Symptoms are commonly worse overnight as the patient sleep in a flexed wrist posture and relieved by shaking the wrist.

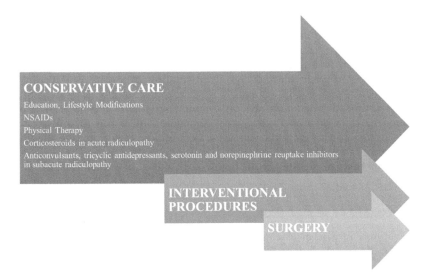

CONSERVATIVE CARE
Education, Lifestyle Modifications
NSAIDs
Physical Therapy
Corticosteroids in acute radiculopathy
Anticonvulsants, tricyclic antidepressants, serotonin and norepinephrine reuptake inhibitors in subacute radiculopathy

INTERVENTIONAL PROCEDURES

SURGERY

FIG. 6.9 Radiculopathy treatment progression.

Ulnar entrapment neuropathy most commonly occurs at the cubital tunnel: between the medial epicondyle and olecranon and two heads of the flexor carpi ulnaris. Patients will complain of paresthesia in medial palmar hand and fourth and fifth digits. With more advanced compression of the median or ulnar nerves, weakness can manifest as difficulty with fine motor movements or perceived grip strength.[145]

Fibular (peroneal) nerve entrapment is the most prevalent neuropathy in the lower extremity. The soleus tendon and peroneus longus tendon overlie the common fibular nerve as it wraps around the fibular head. Patients will report paresthesia in the lateral leg and dorsal foot or ankle dorsiflexion weakness causing foot drop and an impaired gait.

Entrapment neuropathies can be diagnosed clinically but electrodiagnostic confirmation is critical. Electrodiagnostic testing (NCS/EMG) is highly specific for diagnosis and can localize the nerve injury, differentiate between peripheral neuropathy or radiculopathy, and demonstrate timing and severity of injury.[146] NCS/EMG will also confirm whether the process is resulting in a primarily demyelinating or axonal injury. If a patient cannot tolerate NCS/EMG, ultrasound may be a useful adjunctive diagnostic tool. Nerves are typically enlarged at or just proximal to compression sites, and there may be changes in nerve echotexture, shape, and vascularity.[147]

Conservative treatments include rest and/or splinting.[140] Splinting of the wrist in a neutral position for carpal tunnel syndrome maximizes the area under the flexor retinaculum.[148] In ulnar neuropathy, activity modification such as avoidance of resting on elbows and repetitive elbow flexion in combination with elbow pads provides relief to the majority of patients.[140] Corticosteroid injections can provide relief in 70% of carpal tunnel cases, but do not appear effective in ulnar neuropathy.[140,146] Surgical decompression is offered to patients with pain and symptoms who failed conservative management. Surgical referral is also warranted for severe entrapment neuropathy demonstrated on either physical exam (muscle weakness/atrophy) or NCS/EMG to prevent further axonal loss. Surgery typically prevents further nerve injury but motor recovery and resolution of numbness/paresthesias may be limited.[140]

FIBROMYALGIA

Fibromyalgia is a syndrome of persistent widespread pain, stiffness, fatigue, disrupted and unrefreshing sleep, and cognitive difficulties, often accompanied by multiple other unexplained symptoms, anxiety and/or depression, and functional impairment of activities of daily living.[149] Its prevalence is high, and likely underreported. Depending on the diagnostic criteria used, its prevalence has ranged from 2% to 8% of the general population.[150–152]

Fibromyalgia is currently considered a disorder of central pain processing or a syndrome of central sensitivity. Its pathogenesis is incompletely understood but appears to be primarily mediated by abnormalities within the central nervous system. This includes dopamine dysregulation in the brain,[153,154] excess amount of excitatory neurotransmitters (e.g., substance P, glutamate levels) in the insula, and low levels of inhibitory neurotransmitters (e.g., serotonin and norepinephrine) in descending antinociceptive pathways in the spinal cord.[155–158] This combination results in a decreased pain perception threshold. Family studies from the mid-2000s provided substantial evidence of a genetic linkage to fibromyalgia.[159] More recent advances in genotyping are identifying a series of single-nucleotide polymorphism haplotypes that influence neurotransmitter levels and receptor levels (including serotonin) in the brain and thus contribute to the various abnormalities in pain processing.

Patients with fibromyalgia will report that their pains are diffuse, wax, and wane in severity, and are migratory in nature. Pain and muscle tenderness are usually seen on both sides of the body, above and below the waste, while predominately involving paraspinal muscles. Pain is commonly accompanied by trunk and extremity paresthesias, diffuse stiffness, fatigue, sleep disturbances, memory, and mood difficulties.[160]

Fibromyalgia is known as diagnosis of exclusion and disorders that could present with similar symptoms should be ruled out prior to giving a formal diagnosis. These include diseases of the endocrine system (hypothyroidism, hypogonadism), neurologic system (multiple sclerosis, autonomic dysfunction, myopathies), and immune system (inflammatory arthropathies and myopathies). An appropriate history, physical examination, and laboratory testing should be performed on all patients.

In 1990, the American College of Rheumatology (ACR) developed diagnostic criteria for Fibromyalgia to help better diagnose and research patients with this atypical collection of symptoms. This original classification criterion depended on a specialized physical examination to quantify tender points.[161]

A revision of this landmark criterion was subsequently made in 2010 and 2011. The 2010/2011 ACR

Widespread Pain Index
(1 point per check box; score range: 0-19 points)

(1) Please indicate if you have had pain or tenderness **during the past 7 days** in the areas shown below.
   Check the boxes in the diagram for each area in which you have had pain or tenderness.

Right jaw ☐
Neck ☐
Left jaw ☐
Right shoulder ☐
Left shoulder ☐
Chest or breast ☐
Upper back ☐
Right upper arm ☐
Left upper arm ☐
Right lower arm ☐
Abdomen ☐
Left lower arm ☐
Lower back ☐
Right hip or buttocks ☐
Left hip or buttocks ☐
Right upper leg ☐
Left upper leg ☐
Right lower leg ☐
Left lower leg ☐

Symptom Severity
(score range: 0-12 points)

(2) For each symptom listed below, use the following scale to indicate the severity of the symptom **during the past 7 days**.
   • **No problem**
   • **Slight or mild problem:** generally mild or intermittent
   • **Moderate problem:** considerable problems; often present and/or at a moderate level
   • **Severe problem:** continuous, life-disturbing problems

	No problem	Slight or mild problem	Moderate problem	Severe problem
Points	0	1	2	3
A. Fatigue	☐	☐	☐	☐
B. Trouble thinking or remembering	☐	☐	☐	☐
C. Waking up tired (unrefreshed)	☐	☐	☐	☐

(3) During the **past 6 months** have you had any of the following symptoms?

Points	0	1
A. Pain or cramps in lower abdomen	☐ No	☐ Yes
B. Depression	☐ No	☐ Yes
C. Headache	☐ No	☐ Yes

Additional criteria (no score)

(4) Have the symptoms in questions 2 and 3 and widespread pain been present at a similar level for at **least 3 months**?
   ☐ No   ☐ Yes

(5) Do you have a disorder that would otherwise explain the pain?
   ☐ No   ☐ Yes

FIG. 6.10 American College of Rheumatology 2010 fibromyalgia diagnostic criteria.

diagnostic moved away from the use of tender points and incorporated broader clinical symptoms and scales.[162] The 2010/2011 ACR diagnostic criteria included both a physician-driven diagnostic tool (published in 2010) and a self-administered patient questionnaire (published in 2011). The patient questionnaire version was created in order to speed clinical assessment and limit possible physician underreporting of symptoms (Fig. 6.10).[163] This questionnaire is divided into three sections. The first section assesses the distribution of bodily pain using the same 19 body areas with patients marking "yes" or "no" to each area to indicate if they had pain or tenderness in that area over the past week. Patients score 1 point for each painful or tender body area, yielding a self-report widespread pain index (WPI) score between 0 and 19. The second section evaluates the severity of problems with daytime fatigue, nonrestorative sleep, and cognitive dysfunction using separate questions scored on a 0–3 scale with 0 representing no problem

and 3 representing a severe problem. The third section asks patients whether they have experienced pain or cramps in the lower abdomen, depression, or headache during the past 6 months. Patients score 1 point for each positive symptom. Scores from the second and third sections are summed to yield a 0–12 SS scale score.

The most recent ACR update of the diagnostic criteria was made in 2016 incorporating the 2010/2011scales with slight modifications. As per this update, patients need to meet the following criteria for a diagnosis of fibromyalgia:[164]

• Generalized pain, defined as pain in at least four of five regions is present (left upper, right upper, left lower, right lower, and axial)
• Symptoms have been present at a similar level for at least 3 months
• WPI ≥ 7 and symptom severity scale (SSS) score ≥ 5
OR
WPI of 4–6 and SSS score ≥ 9

- A diagnosis of fibromyalgia is valid irrespective of other diagnoses. A diagnosis of fibromyalgia does not exclude the presence of other clinically important illnesses

Treatment of fibromyalgia is best approached by integrating pharmacological and nonpharmacological treatments. Treatment guidelines generally recommend that all patients receive education about the nature of their condition and the need to play an active role in their own care.[165] This includes the importance of stress reduction, sleep regulation, and incorporation of exercise into their daily life. These core concepts should be continually reinforced at each patient encounter.

Pharmacological therapies can be helpful in alleviating some symptoms, but patients rarely achieve meaningful improvements without integrating the core components of self-care. Effective pharmacological therapies generally work in by reducing the activity of pain facilitating neurotransmitters (i.e., glutamate) or by increasing the activity of inhibitory neurotransmitters (i.e., norepinephrine and serotonin). Several drugs or classes of drugs have strong evidence (level 1A evidence) for efficacy in treating fibromyalgia, including tricyclic compounds[166] (amitriptyline, nortriptyline), gabapentinoids[167] (pregabalin, gabapentin), SNRIs[168,169] (duloxetine, milnacipran), and γ-hydroxybutyrate.[170]

Nonpharmacologic therapies have equally strong evidence (level 1A) as pharmacologic treatments and often exceed them in efficacy. These include patient education,[171] graded aerobic exercise,[172] and cognitive behavior therapy.[173] Complementary and alternative therapies can be useful as treatment adjuncts for fibromyalgia but have limited efficacy.[174] These include chiropractic manipulation, trigger-point injections, tai chi, yoga, acupuncture, and myofascial release therapy.

CONCLUSION

With the expected rise in the prevalence of MSK pain conditions, it is essential that Pain Medicine providers feel confident in treating these disorders. Gaining an understanding of each condition's underlying pathophysiology will allow you to better diagnose and treat your patients.

As advancements are made in research and technology, alterations will need to be made to the diagnostic and therapeutic strategies discussed in this chapter. Continued lifelong learning is critical to providing excellent care to our growing number of patients with MSK pain conditions.

REFERENCES

1. Vos T, Flaxman AD, Naghavi M, et al. Years lived with disability (YLDs) for 1160 sequelae of 289 diseases and injuries 1990–2010: a systematic analysis for the Global Burden of Disease Study 2010. *Lancet.* 2012;380(9859): 2163–2196.
2. Rui P, Kang K, Ashman JJ. *National Hospital Ambulatory Medical Care Survey: 2016 Emergency Department Summary Tables.* 2016.
3. Rui P, Okeyode T. *National Ambulatory Medical Care Survey: 2016 National Summary Tables.* 2016.
4. Silverman S. The clinical consequences of vertebral compression fracture. *Bone.* 1992;13:S27–S31.
5. Wasnich R. Vertebral fracture epidemiology. *Bone.* 1996; 18(3):S179–S183.
6. Adinoff AD, Hollister JR. Steroid-induced fractures and bone loss in patients with asthma. *N Engl J Med.* 1983; 309(5):265–268.
7. Houston LA, Grant SF, Reid DM, Ralston SH. Vitamin D receptor polymorphism, bone mineral density, and osteoporotic vertebral fracture: studies in a UK population. *Bone.* 1996;18(3):249–252.
8. Ahn TK, Kim JO, Kumar H, et al. Polymorphisms of miR-146a, miR-149, miR-196a2, and miR-499 are associated with osteoporotic vertebral compression fractures in Korean postmenopausal women. *J Orthop Res.* 2018; 36(1):244–253.
9. Liu CT, Karasik D, Zhou Y, et al. Heritability of prevalent vertebral fracture and volumetric bone mineral density and geometry at the lumbar spine in three generations of the Framingham study. *J Bone Miner Res.* 2012;27(4). 954–958.
10. Huang C, Ross PD, Wasnich RD. Vertebral fracture and other predictors of physical impairment and health care utilization. *Arch Intern Med.* 1996;156(21). 2469–2475.
11. Rapado A. General management of vertebral fractures. *Bone.* 1996;18(3):S191–S196.
12. Lindsay R, Silverman SL, Cooper C, et al. Risk of new vertebral fracture in the year following a fracture. *J Am Med Assoc.* 2001;285(3):320–323.
13. Longo UG, Loppini M, Denaro L, Maffulli N, Denaro V. Osteoporotic vertebral fractures: current concepts of conservative care. *Br Med Bull.* 2012;102(1):171.
14. Urrutia J, Besa P, Piza C. Incidental identification of vertebral compression fractures in patients over 60 years old using computed tomography scans showing the entire thoraco-lumbar spine. *Arch Orthop Trauma Surg.* 2019; 139(11):1497–1503.
15. Cuccurullo SJ. *Physical Medicine and Rehabilitation Board Review.* Demos Medical Publishing; 2014.
16. Panda A, Das CJ, Baruah U. Imaging of vertebral fractures. *Indian J Endocrinol Metab.* 2014;18(3):295–303.
17. Cicala D, Briganti F, Casale L, et al. Atraumatic vertebral compression fractures: differential diagnosis between benign osteoporotic and malignant fractures by MRI. *Musculoskelet Surg.* 2013;97(Suppl 2):S169–S179.

18. Lee HM, Park SY, Lee SH, Suh SW, Hong JY. Comparative analysis of clinical outcomes in patients with osteoporotic vertebral compression fractures (OVCFs): conservative treatment versus balloon kyphoplasty. *Spine J.* 2012; 12(11):998−1005.

19. Lyritis GP, Paspati I, Karachalios T, Ioakimidis D, Skarantavos G, Lyritis PG. Pain relief from nasal salmon calcitonin in osteoporotic vertebral crush fractures: a double blind, placebo-controlled clinical study. *Acta Orthop Scand.* 1997;68(suppl 275):112−114.

20. Lyritis GP, Paspati I, Karachalios T, Ioakimidis D, Skarantavos G, Lyritis PG. Pain relief from nasal salmon calcitonin in osteoporotic vertebral crush fractures. A double blind, placebo-controlled clinical study. *Acta Orthop Scand Suppl.* 1997;275:112−114.

21. Chesnut 3rd CH, Silverman S, Andriano K, et al. A randomized trial of nasal spray salmon calcitonin in postmenopausal women with established osteoporosis: the prevent recurrence of osteoporotic fractures study. PROOF Study Group. *Am J Med.* 2000;109(4):267−276.

22. Knopp-Sihota JA, Newburn-Cook CV, Homik J, Cummings GG, Voaklander D. Calcitonin for treating acute and chronic pain of recent and remote osteoporotic vertebral compression fractures: a systematic review and meta-analysis. *Osteoporos Int.* 2012;23(1):17−38.

23. Agulnek AN, O'Leary KJ, Edwards BJ. Acute vertebral fracture. *J Hosp Med.* 2009;4(7):E20−E24.

24. Sinaki M. Exercise for patients with osteoporosis: management of vertebral compression fractures and trunk strengthening for fall prevention. *PM R.* 2012;4(11): 882−888.

25. Chang V, Holly LT. Bracing for thoracolumbar fractures. *Neurosurg Focus.* 2014;37(1):E3.

26. Anderson PA, Froyshteter AB, Tontz Jr WL. Meta-analysis of vertebral augmentation compared with conservative treatment for osteoporotic spinal fractures. *J Bone Miner Res.* 2013;28(2):372−382.

27. Goldman L, Schafer AI. *Goldman-Cecil Medicine E-Book.* Elsevier Health Sciences; 2015.

28. Sinusas K. Osteoarthritis: diagnosis and treatment. *Am Fam Physician.* 2012;85(1):49−56.

29. Liu-Bryan R, Terkeltaub R. Emerging regulators of the inflammatory process in osteoarthritis. *Nat Rev Rheumatol.* 2015;11(1):35−44.

30. Blagojevic M, Jinks C, Jeffery A, Jordan KP. Risk factors for onset of osteoarthritis of the knee in older adults: a systematic review and meta-analysis. *Osteoarthritis Cartilage.* 2010;18(1):24−33.

31. National CGCU. *Osteoarthritis: Care and Management in Adults.* 2014.

32. Brandt KD. A pessimistic view of serologic markers for diagnosis and management of osteoarthritis. Biochemical, immunologic and clinicopathologic barriers. *J Rheumatol Suppl.* 1989;18:39−42.

33. Boesen M, Ellegaard K, Henriksen M, et al. Osteoarthritis year in review 2016: imaging. *Osteoarthritis Cartilage.* 2017;25(2):216−226.

34. Brosseau L, Wells GA, Pugh AG, et al. Ottawa Panel evidence-based clinical practice guidelines for therapeutic exercise in the management of hip osteoarthritis. *Clin Rehabil.* 2016;30(10):935−946.

35. Brosseau L, Taki J, Desjardins B, et al. The Ottawa panel clinical practice guidelines for the management of knee osteoarthritis. Part two: strengthening exercise programs. *Clin Rehabil.* 2017;31(5):596−611.

36. Hochberg MC, Altman RD, April KT, et al. American College of Rheumatology 2012 recommendations for the use of nonpharmacologic and pharmacologic therapies in osteoarthritis of the hand, hip, and knee. *Arthritis Care Res.* 2012;64(4):465−474.

37. Jüni P, Hari R, Rutjes AW, et al. Intra-articular corticosteroid for knee osteoarthritis. *Cochrane Database Syst Rev.* 2015;(10).

38. Laudy AB, Bakker EW, Rekers M, Moen MH. Efficacy of platelet-rich plasma injections in osteoarthritis of the knee: a systematic review and meta-analysis. *Br J Sports Med.* 2015;49(10):657−672.

39. Jevsevar D, Donnelly P, Brown GA, Cummins DS. Viscosupplementation for osteoarthritis of the knee: asystematic review of the evidence. *J Bone Jt Surg Am.* 2015; 97(24):2047−2060.

40. McAlindon TE, Bannuru RR, Sullivan MC, et al. OARSI guidelines for the non-surgical management of knee osteoarthritis. *Osteoarthritis Cartilage.* 2014;22(3):363−388.

41. Krebs EE, Gravely A, Nugent S, et al. Effect of opioid vs nonopioid medications on pain-related function in patients with chronic back pain or hip or knee osteoarthritis pain: the SPACE randomized clinical trial. *J Am Med Assoc.* 2018;319(9):872−882.

42. Reid D. The management of greater trochanteric pain syndrome: a systematic literature review. *J Orthop.* 2016; 13(1):15−28.

43. Fearon AM, Scarvell JM, Neeman T, Cook JL, Cormick W, Smith PN. Greater trochanteric pain syndrome: defining the clinical syndrome. *Br J Sports Med.* 2013;47(10): 649−653.

44. Hirschmann A, Falkowski AL, Kovacs B. *Greater Trochanteric Pain Syndrome: Abductors, External Rotators.* Paper presented at: Seminars in musculoskeletal radiology. 2017.

45. Segal NA, Felson DT, Torner JC, et al. Greater trochanteric pain syndrome: epidemiology and associated factors. *Arch Phys Med Rehabil.* 2007;88(8):988−992.

46. Braddom RL. *Physical Medicine and Rehabilitation E-Book.* Elsevier Health Sciences; 2010.

47. Lustenberger DP, Ng VY, Best TM, Ellis TJ. Efficacy of treatment of trochanteric bursitis: a systematic review. *Clin J Sport Med.* 2011;21(5):447−453.

48. Brinks A, van Rijn RM, Willemsen SP, et al. Corticosteroid injections for greater trochanteric pain syndrome: a randomized controlled trial in primary care. *Ann Fam Med.* 2011;9(3):226−234.

49. Mellor R, Bennell K, Grimaldi A, et al. Education plus exercise versus corticosteroid injection use versus a wait and see approach on global outcome and pain from gluteal

tendinopathy: prospective, single blinded, randomised clinical trial. *BMJ.* 2018;361:k1662.

50. Brooker Jr AF. The surgical approach to refractory trochanteric bursitis. *Johns Hopkins Med J.* 1979;145(3): 98–100.

51. Barnthouse NC, Wente TM, Voos JE. Greater trochanteric pain syndrome: endoscopic treatment options. *Operat Tech Sports Med.* 2012;20(4):320–324.

52. Neviaser AS, Hannafin JA. Adhesive capsulitis: a review of current treatment. *Am J Sports Med.* 2010;38(11):2346–2356.

53. Evans JP, Guyver PM, Smith CD. Frozen shoulder after simple arthroscopic shoulder procedures: what is the risk? *Bone Jt J.* 2015;97-B(7):963–966.

54. Wohlgethan JR. Frozen shoulder in hyperthyroidism. *Arthritis Rheum.* 1987;30(8):936–939.

55. Zreik NH, Malik RA, Charalambous CP. Adhesive capsulitis of the shoulder and diabetes: a meta-analysis of prevalence. *Muscles Ligaments Tendons J.* 2016;6(1): 26–34.

56. Neviaser TJ. Adhesive capsulitis. *Orthop Clin N Am.* 1987; 18(3):439–443.

57. Bunker TD, Anthony PP. The pathology of frozen shoulder. A Dupuytren-like disease. *J Bone Jt Surg Br.* 1995; 77(5):677–683.

58. Neviaser AS, Neviaser RJ. Adhesive capsulitis of the shoulder. *J Am Acad Orthop Surg.* 2011;19(9):536–542.

59. Speed CA, Hazleman BL. In: *Calcific Tendinitis of the Shoulder.* Mass Medical Soc; 1999.

60. Frontera WR, Silver JK, Rizzo TD. *Essentials of Physical Medicine and Rehabilitation E-Book: Musculoskeletal Disorders, Pain, and Rehabilitation.* Elsevier Health Sciences; 2014.

61. Manske RC, Prohaska D. Diagnosis and management of adhesive capsulitis. *Curr Rev Musculoskelet Med.* 2008; 1(3–4):180–189.

62. Antoniou J, Duckworth DT, Harryman DT. Capsulolabral augmentation for the management of posteroinferior instability of the shoulder. *J Bone Jt Surg Am.* 2000; 82(9):1220.

63. Reeves B. The natural history of the frozen shoulder syndrome. *Scand J Rheumatol.* 1975;4(4):193–196.

64. Favejee MM, Huisstede BM, Koes BW. Frozen shoulder: the effectiveness of conservative and surgical interventions—systematic review. *Br J Sports Med.* 2011; 45(1):49–56.

65. Le HV, Lee SJ, Nazarian A, Rodriguez EK. Adhesive capsulitis of the shoulder: review of pathophysiology and current clinical treatments. *Shoulder Elbow.* 2017;9(2):75–84.

66. Fernandes TL, Pedrinelli A, Hernandez AJ. Muscle injury – physiopathology, diagnosis, treatment and clinical presentation. *Rev Bras Ortop.* 2011;46(3):247–255.

67. Jarvinen TA, Jarvinen TL, Kaariainen M, Kalimo H, Jarvinen M. Muscle injuries: biology and treatment. *Am J Sports Med.* 2005;33(5):745–764.

68. Jarvinen TA, Jarvinen TL, Kaariainen M, et al. Muscle injuries: optimising recovery. *Best Pract Res Clin Rheumatol.* 2007;21(2):317–331.

69. Morelli KM, Brown LB, Warren GL. Effect of NSAIDs on recovery from acute skeletal muscle injury: a systematic review and meta-analysis. *Am J Sports Med.* 2018;46(1): 224–233.

70. Jarvinen M. Healing of a crush injury in rat striated muscle. 4. Effect of early mobilization and immobilization on the tensile properties of gastrocnemius muscle. *Acta Chir Scand.* 1976;142(1):47–56.

71. Jarvinen TA, Jarvinen M, Kalimo H. Regeneration of injured skeletal muscle after the injury. *Muscles Ligaments Tendons J.* 2013;3(4):337–345.

72. Maffulli N, Khan KM, Puddu G. Overuse tendon conditions: time to change a confusing terminology. *Arthroscopy.* 1998;14(8):840–843.

73. Thorpe CT, Chaudhry S, Lei II, et al. Tendon overload results in alterations in cell shape and increased markers of inflammation and matrix degradation. *Scand J Med Sci Sports.* 2015;25(4):e381–391.

74. Scott A, Backman LJ. Speed C. Tendinopathy: update on pathophysiology. *J Orthop Sports Phys Ther.* 2015; 45(11):833–841.

75. Astrom M, Rausing A. Chronic Achilles tendinopathy. A survey of surgical and histopathologic findings. *Clin Orthop Relat Res.* 1995;(316):151–164.

76. Riley G. Tendinopathy—from basic science to treatment. *Nat Clin Pract Rheumatol.* 2008;4(2):82–89.

77. Andersson G, Backman LJ, Scott A, Lorentzon R, Forsgren S, Danielson P. Substance P accelerates hypercellularity and angiogenesis in tendon tissue and enhances paratendinitis in response to Achilles tendon overuse in a tendinopathy model. *Br J Sports Med.* 2011; 45(13):1017–1022.

78. Dean BJ, Snelling SJ, Dakin SG, Murphy RJ, Javaid MK, Carr AJ. Differences in glutamate receptors and inflammatory cell numbers are associated with the resolution of pain in human rotator cuff tendinopathy. *Arthritis Res Ther.* 2015;17:176.

79. Rio E, Moseley L, Purdam C, et al. The pain of tendinopathy: physiological or pathophysiological? *Sports Med.* 2014;44(1):9–23.

80. Dean BJF, Dakin SG, Millar NL, Carr AJ. Review: emerging concepts in the pathogenesis of tendinopathy. *Surgeon.* 2017;15(6):349–354.

81. Ooi CC, Schneider ME, Malliaras P, Chadwick M, Connell DA. Diagnostic performance of axial-strain sonoelastography in confirming clinically diagnosed Achilles tendinopathy: comparison with B-mode ultrasound and color Doppler imaging. *Ultrasound Med Biol.* 2015;41(1):15–25.

82. Chen DJ, Caldera FE, Kim W. Acute achilles tendinopathy diagnosed with ultrasound. *Am J Phys Med Rehabil.* 2014; 93(6):548–549.

83. Movin T, Kristoffersen-Wiberg M, Shalabi A, Gad A, Aspelin P, Rolf C. Intratendinous alterations as imaged by ultrasound and contrast medium-enhanced magnetic resonance in chronic achillodynia. *Foot Ankle Int.* 1998; 19(5):311–317.

84. Neuhold A, Stiskal M, Kainberger F, Schwaighofer B. Degenerative Achilles tendon disease: assessment by magnetic resonance and ultrasonography. *Eur J Radiol.* 1992;14(3):213−220.

85. Forslund C, Bylander B, Aspenberg P. Indomethacin and celecoxib improve tendon healing in rats. *Acta Orthop Scand.* 2003;74(4):465−469.

86. Thomas J, Taylor D, Crowell R, Assor D. The effect of indomethacin on Achilles tendon healing in rabbits. *Clin Orthop Relat Res.* 1991;(272):308−311.

87. Cabuk H, Avci A, Durmaz H, Cabuk FK, Ertem F, Muhittin Sener I. The effect of diclofenac on matrix metalloproteinase levels in the rotator cuff. *Arch Orthop Trauma Surg.* 2014;134(12):1739−1744.

88. Chechik O, Dolkart O, Mozes G, Rak O, Alhajajra F, Maman E. Timing matters: NSAIDs interfere with the late proliferation stage of a repaired rotator cuff tendon healing in rats. *Arch Orthop Trauma Surg.* 2014;134(4):515−520.

89. Connizzo BK, Yannascoli SM, Tucker JJ, et al. The detrimental effects of systemic Ibuprofen delivery on tendon healing are time-dependent. *Clin Orthop Relat Res.* 2014;472(8):2433−2439.

90. Hart L. Corticosteroid and other injections in the management of tendinopathies: a review. *Clin J Sport Med.* 2011;21(6):540−541.

91. Coombes BK, Bisset L, Vicenzino B. Efficacy and safety of corticosteroid injections and other injections for management of tendinopathy: a systematic review of randomised controlled trials. *Lancet.* 2010;376(9754):1751−1767.

92. Mohamadi A, Chan JJ, Claessen FM, Ring D, Chen NC. Corticosteroid injections give small and transient pain relief in rotator cuff tendinosis: ameta-analysis. *Clin Orthop Relat Res.* 2017;475(1):232−243.

93. Mellor R, Bennell K, Grimaldi A, et al. Education plus exercise versus corticosteroid injection use versus a wait and see approach on global outcome and pain from gluteal tendinopathy: prospective, single blinded, randomised clinical trial. *Br J Sports Med.* 2018;52(22):1464−1472.

94. Fritz JM, Thackeray A, Brennan GP, Childs JD. Exercise only, exercise with mechanical traction, or exercise with over-door traction for patients with cervical radiculopathy, with or without consideration of status on a previously described subgrouping rule: a randomized clinical trial. *J Orthop Sports Phys Ther.* 2014;44(2):45−57.

95. Lim HY, Wong SH. Effects of isometric, eccentric, or heavy slow resistance exercises on pain and function in individuals with patellar tendinopathy: a systematic review. *Physiother Res Int.* 2018;23(4):e1721.

96. Pearson SJ, Stadler S, Menz H, et al. Immediate and short-term effects of short- and long-duration isometric contractions in patellar tendinopathy. *Clin J Sport Med.* 2018. Aug 8. Epub ahead of print.

97. Rio E, Kidgell D, Purdam C, et al. Isometric exercise induces analgesia and reduces inhibition in patellar tendinopathy. *Br J Sports Med.* 2015;49(19):1277−1283.

98. Rompe JD, Nafe B, Furia JP, Maffulli N. Eccentric loading, shock-wave treatment, or a wait-and-see policy for tendinopathy of the main body of tendo Achillis: a randomized controlled trial. *Am J Sports Med.* 2007;35(3):374−383.

99. Chester R, Costa ML, Shepstone L, Cooper A, Donell ST. Eccentric calf muscle training compared with therapeutic ultrasound for chronic Achilles tendon pain−a pilot study. *Man Ther.* 2008;13(6):484−491.

100. Andres BM, Murrell GA. Treatment of tendinopathy: what works, what does not, and what is on the horizon. *Clin Orthop Relat Res.* 2008;466(7):1539−1554.

101. Paoloni JA, Appleyard RC, Nelson J, Murrell GA. Topical glyceryl trinitrate treatment of chronic noninsertional achilles tendinopathy. A randomized, double-blind, placebo-controlled trial. *J Bone Jt Surg Am.* 2004;86(5):916−922.

102. Paoloni JA, Appleyard RC, Nelson J, Murrell GA. Topical glyceryl trinitrate application in the treatment of chronic supraspinatus tendinopathy: a randomized, double-blinded, placebo-controlled clinical trial. *Am J Sports Med.* 2005;33(6):806−813.

103. Paoloni JA, Appleyard RC, Nelson J, Murrell GA. Topical nitric oxide application in the treatment of chronic extensor tendinosis at the elbow: a randomized, double-blinded, placebo-controlled clinical trial. *Am J Sports Med.* 2003;31(6):915−920.

104. Carlisi E, Cecini M, Di Natali G, Manzoni F, Tinelli C, Lisi C. Focused extracorporeal shock wave therapy for greater trochanteric pain syndrome with gluteal tendinopathy: a randomized controlled trial. *Clin Rehabil.* 2019;33(4):670−680.

105. Mani-Babu S, Morrissey D, Waugh C, Screen H, Barton C. The effectiveness of extracorporeal shock wave therapy in lower limb tendinopathy: a systematic review. *Am J Sports Med.* 2015;43(3):752−761.

106. Hoksrud A, Ohberg L, Alfredson H, Bahr R. Ultrasound-guided sclerosis of neovessels in painful chronic patellar tendinopathy: a randomized controlled trial. *Am J Sports Med.* 2006;34(11):1738−1746.

107. Ohberg L, Alfredson H. Ultrasound guided sclerosis of neovessels in painful chronic Achilles tendinosis: pilot study of a new treatment. *Br J Sports Med.* 2002;36(3):173−175. discussion 176-177.

108. Mautner K, Colberg RE, Malanga G, et al. Outcomes after ultrasound-guided platelet-rich plasma injections for chronic tendinopathy: a multicenter, retrospective review. *PM R.* 2013;5(3):169−175.

109. Kazemi M, Azma K, Tavana B, Rezaiee Moghaddam F, Panahi A. Autologous blood versus corticosteroid local injection in the short-term treatment of lateral elbow tendinopathy: a randomized clinical trial of efficacy. *Am J Phys Med Rehabil.* 2010;89(8):660−667.

110. Radiculopathy. In: Binder MD, Hirokawa N, Windhorst U, eds. *Encyclopedia of Neuroscience.* Berlin, Heidelberg: Springer Berlin Heidelberg; 2009:3358.

111. Tolba R. Radiculopathy. In: Pope JE, Deer TR, eds. *Treatment of Chronic Pain Conditions: A Comprehensive Handbook.* New York, NY: Springer New York; 2017:253−255.

112. Bono CM, Ghiselli G, Gilbert TJ, et al. An evidence-based clinical guideline for the diagnosis and treatment of cervical radiculopathy from degenerative disorders. *Spine J.* 2011;11(1):64—72.

113. Kreiner DS, Hwang SW, Easa JE, et al. An evidence-based clinical guideline for the diagnosis and treatment of lumbar disc herniation with radiculopathy. *Spine J.* 2014; 14(1):180—191.

114. Kreiner DS, Shaffer WO, Baisden JL, et al. An evidence-based clinical guideline for the diagnosis and treatment of degenerative lumbar spinal stenosis (update). *Spine J.* 2013;13(7):734—743.

115. Watters 3rd WC, Bono CM, Gilbert TJ, et al. An evidence-based clinical guideline for the diagnosis and treatment of degenerative lumbar spondylolisthesis. *Spine J.* 2009; 9(7):609—614.

116. Nicholson KJ, Guarino BB, Winkelstein BA. Transient nerve root compression load and duration differentially mediate behavioral sensitivity and associated spinal astrocyte activation and mGLuR5 expression. *Neuroscience.* 2012;209:187—195.

117. Kang JD, Stefanovic-Racic M, McIntyre LA, Georgescu HI, Evans CH. Toward a biochemical understanding of human intervertebral disc degeneration and herniation. Contributions of nitric oxide, interleukins, prostaglandin E2, and matrix metalloproteinases. *Spine.* 1997;22(10): 1065—1073.

118. Furusawa N, Baba H, Miyoshi N, et al. Herniation of cervical intervertebral disc: immunohistochemical examination and measurement of nitric oxide production. *Spine.* 2001;26(10):1110—1116.

119. Goupille P, Jayson MI, Valat JP, Freemont AJ. The role of inflammation in disk herniation-associated radiculopathy. *Semin Arthritis Rheum.* 1998;28(1):60—71.

120. Crosby ND, Zaucke F, Kras JV, Dong L, Luo ZD, Winkelstein BA. Thrombospondin-4 and excitatory synaptogenesis promote spinal sensitization after painful mechanical joint injury. *Exp Neurol.* 2015;264:111—120.

121. Dong L, Quindlen JC, Lipschutz DE, Winkelstein BA. Whiplash-like facet joint loading initiates glutamatergic responses in the DRG and spinal cord associated with behavioral hypersensitivity. *Brain Res.* 2012;1461:51—63.

122. Majlesi J, Togay H, Unalan H, Toprak S. The sensitivity and specificity of the Slump and the Straight Leg Raising tests in patients with lumbar disc herniation. *J Clin Rheumatol.* 2008;14(2):87—91.

123. Shabat S, Leitner Y, David R, Folman Y. The correlation between Spurling test and imaging studies in detecting cervical radiculopathy. *J Neuroimaging.* 2012;22(4): 375—378.

124. Rubinstein SM, Pool JJ, van Tulder MW, Riphagen II, de Vet HC. A systematic review of the diagnostic accuracy of provocative tests of the neck for diagnosing cervical radiculopathy. *Eur Spine J.* 2007;16(3):307—319.

125. Thoomes EJ, van Geest S, van der Windt DA, et al. Value of physical tests in diagnosing cervical radiculopathy: a systematic review. *Spine J.* 2018;18(1):179—189.

126. Ekedahl H, Jonsson B, Annertz M, Frobell RB. Accuracy of clinical tests in detecting disk herniation and nerve root compression in subjects with lumbar radicula symptoms. *Arch Phys Med Rehabil.* 2018;99(4):726—735.

127. Wilbourn AJ, Aminoff MJ. AAEM minimonograph 32: the electrodiagnostic examination in patients with radiculopathies. American Association of Electrodiagnostic Medicine. *Muscle Nerve.* 1998;21(12):1612—1631.

128. Radhakrishnan K, Litchy WJ, O'Fallon WM, Kurland LT. Epidemiology of cervical radiculopathy. A population-based study from Rochester, Minnesota, 1976 through 1990. *Brain.* 1994;117(Pt 2):325—335.

129. da CMCL, Maher CG, Hancock MJ, McAuley JH, Herbert RD, Costa LO. The prognosis of acute and persistent low-back pain: a meta-analysis. *Can Med Assoc J* 2012;184(11):E613—E624.

130. Goldberg H, Firtch W, Tyburski M, et al. Oral steroids for acute radiculopathy due to a herniated lumbar disk: a randomized clinical trial. *J Am Med Assoc.* 2015; 313(19):1915—1923.

131. Handa J, Sekiguchi M, Krupkova O, Konno S. The effect of serotonin-noradrenaline reuptake inhibitor duloxetine on the intervertebral disk-related radiculopathy in rats. *Eur Spine J.* 2016;25(3):877—887.

132. Chou R, Deyo R, Friedly J, et al. Systemic pharmacologic therapies for low back pain: a systematic review for an American College of Physicians Clinical Practice Guideline. *Ann Intern Med.* 2017;166(7):480—492.

133. Zhu L, Wei X, Wang S. Does cervical spine manipulation reduce pain in people with degenerative cervical radiculopathy? A systematic review of the evidence, and a meta-analysis. *Clin Rehabil.* 2016;30(2):145—155.

134. Hahne AJ, Ford JJ, McMeeken JM. Conservative management of lumbar disc herniation with associated radiculopathy: a systematic review. *Spine.* 2010;35(11):E488—E504.

135. Pandey RA. Efficacy of epidural steroid injection in management of lumbar prolapsed intervertebral disc: a comparison of caudal, transforaminal and interlaminar routes. *J Clin Diagn Res.* 2016;10(7):RC05—11.

136. Manchikanti L, Knezevic NN, Boswell MV, Kaye AD, Hirsch JA. Epidural injections for lumbar radiculopathy and spinal stenosis: a comparative systematic review and meta-analysis. *Pain Physician.* 2016;19(3): E365—E410.

137. Kwon JW, Lee JW, Kim SH, et al. Cervical interlaminar epidural steroid injection for neck pain and cervical radiculopathy: effect and prognostic factors. *Skeletal Radiol* 2007;36(5):431—436.

138. Lee SH, Kim KT, Kim DH, Lee BJ, Son ES, Kwack YH. Clinical outcomes of cervical radiculopathy following epidural steroid injection: a prospective study with follow-up for more than 2 years. *Spine.* 2012;37(12):1041—1047.

139. Gutman G, Rosenzweig DH, Golan JD. Surgical treatment of cervical radiculopathy: meta-analysis of randomized controlled trials. *Spine.* 2018;43(6):E365—E372.

140. Hobson-Webb LD, Juel VC. Common entrapment neuropathies. *Continuum.* 2017;23(2):487—511. Selected Topics in Outpatient Neurology.

141. Mackinnon SE, Dellon AL, Hudson AR, Hunter DA. Chronic nerve compression—an experimental model in the rat. *Ann Plast Surg.* 1984;13(2):112—120.

142. Mackinnon SE, Dellon AL, Hudson AR, Hunter DA. Chronic human nerve compression–a histological assessment. *Neuropathol Appl Neurobiol.* 1986;12(6): 547−565.

143. Mackinnon SE, O'Brien JP, Dellon AL, McLean AR, Hudson AR, Hunter DA. An assessment of the effects of internal neurolysis on a chronically compressed rat sciatic nerve. *Plast Reconstr Surg.* 1988;81(2):251−258.

144. Aboonq MS. Pathophysiology of carpal tunnel syndrome. *Neurosciences.* 2015;20(1):4−9.

145. Elhassan B, Steinmann SP. Entrapment neuropathy of the ulnar nerve. *J Am Acad Orthop Surg.* 2007;15(11):672−681.

146. Doughty CT, Bowley MP. Entrapment neuropathies of the upper extremity. *Med Clin N Am.* 2019;103(2):357−370.

147. Cartwright MS, Walker FO. Neuromuscular ultrasound in common entrapment neuropathies. *Muscle Nerve.* 2013; 48(5):696−704.

148. Walker WC, Metzler M, Cifu DX, Swartz Z. Neutral wrist splinting in carpal tunnel syndrome: a comparison of night-only versus full-time wear instructions. *Arch Phys Med Rehabil.* 2000;81(4):424−429.

149. Lopez-Pousa S, Garre-Olmo J, de Gracia M, Ribot J, Calvo-Perxas L, Vilalta-Franch J. Development of a multi-dimensional measure of fibromyalgia symptomatology: the comprehensive rating scale for fibromyalgia symptomatology. *J Psychosom Res.* 2013;74(5):384−392.

150. McBeth J, Jones K. Epidemiology of chronic musculoskeletal pain. *Best Pract Res Clin Rheumatol.* 2007;21(3): 403−425.

151. Vincent A, Lahr BD, Wolfe F, et al. Prevalence of fibromyalgia: a population-based study in olmsted county, Minnesota, utilizing the rochester epidemiology project. *Arthritis Care Res.* 2013;65(5):786−792.

152. Wolfe F, Ross K, Anderson J, Russell IJ, Hebert L. The prevalence and characteristics of fibromyalgia in the general population. *Arthritis Rheum.* 1995;38(1):19−28.

153. Wood PB, Schweinhardt P, Jaeger E, et al. Fibromyalgia patients show an abnormal dopamine response to pain. *Eur J Neurosci.* 2007;25(12):3576−3582.

154. Staud R, Spaeth M. Psychophysical and neurochemical abnormalities of pain processing in fibromyalgia. *CNS Spectr.* 2008;13(3 Suppl 5):12−17.

155. Docampo E, Escaramis G, Gratacos M, et al. Genome-wide analysis of single nucleotide polymorphisms and copy number variants in fibromyalgia suggest a role for the central nervous system. *Pain.* 2014;155(6):1102−1109.

156. Clauw DJ. Fibromyalgia: update on mechanisms and management. *J Clin Rheumatol.* 2007;13(2):102−109.

157. Russell IJ, Orr MD, Littman B, et al. Elevated cerebrospinal fluid levels of substance P in patients with the fibromyalgia syndrome. *Arthritis Rheum.* 1994;37(11):1593−1601.

158. Sarchielli P, Di Filippo M, Nardi K, Calabresi P. Sensitization, glutamate, and the link between migraine and fibromyalgia. *Curr Pain Headache Rep.* 2007;11(5): 343−351.

159. Arnold LM, Hudson JI, Hess EV, et al. Family study of fibromyalgia. *Arthritis Rheum.* 2004;50(3):944−952.

160. Clauw DJ. Fibromyalgia: a clinical review. *J Am Med Assoc.* 2014;311(15):1547−1555.

161. Wolfe F, Smythe HA, Yunus MB, et al. The American College of Rheumatology 1990 criteria for the classification of fibromyalgia. Report of the Multicenter Criteria Committee. *Arthritis Rheum.* 1990;33(2):160−172.

162. Wolfe F, Clauw DJ, Fitzcharles MA, et al. The American College of Rheumatology preliminary diagnostic criteria for fibromyalgia and measurement of symptom severity. *Arthritis Care Res.* 2010;62(5):600−610.

163. Wolfe F, Clauw DJ, Fitzcharles MA, et al. Fibromyalgia criteria and severity scales for clinical and epidemiological studies: a modification of the ACR preliminary diagnostic criteria for fibromyalgia. *J Rheumatol.* 2011;38(6): 1113−1122.

164. Wolfe F, Clauw DJ, Fitzcharles MA, et al. 2016 Revisions to the 2010/2011 fibromyalgia diagnostic criteria. *Semin Arthritis Rheum.* 2016;46(3):319−329.

165. Fitzcharles MA, Ste-Marie PA, Goldenberg DL, et al. 2012 Canadian Guidelines for the diagnosis and management of fibromyalgia syndrome: executive summary. *Pain Res Manag.* 2013;18(3):119−126.

166. Arnold LM. Duloxetine and other antidepressants in the treatment of patients with fibromyalgia. *Pain Med.* 2007;8(Suppl 2):S63−S74.

167. Tzellos TG, Toulis KA, Goulis DG, et al. Gabapentin and pregabalin in the treatment of fibromyalgia: a systematic review and a meta-analysis. *J Clin Pharm Therapeut.* 2010; 35(6):639−656.

168. Arnold LM, Clauw DJ, Wohlreich MM, et al. Efficacy of duloxetine in patients with fibromyalgia: pooled analysis of 4 placebo-controlled clinical trials. *Prim Care Companion J Clin Psychiatry.* 2009;11(5):237−244.

169. Geisser ME, Palmer RH, Gendreau RM, Wang Y, Clauw DJ. A pooled analysis of two randomized, double-blind, placebo-controlled trials of milnacipran monotherapy in the treatment of fibromyalgia. *Pain Pract.* 2011;11(2):120−131.

170. Russell IJ, Holman AJ, Swick TJ, et al. Sodium oxybate reduces pain, fatigue, and sleep disturbance and improves functionality in fibromyalgia: results from a 14-week, randomized, double-blind, placebo-controlled study. *Pain.* 2011;152(5):1007−1017.

171. Hauser W, Bernardy K, Arnold B, Offenbacher M, Schiltenwolf M. Efficacy of multicomponent treatment in fibromyalgia syndrome: a meta-analysis of randomized controlled clinical trials. *Arthritis Rheum.* 2009; 61(2):216−224.

172. Hauser W, Klose P, Langhorst J, et al. Efficacy of different types of aerobic exercise in fibromyalgia syndrome: a systematic review and meta-analysis of randomised controlled trials. *Arthritis Res Ther.* 2010;12(3):R79.

173. Bernardy K, Fuber N, Kollner V, Hauser W. Efficacy of cognitive-behavioral therapies in fibromyalgia syndrome - a systematic review and metaanalysis of randomized controlled trials. *J Rheumatol.* 2010;37(10):1991−2005.

174. Porter NSJL, Boulton A, Bothne N, Coleman B. Alternative medical interventions used in the treatment and management of myalgic encephalomyelitis/chronic fatigue syndrome and fibromyalgia. *J Alternative Compl Med.* 2010;16(3):235−249.

CHAPTER 7

Palliative Care and Cancer Pain

ERIC PROMMER, MD, FAAHPM, HMDC • PATRICIA JACOBS, MD •
AMBEREEN K. MEHTA, MD

PALLIATIVE APPROACH TO ADVANCED ILLNESS

Palliative care is the interdisciplinary specialty focusing on improving quality of life for those with serious illness and their families. Over the past decade, palliative care has experienced an expanded evidence base, novel care-delivery models, creative payment mechanisms, and increasing public and professional awareness.[1] Currently, palliative care and hospice have different meanings. Palliative care is interdisciplinary care (medicine, nursing, social work, chaplaincy, and other specialties when appropriate) that focusing on improving quality of life for patients who are living with any serious illness and for their families.[2] Palliative care treats pain, nonpain symptoms, addresses psychological and spiritual distress, and uses advanced communication skills to establish goals of care and help match treatments to patients personal goals. It also provides sophisticated care coordination, thus adding another layer of support to patients, their loved ones, and treating clinicians. Palliative care should be started at the time of diagnosis and is provided concurrently with all other disease-directed or curative treatments. Hospice is viewed as a formal system of interdisciplinary care that provides palliative care services to the dying in the last months of life.

SYMPTOM MANAGEMENT

Many patients with chronic and severe illness experience nonpain symptoms.[3] Nausea affects as many as 70% of patients with advanced cancer and up to 50% of patients with congestive heart failure (CHF), chronic obstructive lung disease (COPD), and renal failure.[4] Delirium occurs in up to 85% of terminally ill cancer patients. Delirium affects not only the quality of life of patients but causes lingering emotional effects on family and caregivers.[5,6] Fatigue affects two-thirds of patients with advanced CHF,[7] more than 70% of patients with advanced COPD,[8] and 80% of advanced cancer patients receiving chemotherapy and/or radiotherapy.[9] Dyspnea affects up to 90% of patients with end-stage lung disease,[8] 70% of patients with advanced cancer,[10] nearly 50% of patients with end-stage renal disease,[11] and more than 60% of patients with end-stage CHF.[12]

ADVANCED DIRECTIVES (DISCUSSION OF CODE STATUS, GOALS OF CARE, ADVANCED DIRECTIVES, AND CARE PLANNING)

As patients near the end of life, communication about goals of care and planning helps assure that patients receive the care they want, alleviates anxiety, and supports families.[13] Effective communication also supports quality of life throughout the illness trajectory, even if death is not an imminent. While goals of care discussions take time,[14] absent, delayed, or inadequate communication about end-of-life preferences leads to poor quality of life, anxiety, family distress,[15] prolongation of the dying process, undesired hospitalizations, patient mistrust of the healthcare system,[16] physician burnout,[17] and high costs.[18] Patients having end-of-life conversations are more likely to know their disease severity, to report less anxiety, and receive less-invasive care.[19] Quality end-of-life conversations lead to better bereavement adjustment for families.[15] Overall, existing evidence does not support the commonly held belief that communication that goals of care and end-of-life issues increase patient anxiety, depression, and/or hopelessness.[20]

EMOTIONAL, PSYCHOLOGICAL, AND SPIRITUAL SUPPORT

Psychological distress is common in patients with a serious illness and correlates with impaired quality of life.[21] While clinical depression is not a normal part of the dying process, preparatory grief contributes to distress experienced by most dying patients. Preparatory

Pain Care Essentials and Innovations. https://doi.org/10.1016/B978-0-323-72216-2.00007-7

grief occurs as people prepare for death and manifests by mourning impending losses, including loss of function, anticipating missed events (such as a child's graduation or wedding), and separation from loved ones.[21] Palliative care teams help distinguish between normal preparatory grieving and clinical depression which can be complicated by the neurovegetative symptoms that are part of the severe illness presentation.[21] Palliative care teams help providers identify these differences, allowing for earlier interventions leading to improved symptom control.[21] Palliative care teams also work to improve mood through psychosocial and spiritual support. Palliative care teams also recognize that the management of other symptoms, such as severe pain or intractable nausea, can improve a patient's mood and quality of life.[21] Many policy-leading organizations advocate the need to integrate physical, psychosocial, and spiritual aspects within palliative care. As patients progress toward the terminal or end-of-life stage, confronting death may prompt a person to engage in spiritual reflection.[22] The palliative care movement has led the way in including the spiritual dimension as a part of total person care defines spirituality as a more comprehensive term than "religiosity." Spirituality is defined as "a dynamic and intrinsic aspect of humanity through which persons seek ultimate meaning, purpose and transcendence, and experience relationship to self, family, others, community, society, nature, and the significant or sacred. Spirituality is expressed through beliefs, values, traditions, and practices."[23] Healthcare chaplains typically provide spiritual care,[2] but often, due to insufficient numbers of healthcare chaplains, other members of the palliative care team can help address spiritual concerns. Spiritual care can be given in the manner in which physical care is given, focusing on presence, journeying together, listening, connecting, creating openings, and engaging in reciprocal sharing and common nurturing. Quantitative studies show that 87% of patients consider spirituality to be important in their lives,[24] and between 51% and 77% of patients consider religion to be important.[24] Studies show that spiritual support is associated with better quality of life in seriously ill patients and it is important to identify these needs.[25] An observational study by Winkelman et al. showed that cancer patients with unmet spiritual concerns are more likely to have significantly worse psychological quality of life than those whose spiritual concerns were addressed.[26] A multisite cohort study involving 343 patients with advanced cancer showed that the patients whose spiritual needs were supported received more hospice care and better higher quality-of-life scores.[27] In the same cohort, patients relying on religious faith to cope with cancer were less likely than those with a low level of religious coping to receive mechanical intubation and intensive care unit care near the end of life.[28]

FAMILY AND PATIENT UNDERSTANDING OF SERIOUS ILLNESS

Patient emotions such as anxiety as well as denial are two critical patient-related factors contributing to challenges in discussing serious illness care goals. Anxiety is common in those with serious illness; one-quarter to one-half of all patients with advanced cancer experience significant anxiety symptoms, and 2%–14% have anxiety disorders.[29] Denial of terminal illness is common and can be "healthy" if it facilitates adaptation. Denial that impairs patients' ability to appreciate reality and engage in an informed manner with key decisions becomes a challenge. Denial is amplified in situations of high anxiety and crisis, such as hospitalization; in these situations, patients lack cognitive and emotional resources to manage strong feelings and difficult decisions, such as those related to end-of-life care.[20] One recent study of patients with either metastatic lung or colorectal cancer, most (69% of those with lung cancer and 81% of those with colon cancer) failed to understand that chemotherapy was noncurative.[30] Clearly, anxiety, denial, and misunderstanding may make it difficult for patients to consider end-of-life care options such as hospice, even when hospice is consistent with the patients' goals.[31] Data suggest that by engaging in discussions about one's illness, wishes, benefits, and burdens of disease-modifying therapies, patients achieve better understanding of their illness, which leads to better decision-making about the types of healthcare they wish to receive.

DISCHARGE PLANNING

Palliative care consultation helps with discharge planning.[32] Palliative care consultants provide critical support through prognostication, symptom management, goals of care clarification, and addressing psychosocial and spiritual concerns. Approaching discharge, hospital-based palliative care teams identify gaps in care occurring during "care transitions" from the hospital to the next care setting, which could be a private home or care facility. Palliative care helps patient and families know whom to call when problems arise. Deficits in these areas are potentially preventable and can be addressed before a patient leaves the hospital. However, they require complex interdisciplinary participation, so responsibility for addressing them is often ambiguous. Studies have shown that many families want to be informed of prognosis and disease progression so that they can prepare emotionally and logistically for a loved one's death.[33]

MANAGEMENT OF CANCER PAIN

Pain occurs in 50% of patients with cancer at the time of diagnosis, increasing to 80% of patients with advanced-stage cancer. Pain impacts quality of life, limits function, and affects mood. Untreated pain leads to unwanted outcomes such as requests for physician-assisted suicide or unnecessary visits to the emergency department and hospital admissions.[34,35] Opioids remain the cornerstone of treatment for moderate to severe pain associated with cancer because they decrease pain and improve function.[36] Strong opioids are recommended for moderate to severe pain associated with cancer. The World Health Organization (WHO) developed a pain ladder, which is a step-by-step approach for the management of chronic pain based on pain intensity.[37,38]

EPIDEMIOLOGY

Pain occurs at diagnosis in 20%–50% of patients with cancer.[39] Cancer-related pain results from the cancer itself, oncology treatments, and coexisting nonmalignant pain.[40] Cancer types determine pain prevalence; for example, patients with head and neck cancer have the highest prevalence of cancer pain.[41] Age affects cancer pain presentation; younger patients experience more pain and more pain flares than older patients.[42] Of concern is that elderly patients receive less opioids than their younger counterparts.[43] Patients with cancer most commonly experience pain in the back—which should prompt healthcare professionals to exclude spinal cord metastasis—as well as in the abdomen, shoulders, and hips.[44]

WORLD HEALTH ORGANIZATION PAIN LADDER

WHO guidelines form the basis of cancer pain management, using a step-by-step approach to managing cancer pain based on pain intensity.[45] The pain ladder starts with nonopioid analgesics, such as acetaminophen or nonsteroidal antiinflammatory drugs (NSAIDs), for mild pain, then adds a so-called weak opioid if pain persists or increases, and then replaces the weak opioid with a Step 3 opioid for severe pain. Some research recommends elimination of Step 2 altogether and starting low dose Step 3 opioids.[46] Morphine remains the first-line opioid to relieve cancer-related pain; however, the evidence level for morphine as a first-line opioid is not strong.[38] Other Step 3 options for moderate to severe pain include methadone, oxycodone, fentanyl, and hydromorphone.

These opioids are considered equivalent to morphine. Successfully using the WHO pain ladder helps to provide effective analgesia in 90% of patients in certain settings, although results from randomized control trials show success rates of 70%–80%.[47,48]

STEP 1 ANALGESICS

Step 1 analgesics include acetaminophen (analgesic only) and NSAIDs (analgesic and antiinflammatory).[49,50] Dosing of acetaminophen and NSAIDs is limited by a ceiling effect, which means that further dose escalation will not improve analgesia. Acetaminophen dosing is limited by concerns of hepatic toxicity at a total dose of more than 4 g/day.[51] Recent studies suggest no benefit of intravenous acetaminophen on opioid consumption.[52] Acetaminophen works by various postulated mechanisms including central inhibition of the cyclooxygenase system, nitric oxide synthetase, the endocannabinoid system, and the descending serotonin pathways.[50] NSAIDs target and inhibit the enzyme cyclooxygenase, lowering inflammatory prostaglandins which cause nociceptive responses by lowering pain thresholds in nociceptive, neuropathic, and possibly visceral pain through a process called peripheral sensitization.[53] One major action of NSAIDs is the prevention of peripheral sensitization.[54] When considering the use of NSAIDs, choices should be based on experience and the toxicity profile, which depends on the cyclooxygenase 1:2 ratio. There is no ideal NSAID. NSAIDs are orally administered, with the exception of ketorolac, diclofenac, and ibuprofen which are available parenterally.[55] At the end of life, NSAIDs are usually replaced by stronger analgesics in the setting of moderate to severe pain. It may be advisable to continue NSAIDs as long as possible, because clinical trials show additive analgesia when combined with opioids as well as an opioid-sparing effect.[56] Ketorolac is useful for the treatment of cancer pain syndromes not uniformly responsive to opioid therapy.[55] Ketorolac use in the advanced patient with cancer is not recommended beyond 1 week.[57] Oral acetaminophen has not been shown to work synergistically with opioids but has not been shown to be opioid sparing with opioid doses of more than 200 mg of morphine equivalents.[55] NSAIDs treat pain originating in tissues such as connective tissue, joints, serous membranes, and the periosteum; in addition, visceral pain may also respond to NSAIDs.[58]

STEP 2 ANALGESICS

Step 2 on the WHO pain ladder is for mild to moderate cancer pain and includes recommendations for acetaminophen products containing hydrocodone, oxycodone, codeine, and tramadol, as well as propoxyphene and dihydrocodeine (not available in the United States).[1] Propoxyphene is not recommended for use in cancer pain.[59]

HYDROCODONE

Hydrocodone is structurally similar to morphine, differing by having a single bond at carbons 7 and 8 and a keto (=O) group at 6-carbon. Hydrocodone is metabolized by both cytochrome P450-dependent oxidative metabolism and glucuronides. CYP3A4 and CYP2D6 generate hydrocodone metabolites: norhydrocodone and hydromorphone, respectively.[60] Polymorphisms of CYP2D6 potentially affect hydrocodone metabolism and therapeutic efficacy.[61] Hydrocodone has equivalent potency as morphine on a milligram-for-milligram basis.[61] Reddy and coworkers found hydrocodone to be more potent than morphine.[62] Rodriguez et al. evaluated 118 study patients with cancer pain and compared hydrocodone/acetaminophen with tramadol in a double-blind, randomized-controlled trial (RCT). A total of 62 study patients received hydrocodone/acetaminophen and 56 received tramadol.[63] Hydrocodone/acetaminophen decreased pain in 57% of participants at a starting dose of 25 mg/2500 mg/day (5 doses per day).[63] Analgesic responses increased by 15% with dose doubling. Pain did not respond to hydrocodone/acetaminophen administration in 29% of study patients.[63] There was no superior analgesic efficacy with the administration of hydrocodone/acetaminophen when compared with patients receiving tramadol in the relief of cancer pain. Another multicenter, double-blind, randomized, parallel-group study compared codeine/acetaminophen phosphate with hydrocodone/acetaminophen for moderate to severe pain.[64] Study patients had chronic moderate to severe cancer pain (>3 on a 10-cm visual analog scale and >1 on a 4-point verbal intensity scale). A total of 88% of study patients had moderate pain and 12% had severe pain; 121 participants received either one tablet of codeine/acetaminophen 30/500 mg or hydrocodone/acetaminophen 5/500 mg orally every 4 h (total daily doses, 150/2500 and 25/2500 mg, respectively) for 23 days. Dose escalation occurred after 1 week if participants experienced severe pain. The primary endpoint was the percentage of study patients achieving a decrease in their pain score by 1 point on a 5-point verbal intensity scale. The secondary endpoint was the percentage of study patients whose pain decreased by at least 3 cm on the 10-point scale. Of the 121 participants, 59 received codeine/acetaminophen and 62 received hydrocodone/acetaminophen. Of the total number of cases, 59 had ages ranging from 60 to 89 years. A total of 58% of patients in the codeine/acetaminophen arm of the study experienced pain relief, and an additional 8% achieved pain relief with a doubling of the dose. Approximately one-third had unresponsive pain. In the hydrocodone/acetaminophen arm of the study, 56% experienced pain relief with a starting dose of 25/2500 mg/day. A total of 15% more achieved pain relief doubling of the initial dose, and one-third of patients did not respond to hydrocodone/acetaminophen. Analgesic efficacy was the same between the two arms of the study.[64]

TRAMADOL

Tramadol is a synthetic opioid from the aminocyclohexanol group. Tramadol has opioid-agonist properties and prevents the uptake of neurotransmitters norepinephrine and serotonin, making it useful for neuropathic pain.[65] Tramadol has low affinity for opioid receptors, with an affinity to μ receptors 10 times weaker than codeine, and 6000 times weaker than morphine.[32] Tramadol requires conversion to an active metabolite by CYP2D6. This metabolite has affinity for opioid receptors, but less so than Step 3 opioids.[66] Patients who are poor metabolizers of CYP2D6 may experience poor analgesia.[67] Adverse events of tramadol include constipation, dizziness, nausea, sedation, dry mouth, and vomiting.[68] Rodriguez et al. (see above) evaluated 118 participants with chronic cancer pain and compared hydrocodone/acetaminophen and tramadol in a double-blind, RCT.[63] In addition, Wilder-Smith et al. compared tramadol with morphine in a randomized, crossover, double-blind study for severe cancer pain (N = 20). Initially, participants received either tramadol 50 mg or morphine 16 mg every 4 h, with dose titration to achieve pain control.[69] After 4 days, pain intensities did not differ between the groups, although adverse events appeared to differ, with less-intense nausea and constipation noted in the tramadol group.[69] The authors estimated equianalgesic doses of morphine and tramadol and found a ratio of morphine to tramadol of 1:4.[69] Tawfik et al.[70] compared oral tramadol with sustained release morphine for cancer pain in 64 participants with severe cancer pain in a randomized, double-blind study. Tramadol worked best in participants with lesser pain intensity, and morphine worked more effectively and was preferred for participants experiencing severe pain intensity. Good analgesia was achieved in 2 weeks of treatment in 88% of study patients receiving tramadol and 100% of study patients receiving sustained-release morphine. Participants receiving tramadol experienced fatigue (15%), nausea (8%), and sweating (8%). In those receiving morphine, adverse events included constipation (35%), rash (14%), and drowsiness (14%). Bono and Cuffari[71] compared tramadol with buprenorphine in a randomized, crossover trial in study patients with cancer pain. All 60 study patients received either drug for 1 week and then, after a 24-hour wash-out period, were switched to the other drug. The tramadol dose was 300 mg/day and the buprenorphine dose was 0.2 mg 3 times a day. Tramadol was associated with better analgesia ($P < 0.05$) and was associated with higher acceptance among study patients.[37] Tramadol was better tolerated than buprenorphine and caused less frequent and milder adverse events, and more study drug withdrawals occurred in the buprenorphine arm.

CODEINE

Codeine is a prodrug whose analgesia is mediated through the μ receptor by its metabolite, morphine. A total of 10% of codeine is broken down to morphine by CYP2D6, an enzyme lacking in 5%−10% of white populations.[72] Codeine use is not recommended in the setting of renal failure.[73] One placebo-controlled study has evaluated codeine for cancer pain involving a sustained-release formulation.[74] Thirty study patients with chronic cancer pain completed the study and received either sustained-release codeine every 12 h or placebo in a double-blind study. Crossover occurred after 7 days. Pain intensity was measured using a visual analog scale as well as a 5-point categorical scale. Rescue analgesia (acetaminophen/codeine 300 mg/30 mg every 4 h as needed) was recorded. The median doses of controlled-release codeine doses were 277 ± 77 mg (range, 200−400 mg). Pain intensity scores on a visual analog scale, categorical pain intensity scores when assessed by day of treatment and by time of day, and need for breakthrough pain were significantly lower in the codeine arm ($P < 0.0001$).

STEP 3 OPIOIDS

The WHO pain ladder recommends Step 3 opioids as first-line therapy for moderate to severe pain (morphine, oxycodone, hydromorphone, fentanyl, levorphanol, methadone, and tapentadol).[75] Step 3 opioids differ from those in Step 2 medications in terms of potency and dosing. Although many Step 2 medications often have a ceiling dose due to fixed formulations

with acetaminophen, Step 3 opioids do not have this ceiling allowing dose flexibility. Dosing can increase to achieve adequate analgesia as long as adverse events are tolerated. Step 3 opioids interact with opioid receptors found throughout the central nervous system and peripheral tissues, resulting in analgesic effects, as well potential adverse events, including sedation, respiratory depression, and constipation. Constipation results from opioid receptor activation in the intestinal tract leading to decreased bowel motility and interference with peristalsis.[76] Varying degrees of activation and affinity for each receptor subtype may account for the differences in efficacy and activity between opioids.[77] In addition, interindividual variation is significant in analgesic response and toxicities based on genetic disparities.[78]

However, a reliable method to predict an individual patient's response does not exist and a paucity of evidence suggests superiority of one opioid over another in terms of efficacy or tolerability.

MORPHINE

WHO considers morphine the drug of choice for moderate to severe cancer pain.[79] Morphine is glucoronidated in the liver.[80] There is a small contribution (30%) to glucuronidation from the kidneys.[81] First-pass metabolism of oral morphine determines its systemic bioavailability which is 25%.[82] Morphine has three major metabolites: normorphine, morphine-3-glucuronide, and morphine-6-glucuronide. Metabolites are principally eliminated by the kidney and accumulate in renal failure contributing to adverse effects.[82] The elimination half-life of morphine is approximately 2 h and is independent of route of administration or formulation.[83] Morphine administered by sublingual and buccal routes has a delayed onset of action compared with oral morphine (smaller peak plasma levels, lower bioavailability, and larger interpatient variability).[83] Intrathecal morphine is 100 times as potent as its oral form, and epidural morphine is 10 times as potent (0.5 mg intrathecally equals 5 mg epidurally).[83] Morphine dosing is minimally affected by hepatic failure but is greatly affected by renal failure. A linear relationship exists between creatinine clearance and renal clearance of morphine and metabolites morphine-3-glucuronide, and morphine-6-glucuronide.[84] Kidney failure impairs glucuronide excretion more than morphine excretion, increasing the duration of action of morphine-6-glucuronide and morphine-3-glucuronide, thus leading to adverse events such as sedation and/or myoclonus.[85] Glucuronidation is largely unaffected by cirrhosis. Morphine should be avoided when creatinine clearance is less than 30 mL/

min.[83] Morphine continues to be considered the standard medication for the treatment of cancer pain partly due to familiarity with the product as well as cost. However, it may not always be the ideal product due to issues associated with its metabolism and adverse-event profile.[44] Almost all randomized controlled comparisons of potent opioids show equivalence (i.e., noninferiority) to morphine.[86]

METHADONE

Methadone is unique in that it works at three levels to provide analgesia. It is a potent opioid with strong interactions with the μ opioid receptor, it is an N-methyl-D-aspartate (NMDA) receptor antagonist, which is activated in chronic pain, and when blocked, enhances analgesia and reverses opioid tolerance. Methadone inhibits the uptake of neurotransmitters, such as norepinephrine and serotonin, which play a role in descending pain modulation.[87] Methadone is a second-line analgesic for pain poorly responsive to other opioids.[87] It shows promise as a first-line analgesic for cancer pain, neuropathic pain, and as a breakthrough agent. Methadone is available in oral, sublingual, and intravenous formulations. Methadone has different pharmacokinetics from other opioids. Methadone has a long half-life that varies between 60 and 120 h.[87] High-dose intravenous methadone is associated with QT prolongation and torsades de pointes.[88] The risk for QT prolongation is less with oral methadone. A retrospective study found that oral methadone can cause QT prolongation in 16% of patients.[89] Dosing of methadone is complicated. Methadone shows an inverse relationship of its starting dose to the total morphine equivalent daily dose (MEDD). As the MEDD increases, the equianalgesic dose of methadone progressively decreases.[90] Clinical trials comparing methadone to morphine have not shown superiority of methadone; in fact, three studies have compared morphine and methadone as first-line therapy for cancer-related pain.[38,91,92] Ventafridda et al.[91] Reinhart[57] compared methadone with morphine for moderate to severe cancer pain in 54 study patients who had previously been taking Step 2 opioids. Patients received either morphine or methadone by mouth for 14 days. While both therapies provided clear reductions in pain intensity, analgesia was less stable in the morphine arm, and study patients receiving morphine had a higher incidence of dry mouth. Otherwise, no other differences in toxicities or the ability to achieve pain relief were seen. Mercadante et al.[92] conducted a prospective randomized study in 40 study patients with advanced cancer who

required strong opioids for their pain management and receiving home hospice care. Study patients were treated with sustained-release morphine or methadone in doses titrated to pain relief and administered two or three times daily according to clinical need. Results suggested that methadone achieved analgesia more rapidly and that methadone analgesia was more stable than that achieved with morphine. Bruera and coworkers[38] compared the effectiveness and adverse events of methadone and morphine as first-line treatment with opioids for cancer pain. In this multicenter, international study, 103 participants with pain requiring strong opioids were randomly assigned to receive either methadone or morphine for 4 weeks. Participants having a 20% or more reduction in pain scores were equal in both groups. Patients in both arms reported satisfaction with their therapies. The methadone arm had a higher number of dropouts and required fewer dose adjustments to achieve analgesia than those in the morphine arm.

HYDROMORPHONE

Hydromorphone is similar in structure to morphine and is available as parenteral and oral products. It is the best opioid for subcutaneous administration.[93] The oral formulation is available in an immediate-release formulation, and a single, daily dose, extended-release formulation has been shown to be effective in patients with cancer.[94,60] Administered orally, hydromorphone has a bioavailability of 50% and its plasma elimination half-life is 2.5 h.[95] Metabolism in the liver produces hydromorphone-3-glucuronide, which has no analgesic properties but can cause neurotoxicity.[96] Hydromorphone is effective in treating pain in patients with renal impairment. Hydromorphone metabolites accumulate in patients receiving chronic infusions.[97,63] A double-blind, randomized comparison of sustained-release hydromorphone with sustained-release morphine showed equivalence in pain relief.[64] Systematic reviews involving 11 studies and 645 study patients show that hydromorphone equals morphine in analgesic effect.[98] More recent systematic reviews confirm equivalency.[99]

OXYCODONE

Oxycodone is available as immediate-release and sustained-release formulations. (Intravenous formulations are available in Europe.) The immediate-release formulation has a half-life of approximately 2–4 h and a bioavailability of 50%–60%.[100] The primary difference between oxycodone and morphine is its bioavailability: its half-life is longer than normal in renal failure and liver failure.[101] Oxycodone is metabolized to noroxycodone and oxymorphone via CYP 2D6.[102] Multiple studies show therapeutic equivalency with morphine for cancer pain.[100,103,104] Minor differences in adverse events have been described.[70] Hallucinations and nausea are less common with oxycodone treatment.[105,73] However, because of its cost and lack of versatility, morphine remains the preferred analgesic.[106,74] Bruera et al. demonstrated that oxycodone is 1.5 times as potent as morphine when comparing analgesic potency.[103]

OXYMORPHONE

Oxymorphone is a semisynthetic μ opioid agonist 1.2 times as potent as morphine.[107] Until recently, oxymorphone was available as parenteral injection and in suppository form; however, immediate-release and long-acting oral formulations were developed that make oxymorphone another option for treating moderate to severe pain. Trials in malignant and nonmalignant pain confirm its potential as another Step 3 option.[107] Oxymorphone is more lipid soluble than morphine. The oral bioavailability of oxymorphone is approximately 10%, which is the lowest of the oral Step 3 opioids.[107] In healthy volunteers, the half-life ranges from 7.2 to 9.4 h. The half-life of immediate-release oxymorphone is longer than that of morphine, hydromorphone, and oxycodone.[108] Immediate-release oxymorphone tablets may be given at 6-hour intervals, whereas the extended-release formula is dosed twice daily. Steady-state conditions are achieved after 3−4 days. Oxymorphone is subject to hepatic first-pass effects and is excreted by the kidneys. Oxymorphone accumulates in renal failure. Oxymorphone has a prolonged half-life in renal failure.[109] In the setting of hepatic insufficiency, increasing the dosing interval is recommended.[110] Sloan et al.[107] conducted a pilot study comparing extended-release oxymorphone and controlled-release oxycodone in 86 study patients with moderate to severe cancer pain. The tolerability and safety profiles (e.g., nausea, drowsiness, somnolence) were similar between the two drugs, and no significant differences in daily pain intensity scores were seen between extended-release oxymorphone and oxycodone.

FENTANYL

Fentanyl, a lipid-soluble, synthetic opioid, is available as parenteral, transdermal, and transmucosal products. Its lipophilic properties allow it to cross both the skin and oral mucosa.[111]

The transdermal formulation delivers fentanyl from the reservoir into the stratum corneum where it then slowly diffuses into the blood. Another formulation on the market is a matrix-delivery system in which fentanyl is dissolved in a polyacrylate adhesive. This formulation can be cut.[112] Both the reservoir and matrix-based patches have similar kinetics and clinical effectiveness.[112] Fentanyl is metabolized to norfentanyl under the influence of CYP3A4.[113] The concomitant use of fentanyl with potent CYP3A4 inhibitors (e.g., ritonavir, ketoconazole) may affect its metabolism. Fentanyl is safe to use in patients with renal failure.[86] Absorption of transdermal fentanyl may be impaired in cachectic patients.[114] The elimination half-life of transdermal fentanyl is approximately 12 h. Conversions to fentanyl are made by calculating the MEDD and the using the ratio of 2 mg:1 μg to reach the starting fentanyl dose.[111] Most experts do not recommend using transdermal fentanyl for acute titration.[115,83] Compared with morphine, constipation is less frequent with fentanyl.[116] Comparisons between morphine and transdermal fentanyl have shown equal analgesic efficacy.[117] When compared with morphine, daytime drowsiness and interference with daytime activity occur at lower rates.[117,85] The oral transmucosal administration of fentanyl has been extensively explored. In one study, 25% of the delivered drug was transmucosally absorbed, with another 25% delivered through the gastrointestinal tract.[111] RCTs of oral transmucosal fentanyl citrate show increased analgesic efficacy and patient preference over placebo and morphine.[118] Administration of fentanyl is being explored through other routes (e.g., intranasal).[119] Rapid intravenous administration of fentanyl in the emergency department can result in rapid improvement in pain control.[120]

Buprenorphine is emerging as another option for cancer pain. Well known as a strong analgesic, the development of a transdermal formulation makes it a possible option for cancer pain.[121] Buprenorphine is also available in intravenous and sublingual formulations, with the sublingual formulation having a bioavailability of 50%−65% and a half-life of more than 24 h.[122] After application of the transdermal formulation, plasma concentrations steadily increase. The larger-dose transdermal formulations achieve the minimum effective therapeutic dose sooner. Open-label, randomized, parallel-group, multiple dose pharmacokinetic studies show that the minimum effective concentrations are reached after 31, 14, and 13 h, respectively, with the 35, 52.5, and 70 mg/h patches (not available in the United States).[123] Patches reach steady state after the third consecutive application.[124] Bioavailability of the transdermal formulation is 60% compared with the intravenous route.[125] Effective plasma levels occur within 12−24 h and last for 72 h. It takes 60 h to reach Cmax. After patch removal, concentrations decrease to one-half in 12 h, then more gradually decline.[123] Metabolism by CYP3A4 and CYP2C8 converts buprenorphine to an active metabolite, norbuprenorphine, which is a weaker but full-opioid agonist. Buprenorphine and its metabolite later experience glucuronidation.[126] Liver disease affects buprenorphine metabolism. With involvement of both cytochrome oxidase system and glucuronidation in metabolism, severe liver disease potentially inhibits formation of norbuprenorphine through effects on the cytochrome oxidase system. Liver disease does not affect glucuronidation as much. Buprenorphine is safe to use in the presence of mild to moderate liver failure as well as in the setting of renal insufficiency and dialysis.[127] Buprenorphine produces adverse events similar to other Step 3 opioids and include constipation, urinary retention, sedation, and cognitive dysfunction. Buprenorphine causes less nausea than transdermal fentanyl.[128] Three Phase 3 placebo-controlled studies confirmed the efficacy of transdermal buprenorphine for cancer pain and also demonstrated the absence of a dose ceiling and opioid antagonist activity.[129−131]

LEVORPHANOL

Levorphanol is a potent Step 3 opioid with similarities to methadone.[132] Structurally similar to morphine, levorphanol has strong affinity for μ, δ, and κ opioid receptors.[133] Levorphanol is also a noncompetitive NMDA receptor antagonist and blocks NMDA with the same potency as ketamine.[134] Levorphanol can be orally, intravenously, subcutaneously, and intramuscularly administered.[132,100] Levorphanol has poor absorption via the sublingual route compared with other opioids such as morphine sulfate (18%), buprenorphine (55%), fentanyl (51%), and methadone (34%).[135] The pharmacokinetics of levorphanol are similar to methadone with a duration of analgesia ranging from 6 to 15 h and a half-life as long as 30 h.[136] First-pass metabolism produces a 3-glucuronide metabolite, which may have neurotoxicity.[136] Metabolites of levorphanol are renally excreted. The high volume of distribution and increased protein binding suggest that levorphanol should not be dialyzable.[73] The predominant mode of metabolism is hepatic. In the setting of hepatic insufficiency, it is advisable to consider an increased dosing interval.[132] Experience and clinical trial results suggest that the type and incidence of adverse events are similar to those seen with strong opioids.[132] Levorphanol has been studied as a treatment for chronic neuropathic pain and has been shown to be effective.[137]

TAPENTADOL

Tapentadol is structurally related to tramadol.[138] Opioid receptor-binding studies show that tapentadol is a strong opioid with high-affinity binding to μ, δ, and κ opioid receptors.[139] In human μ opioid receptor S GTPγS-binding assays, tapentadol shows agonistic activity, with an efficacy of 88% relative to morphine; tapentadol also targets neurotransmitters such as norepinephrine. It provides potent inhibition of norepinephrine uptake.[66] Tmax is achieved in 1.25−1.5 h, the half-life is 24 h, and the plasma protein binding is 20%.[140] Tapentadol metabolism is mainly by glucuronidation, with some contribution from CYP enzymes, especially CYP2D6.[141] Tapentadol has no active metabolites. Excretion is predominantly renal. Tapentadol causes adverse events such as nausea, dizziness, vomiting, headache, and somnolence.[142] Tapentadol has less effect of the gastrointestinal tract than other Step 3 opioids.[143]

The manufacturer recommends against using tapentadol in severe hepatic or renal failure, and dosing above 600 mg/day should be avoided.[144] Equianalgesic dosing studies are unavailable but information from its use in non-cancer-related pain studies suggests morphine 60 mg is equivalent to tapentadol 100−200 mg.[145] The current dosing recommendations is 50, 75, or 100 mg every 4−6 h.[142] Tapentadol does not affect the QTc interval.[146] Prolonged-release tapentadol (100−250 mg twice daily) is effective compared with placebo for managing moderate to severe, chronic, malignant tumor-related pain.[143]

INTERVENTIONAL PAIN MODALITIES

Clinicians consider "Step 4" of the WHO pain ladder when they encounter an inadequate response to Step 3 agents, adjuvants, or both.[147] Treatment options include use of nerve blocks, and/or spinal administration of local anesthetics, opioids, and other adjuvants. Abdominal pain may be controlled by a blockade of the celiac plexus, which, if successful, can block nociceptive input from many structures in the upper abdomen, in particular the pancreas.[148] Use of the superior hypogastric ganglion block for the treatment of malignant pelvic pain was first described by Plancarte et al.[149]

OPIOIDS

Receptor Interactions

Opioids interact with opioid receptors to produce analgesia (as well as adverse events).[150,151] Opioids interaction with receptors leads to receptor phosphorylation by G protein-coupled receptor kinases. Arrestin binding is associated with activation of distal pathways.[151] Opioids differ G protein coupling and in their propensity to drive receptors into the cell. For example, compared with other strong opioids, morphine is inefficient in its ability to promote receptor internalization.[151] Some postulate that noninternalized receptors continue to signal and promote adaptive responses, thus causing cellular tolerance.[151]

OPIOID RESPONSIVENESS

Opioid responsiveness is the degree of analgesia achieved as the opioid dose is titrated to an endpoint, defined either by intolerable side effects or the occurrence of acceptable analgesia.[152] Pain poorly responsive to opioids exists when intolerable adverse events, inadequate analgesia, or both continue during opioid escalation. Pharmacodynamic and nonpharmacodynamic factors affect opioid responsiveness. Identifying pain poorly responsive to opioids should lead the healthcare professional to consider the use of adjuvant analgesics, opioid switching, changing the route of administration, using NMDA antagonists, or interventional pain techniques.[153–155]

ROUTES OF ADMINISTRATION

Opioids are available in many dosage forms and routes of administration including via the oral, rectal, subcutaneous, intramuscular, intravenous, transdermal, transmucosal, and intraspinal routes of administration. Oral administration is simple, cost-effective, and is the preferred route of delivery. Both immediate-release and extended-release preparations are available. Clinicians use the subcutaneous, intravenous, rectal, transdermal, transmucosal, and intraspinal routes when patients cannot take oral medications. Intramuscular administration is contraindicated as it does not confer any pharmacokinetic advantages and is painful.[156] Subcutaneous delivery is easy, effective, and safe.[157] Intravenous routes are useful when pain is severe or pain levels have acutely increased. Transdermal fentanyl preparations are effective for patients unable to take oral medications and have stable pain control. Other short-acting opioids are used to control pain when transdermal fentanyl is initiated, because levels of fentanyl gradually increase during a 12- to 24-hour period until reaching steady state.[158] Transmucosal fentanyl is similar to intravenous administration in its rapid onset, and it can be used for acute breakthrough pain. Historically, dosing of transmucosal fentanyl was not thought to be based on dose proportionality, but this consideration has been challenged.[159] Intraspinal administration of opioids can either be epidural or intrathecal. This method is the most invasive technique and requires a specialist for initiation. This delivery confers advantages in patients with significant dose-limiting adverse events as systemic involvement is circumvented. Intraspinal delivery allows the addition of adjuvant medications to opioids that can be directly administered to the spinal cord.[160]

DOSE TITRATION

Clinicians adjust opioid analgesics to balance adequate pain control and adverse events. Dosage requirements change with cancer progression. Most patients with cancer have chronic daily pain, so analgesics should be given on a scheduled basis.[155] Breakthrough analgesics are ideally given according to the time it takes to reach Cmax. The Cmax depends on the route of administration. Cmax is 1 h for the oral route, 30 min for the subcutaneous route, and 6 min for the intravenous route.[161,162] Once Cmax is reached, another dose should be given if pain is not adequately controlled. Multiple approaches to opioid initiation and titration exist. The European Association for Palliative Care recommends dose titration with immediate-release oral morphine every 4 h, with breakthrough dosing of the same dose given every hour as needed.[163] The scheduled dose should then be adjusted to account for the oral MEDD. Several studies have shown acceptable pain control and adverse event profiles with use of 5 mg every 4 h in study patients naive to opioids and 10 mg every 4 h in patients previously using a Step 2 drug.[164,165] After acceptable pain control occurs, patients can use extended-release preparations as this is convenient and improves compliance.[166] Breakthrough dosing is 10%–20% of the MEDD.[167] Opioid titration with sustained-release formulations is slower than titration with immediate-release formulations.[163] Titration with intravenous medications is effective and tolerated.[168] In patients on established opioid regimens, dosing adjustment should be made according to the level of pain. Adult cancer pain guidelines recommend an increase of 25%–50% in the total MEDD for moderate pain (4–6 out of 10) and 50%–100% for severe pain (7–10 out of 10).[167]

EQUIANALGESIC CONVERSIONS

When converting between opioids, equianalgesic guidelines are followed although they may be modified according to clinical judgment with regard to adequacy of a patient's current pain medication regimen.[169] Opioid rotation may be due to poor analgesia, excessive adverse events, convenience, or patient preference.[170] Incomplete cross tolerance is identified when patients may develop less of a response (e.g., poor analgesia, adverse events) to a particular opioid over time. Patients may not show these characteristics with a new opioid, despite similar action between opioids, and slight variations in opioid structures may account for this.[169] Patients may not show these characteristics with a new opioid, despite similar action between opioids, or slight variations in opioid structures.[171] When calculating the dose of the new opioid, new doses should be reduced by 25%–50% to account for non-cross tolerance especially when current pain is controlled.[172] This is not done for fentanyl or methadone.[172]

ADVERSE EVENTS

The development of adverse events varies between individuals and depends on factors such as age, comorbidities, stage of illness, and genetic differences.[173] Impaired renal function increases the risk of adverse events due to accumulation of active metabolites.[173] The most common adverse events include constipation, nausea, vomiting, and altered cognition. Other adverse events may include xerostomia, urinary retention, respiratory depression, myoclonus, pruritus, and hyperalgesia. Most adverse events from opioid use subside within days to weeks, except for constipation for which patients do not develop tolerance and is not dose related. For those symptoms that persist or are present during the initiation of opioid therapy, symptom management is a key element of care. Constipation is prophylactically managed. Opioids inhibit gastrointestinal peristalsis; thus, all patients should receive a stimulant laxative such as senna.[174] Bowel stimulant dose is typically increased as the opioid dose is increased.[175] Dietary recommendations, such as increasing fiber in the diet, are unrealistic in patients with advanced disease because hydration is necessary to facilitate the action of fiber, often something difficult to achieve in ill patients.[160] Constipation is exacerbated by metabolic abnormalities, including diabetes, hypercalcemia, hypokalemia, and hypothyroidism, that should be corrected if possible.[173] Increased physical activity is often helpful if possible. Use of quaternary opioid antagonists may be needed.[173] The quaternary agents do not cross the blood-brain barrier and do not reverse the analgesic effects of opioids.

Nausea frequently occurs at the start of opioid therapy but seldom persists. Ongoing nausea may occur with advanced disease or as a complication of disease treatments. Opioids can cause nausea through several mechanisms, through direct stimulation of the chemoreceptor trigger zone, increased sensitivity of the vestibular apparatus, or delayed gastric emptying. Management consists of therapies targeting these processes. Dopamine antagonists, such as prochlorperazine or haloperidol, work on the chemoreceptor trigger zone. Antihistamines or anticholinergics can be used in patients who have nausea associated with movement. Metoclopramide is both a dopamine antagonist and promotility agent commonly used for the treatment of nausea in palliative care. Ondansetron, a serotonin receptor antagonist, is also a first-line agent for the management of nausea.[176] If sedation and altered sensorium are present, then management should include evaluation for other sources such as dehydration, drug interactions, or disease progression. Studies have investigated use of stimulants such as methylphenidate and modafinil with varying results.[177,178] If excessive adverse events limit pain control or impair quality of life, opioid rotation is often effective at achieving greater pain control with less adverse events.[170] In addition, this method of adverse-event management is preferable in patients for whom polypharmacy is a concern. Based on pharmacodynamics studies, dose-response relationships exist for central nervous system effects, such as sedation, myoclonus, and delirium, and may improve with dose reduction.[173]

TREATING NEUROPATHIC PAIN

Although adjuvant analgesics are often used in neuropathic pain, healthcare professionals should consider opioids as another option for neuropathic pain. Opioids are recommended as part of neuropathic pain algorithms.[179]

ADJUVANT ANALGESICS

Adjuvant analgesics are drugs with a primary indication other than pain that have analgesic properties.[180] The group includes drugs such as antidepressants, anticonvulsants, corticosteroids, neuroleptics, and other drugs with narrower adjuvant functions. Adjuvant analgesics are particularly useful when evidence of decreased opioid responsiveness is present.

TRICYCLIC ANTIDEPRESSANTS AND SELECTIVE SEROTONIN REUPTAKE INHIBITORS

The tricyclic antidepressants have been studied for use in neuropathic pain syndromes, although study results are conflicting about their analgesic effectiveness.[181-183] Amitriptyline has been shown to decrease chemotherapy-induced neuropathic pain intensity and improvement in quality of life with 10 mg per day up to 50 mg per day for 8 weeks.[183] Side effects of drowsiness, confusion, orthostatic hypotension, and dry mouth may limit the use of this drug especially in the elderly.[184,185] A Cochrane review in 2015 of nortriptyline for neuropathic pain in adults included six studies treating 310 patients from a range of 3−8 weeks found little evidence to support its use for neuropathic pain.[186] Additionally, tricyclic antidepressants should also be cautiously used in patients with coronary artery disease or cardiac rhythm disorders, as well as those with a history of narrow-angle glaucoma and urinary retention.[187] The anticholinergic properties of these drugs contribute to delirium in the elderly or anyone at risk for delirium such as patients whose cancer has metastasized to the central nervous system. These drugs should be started at the lowest dose with cautious escalation. Dose escalations are made every 3−4 days if analgesic response is suboptimal. Selective serotonin reuptake inhibitors have a limited role as adjuvants, although paroxetine and citalopram have been evaluated for nonmalignant neuropathic pain.[188,189] No studies have been performed on cancer pain.

SEROTONIN AND NOREPINEPHRINE DUAL REUPTAKE INHIBITORS

Newer drugs, such as duloxetine, inhibit the uptake of both serotonin and norepinephrine, both considered key neurotransmitters that suppress painful transmission of peripheral pain stimuli to the dorsal horn of the spinal cord.[190] Smith and colleagues[190] conducted a randomized, double-blind, placebo-controlled crossover trial at eight National Cancer Institute (NCI)-funded cooperative research networks enrolling 231 patients receiving primarily paclitaxel and oxaliplatin. Patients were randomized to receive either duloxetine followed by placebo or placebo followed by duloxetine. After 5 weeks of duloxetine (1 week of duloxetine 30 mg and 4 weeks of 60 mg) compared with placebo, patients who received duloxetine had an increased reduction in pain (59% of those initially receiving duloxetine vs. 38% of those initially receiving placebo reported decreased pain of any amount). The drug

was considered safe and well tolerated with fatigue, insomnia, and nausea being the most common adverse effects. Duloxetine seems to work better on patients receiving oxaliplatin. Venlafaxine also inhibits the uptake of serotonin and norepinephrine and is effective for painful neuropathy and neuropathic pain associated with therapy used in breast cancer.[191] It has been found to relieve painful polyneuropathy with as much effectiveness as imipramine.[189]

DOPAMINE AND NOREPINEPHRINE UPTAKE INHIBITORS

Bupropion is a second-generation nontricyclic "atypical" antidepressant that is a specific inhibitor of neuronal noradrenaline reuptake and a weak inhibitor of dopamine reuptake at presynaptic level. It does not affect sodium or calcium channels. Importantly, it does not block histaminergic, alpha-adrenergic, and muscarinic receptors and thus is well tolerated in patients who are having difficulty with tricyclic antidepressants.[192] Bupropion can potentiate seizure activity and is contraindicated in patients with a history of seizures, eating disorder, or abrupt alcohol cessation. Currently, bupropion is indicated for depression, seasonal affective disorder, and smoking cessation.[193] There seems to be evidence in favor of bupropion in neuropathic pain. Semenchuk conducted an open-label pilot study[194] to assess the efficacy of bupropion SR on neuropathic pain. In this study, 22 patients with diagnosis of neuropathic pain underwent treatment with bupropion SR 150 mg once a day for 7 days followed by 150 mg bupropion SR twice a day for 7 weeks. A total of 15 patients (68%) reported significantly decreased symptoms after bupropion therapy. Adverse effects were mild including insomnia, tremor, gastrointestinal upset, and weakness/dizziness. None of the patients dropped out because of adverse effects. A subsequent 12-week, randomized, placebo-controlled, double-blinded, crossover study showed that of the 41 patients who started the study, 30 (73%) reported "improved" or "much improved" pain after 6 weeks of bupropion SR therapy. The mean average pain score at baseline was 5.7, which dropped to 4.0 on bupropion but remained unchanged on placebo. Adverse effects were minimal and quality of life improved.[195]

CORTICOSTEROIDS

Corticosteroids are used to treat bone pain and swelling in the brain and spinal cord due to metastatic disease. Their role as antiinflammatory drugs as a result of reducing proinflammatory cytokines, stimulating lipocortin synthesis, and inhibiting collagenase expression makes them powerful for pain resulting from inflammation such as nerve root inflammation.[196] They are often considered for painful liver metastasis and obstruction of the ureter, although the evidence base for this use is not strong.[197] The most commonly used corticosteroid is dexamethasone, due to its low mineralocorticoid properties resulting in less fluid retention. It is metabolized by the CYP3A4 hepatic enzyme, has many drug interactions, and its effect may be altered by CYP3A4 inhibitors and inducers. Its effects on cancer-induced fatigue, cachexia, nausea, vomiting, and depression provides additional benefits.[196] Optimal dosing for palliation may be 8 mg/day as this dose has no more adverse events than placebo.[198] In the case of spinal cord compression, recommendations exist for either high-dose (96 mg/day) or low-dose (16 mg/day) dexamethasone.[199] Higher doses and longer use of steroids increases the occurrence of adverse events.[200] The management of edema associated with brain metastasis can be treated with dexamethasone 4–6 mg every 6 h with a careful taper during the last phases of palliative radiation therapy. The minimal effective dose for brain metastasis is 8 mg/day.[201] Steroids can be useful to counteract the phenomenon of radiation "flare," which occurs during radiation therapy to painful bony sites.[202]

ANTICONVULSANT DRUGS

Anticonvulsants can be used for managing neuropathic pain.[203] The most often used anticonvulsant for neuropathic pain is gabapentin, which is effective for cancer-related neuropathic pain.[204,205] It is an inhibitor of the alpha-2-delta-1 calcium channel subunit that blocks neurotransmitter release resulting in decreased nociception in neuropathic pain. Gabapentin can have significant adverse events if it is started at too high a dose or titrated too fast. Dosing begins at 150–300 mg at bedtime, with escalations every 3 days if pain control is suboptimal. The chief adverse event is somnolence.[206] Gabapentin must be dose adjusted for renal insufficiency, with the maximum dose for normal renal function of 3600 mg/day. A Phase 3 randomized, double-blind, placebo-controlled, crossover trial by Rao and colleagues found no significant benefit to using gabapentin at 2700 mg per day for 6 weeks for symptoms due to chemotherapy-induced peripheral neuropathy. Another anticonvulsant that may be useful for cancer pain is phenytoin.[207] Agents such as lamotrigine, oxcarbazepine, pregabalin, topiramate, and levetiracetam have been used for nonmalignant neuropathic pain and are considerations in the refractory case, but

they have not been studied in the cancer pain population. Levetiracetam requires further study for cancer-related neuropathy.[208] Lamotrigine is not effective in chemotherapy-related neuropathy.[209]

ORAL AND PARENTERAL AND TRANSDERMAL ANESTHETICS

The parenteral anesthetic commonly used for refractory cancer pain is lidocaine. While there is limited data on its use, some studies suggest its efficacy in opioid-refractory cases of cancer pain.[176] There is less evidence supporting the benefit of lidocaine for neuropathic pain.[210,211] One study in patients with cancer with refractory pain showed improved analgesia with a single dose of lidocaine.[212] The recommended starting dose is 1–5 mg/kg infused for 20–30 min. In patients who are frail, lower doses may be needed. Lidocaine should be avoided in patients with coronary artery disease. One potential benefit of lidocaine is prolonged pain relief that occurs following its infusion[213] Lidocaine can be given in the home or hospice setting.[214] Cognitive impairment, delirium, dizziness, perioral numbness, and somnolence are adverse effects to be aware of.[213] Mexiletine, an oral congener of lidocaine, has been used after lidocaine infusions.[215] Clinical trial results suggest that mexiletine has a distinct adverse-event profile and may not be tolerated by all patients.[216]

TRANSDERMAL LOCAL ANALGESICS

Transdermal lidocaine (5% patch) provides another route for local anesthetics. It can be used to treat post herpetic neuralgia, but its role in cancer-related neuropathy requires further study. A study by Garzon-Rodriguez and colleagues found that it can be a helpful short-term treatment option for painful scars such as postthoracotomy or postmastectomy, and pain from chest wall tumors.[217,218] The patch has minimal systemic absorption, and it can be applied 12 h per day; evidence suggests that increasing the number of patches and extended dosing periods may be safe.[219,220] It may take several weeks to observe a maximal effect. The most frequently reported adverse events are mild to moderate skin redness, rash, and irritation at the patch application site.[220]

KETAMINE

Chronic pain is associated with central nervous system changes, including activation of the NMDA receptor, leading to the development of decreased opioid responsiveness.[221] Pharmacological blockade of the NMDA receptor offers a therapeutic approach in the setting of decreased opioid responsiveness. As an NMDA receptor antagonist, ketamine has been considered in the management of refractory cancer pain and may lead to reduced opioid requirements.[154,218] It is recommended by the WHO for the management of refractory pain.[222] Given at subanesthetic doses (<1 mg/kg), ketamine is an effective analgesic in cancer-related neuropathic pain.[154] Multiple routes exist for administration including oral, intravenous, subcutaneous, and topical routes. It is metabolized via CYP3A4 and no significant drug interactions have been reported.[223] Adverse effects to be aware of are hallucinations, psychomimetic toxicity that improve with haloperidol and diazepam, hypertension, nausea, and vomiting.[154,218,224] Its analgesic effect is due to the norketamine metabolite, which has a duration of action of 8 h, and pharmacologically, no major differences exist in the characteristics between the isomers.[185,225] Ketamine has protein binding of 20%–30%.[226] Its oral bioavailability is 17%, it has an onset of action of 15–20 min, and it has a half-life of 2.5–3 h. Its intravenous onset of action is within seconds and, subcutaneously, the onset of action is 15–20 min. The half-life is 2–3 h for both routes.[223] The results of one trial of subcutaneous ketamine as an add-on option to opioids showed no efficacy in cancer-related nociceptive pain[224] and a Cochrane review found insufficient evidence regarding the use of ketamine as an opioid adjunct for cancer pain relief[227]; however, a recent study by Cheung and colleagues found a favorable response to ketamine in patients using one or more opioid analgesics.[218]

CANNABINOIDS

Formulations of cannabinoids, the cannabinoid extracts, have been studied for cancer-related pain.[228–230] Two RCTs have studied tetrahydrocannabinol (THC)/cannabidiol (CBD) and found significant change in pain compared with placebo and a decrease in breakthrough pain medications.[228,229] A third RCT found no significant difference compared with placebo for chronic neuropathic pain related to taxol-based chemotherapy.[230] The cannabinoid used in these studies is nabiximols, which is an extract that contains THC 2.7 mg and CBD 2.5 mg per dose. It is formulated in ethanol/propylene glycol with peppermint flavoring and is designed as a pump spray for self-administration and titration via the oromucosal route.[231] Another larger study using the same formulation again confirmed this cannabinoid extract as an add-on therapy for advanced cancer.[228] Pain relief with THC has been shown to be dose dependent[232] and one study found a dose of 20 mg to provide significant relief (Noyes).[232] Significant adverse effects include mental clouding, drowsiness, euphoria, somnolence, and nausea.[229]

NEUROLEPTICS

Second-generation (atypical) antipsychotics, such as olanzapine, have been shown to have antinociceptive activity in animal models.[233] Khojainova et al.[234] evaluated the analgesic activity of olanzapine in eight study patients with severe cancer pain unresponsive to increased opioid dosing and who were receiving olanzapine for the treatment of severe anxiety and mild cognitive impairment. Patients reported a decrease in pain scores. The authors note that this decrease may be the result of intrinsic analgesic action but may also be the result of treated anxiety and improved cognitive function. Further studies are needed to explore olanzapine's analgesic potential.

AGENTS SPECIFICALLY USED FOR BONE PAIN

Bone pain is a common problem in the palliative care setting. Radiation therapy can be effective with localized pain. Systemic therapies with NSAIDs, corticosteroids, bisphosphonates, and radiopharmaceuticals can be useful for patients with multifocal lesions.

BISPHOSPHONATES

Bisphosphonates are analogues of inorganic pyrophosphate that inhibit osteoclast activity and can be useful in many types of cancer in which bone resorption leads to complications. Bisphosphonates bind to calcium on bone, become ingested by osteoclasts, and subsequently kill osteoclasts thus preventing bone resorption.[235] The end result of decreased osteoclast activity is increased bone stability and reduced pathological fractures. In the United States, zoledronic acid and pamidronate are used. The most potent bisphosphonate is zoledronic acid, which has been shown to reduce pain and prevent the occurrence of skeletal-related events in breast cancer, prostate cancers, multiple myeloma, and a variety of solid tumors, including lung cancer.[236–238] Breast cancer and multiple myeloma are the most responsive to bisphosphonates. Denosumab is useful when renal insufficiency precludes the use of bisphosphonates.[239] Pain reduction occurs as soon as within a week and can last up to 3 months with redosing every 3–4 weeks for maximum effect. The most common adverse effect is a flu-like syndrome.[240]

RADIOPHARMACEUTICALS

Radionuclides are agents absorbed in areas of metastatic cancer activity. Strontium-89, radium-223, and samarium-153 are effective for diffuse bony metastatic disease (without visceral disease) that bind to areas with rapid bone turnover such as osteoblastic metastases such as in the case of prostate cancer.[241] Pain relief often occurs within 1–2 weeks and may last from 2 to 6 months. Radium-223 has been found to increase survival by 3 months in patients with metastatic prostate cancer with less myelosuppression and adverse effects. This treatment is appropriate for patients who have an expected survival of more than 3 months. It is contraindicated in patients who have preexisting myelosuppression, oncological urgencies or emergencies, renal insufficiency, pregnancy, or disseminated intravascular coagulation.[242]

MUSCLE RELAXANTS

Pain originating from connective tissue injury is common in patients with cancer; however, use of muscle relaxants as adjuvant agents has had limited evaluation in patients with cancer. In a small study of 25 patients with neuropathic cancer pain, baclofen was effective in reducing pain score.[243] Use of muscle relaxants has been associated with psychosis as well as insomnia, decreased appetite, poor concentration, irritability, disorganized thoughts, persecutory delusions, and auditory hallucinations.[244] Muscle relaxants like cyclobenzaprine are structurally related to tricyclic antidepressants and share not only structural similarity but similar adverse effects.[244] Dose tapering after treatment for a prolonged time is necessary to prevent withdrawal.[245] In a review comparing the efficacy and safety of muscle relaxants, Chou and colleagues[245] found limited or inconsistent data to supporting meaningful differences.

OCTREOTIDE

Pain, along with nausea and vomiting, is a common symptom associated with malignant bowel obstruction. Nonsurgical management of malignant bowel obstruction focuses on the management of pain and other obstructive symptoms, such as distension, nausea, and vomiting. The use of parenteral opioids, antiemetics, and antisecretory agents, such as octreotide, are common methods of pharmacological symptom control. Octreotide has been shown to have analgesic properties in specific conditions such as abdominal pain or headaches.[246,247]

ADJUVANT COMBINATIONS

The treatment of neuropathic pain frequently requires several adjuvants. For example, it is not unusual for a patient with severe, cancer-related neuropathic pain to require an opioid or several additional adjuvants. When this occurs, the clinician should monitor the patient for potential drug interactions.[248]

REFERENCES

1. Morrison RS, Meier DE. Palliative care. *N Engl J Med.* 2004;350:2582–2590.
2. *Clinical Practice Guidelines for Quality Palliative Care.* 3rd ed.; 2013. http://www.nationalconsensusproject.org/NCP_Clinical_Practice_Guidelines_3rd_Edition.pdf.
3. Meuser T, Pietruck C, Radbruch L, Stute P, Lehmann KA, Grond S. Symptoms during cancer pain treatment following WHO-guidelines: a longitudinal follow-up study of symptom prevalence, severity and etiology. *Pain.* 2001;93:247–257.
4. Harris DG. Nausea and vomiting in advanced cancer. *Br Med Bull.* 2010;96:175–185.
5. Breitbart W, Bruera E, Chochinov H, Lynch M. Neuropsychiatric syndromes and psychological symptoms in patients with advanced cancer. *J Pain Symptom Manag.* 1995;10:131–141.
6. Buss MK, Vanderwerker LC, Inouye SK, Zhang B, Block SD, Prigerson HG. Associations between caregiver-perceived delirium in patients with cancer and generalized anxiety in their caregivers. *J Palliat Med.* 2007;10:1083–1092.
7. Blinderman CD, Homel P, Billings JA, Portenoy RK, Tennstedt SL. Symptom distress and quality of life in patients with advanced congestive heart failure. *J Pain Symptom Manag.* 2008;35:594–603.
8. Blinderman CD, Homel P, Billings JA, Tennstedt S, Portenoy RK. Symptom distress and quality of life in patients with advanced chronic obstructive pulmonary disease. *J Pain Symptom Manag.* 2009;38:115–123.
9. Henry DH, Viswanathan HN, Elkin EP, Traina S, Wade S, Cella D. Symptoms and treatment burden associated with cancer treatment: results from a cross-sectional national survey in the US. *Support Care Cancer.* 2008;16:791–801.
10. Cachia E, Ahmedzai SH. Breathlessness in cancer patients. *Eur J Cancer.* 2008;44:1116–1123.
11. Janssen D, Spruit M, Wouters E, Schols J. Daily symptom burden in end-stage chronic organ failure: a systematic review. *Palliat Med.* 2008;22:938–948.
12. Levenson JW, McCarthy EP, Lynn J, Davis RB, Phillips RS. The last six months of life for patients with congestive heart failure. *J Am Geriatr Soc.* 2000;48:S101–S109.
13. Detering KM, Hancock AD, Reade MC, Silvester W. The impact of advance care planning on end of life care in elderly patients: randomised controlled trial. *Br Med J.* 2010;340:c1345.

14. Roter DL, Larson S, Fischer GS, Arnold RM, Tulsky JA. Experts practice what they preach: a descriptive study of best and normative practices in end-of-life discussions. *Arch Intern Med.* 2000;160:3477−3485.

15. Wright AA, Zhang B, Ray A, et al. Associations between end-of-life discussions, patient mental health, medical care near death, and caregiver bereavement adjustment. *J Am Med Assoc.* 2008;300:1665−1673.

16. Mack JW, Weeks JC, Wright AA, Block SD, Prigerson HG. End-of-life discussions, goal attainment, and distress at the end of life: predictors and outcomes of receipt of care consistent with preferences. *J Clin Oncol.* 2010;28: 1203.

17. Jackson VA, Mack J, Matsuyama R, et al. A qualitative study of oncologists' approaches to end-of-life care. *J Palliat Med.* 2008;11:893−906.

18. Zhang B, Wright AA, Huskamp HA, et al. Health care costs in the last week of life: associations with end-of-life conversations. *Arch Intern Med.* 2009;169:480−488.

19. Ray A, Block SD, Friedlander RJ, Zhang B, Maciejewski PK, Prigerson HG. Peaceful awareness in patients with advanced cancer. *J Palliat Med.* 2006;9: 1359−1368.

20. Mack JW, Cronin A, Taback N, et al. End-of-life care discussions among patients with advanced cancer: a cohort study. *Ann Intern Med.* 2012;156:204−210.

21. Block SD. Assessing and managing depression in the terminally ill patient. *Ann Intern Med.* 2000;132: 209−218.

22. Byock IR. To life! Reflections on spirituality, palliative practice, and politics. *Am J Hospice Palliat Med.* 2007;23: 436−438.

23. Puchalski CM, Vitillo R, Hull SK, Reller N. Improving the spiritual dimension of whole person care: reaching national and international consensus. *J Palliat Med.* 2014; 17:642−656.

24. Claxton RN, Blackhall L, Weisbord SD, Holley JL. Undertreatment of symptoms in patients on maintenance hemodialysis. *J Pain Symptom Manag.* 2010;39: 211−218.

25. Grant E, Murray SA, Kendall M, Boyd K, Tilley S, Ryan D. Spiritual issues and needs: perspectives from patients with advanced cancer and nonmalignant disease. A qualitative study. *Palliat Support Care.* 2004;2:371−378.

26. Winkelman WD, Lauderdale K, Balboni MJ, et al. The relationship of spiritual concerns to the quality of life of advanced cancer patients: preliminary findings. *J Palliat Med.* 2011;14:1022−1028.

27. Balboni TA, Vanderwerker LC, Block SD, et al. Religiousness and spiritual support among advanced cancer patients and associations with end-of-life treatment preferences and quality of life. *J Clin Oncol.* 2007;25:555.

28. Phelps A, Maciejewski P, Nilsson M, et al. Coping with cancer: associations between coping methods and use of intensive life-prolonging care near death. *J Clin Oncol.* 2009;27:9575.

29. Miovic M, Block S. Psychiatric disorders in advanced cancer. *Cancer.* 2007;110:1665−1676.

30. Weeks JC, Catalano PJ, Cronin A, et al. Patients' expectations about effects of chemotherapy for advanced cancer. *N Engl J Med.* 2012;367:1616−1625.

31. Casarett D, Crowley R, Stevenson C, Xie S, Teno J. Making difficult decisions about hospice enrollment: what do patients and families want to know? *J Am Geriatr Soc.* 2005; 53:249−254.

32. Weissman DE. Consultation in palliative medicine. *Arch Intern Med.* 1997;157:733−737.

33. Apatira L, Boyd EA, Malvar G, et al. Hope, truth, and preparing for death: perspectives of surrogate decision makers. *Ann Intern Med.* 2008;149:861.

34. Foley KM. The relationship of pain and symptom management to patient requests for physician-assisted suicide. *J Pain Symptom Manag.* 1991;6:289−297.

35. Mayer DK, Travers D, Wyss A, Leak A, Waller A. Why do patients with cancer visit emergency departments? Results of a 2008 population study in North Carolina. *J Clin Oncol.* 2011;29:2683.

36. Cherny N. New strategies in opioid therapy for cancer pain. *J Oncol Manag.* 2000;9:8−15.

37. Stjernswärd J. WHO cancer pain relief programme. *Cancer.* 1988;7:195−208.

38. Bruera E, Palmer JL, Bosnjak S, et al. Methadone versus morphine as a first-line strong opioid for cancer pain: a randomized, double-blind study. *J Clin Oncol.* 2004;22: 185−192.

39. Fischer DJ, Villines D, Kim YO, Epstein JB, Wilkie DJ. Anxiety, depression, and pain: differences by primary cancer. *Support Care Cancer.* 2010;18:801−810.

40. Gutgsell T, Walsh D, Zhukovsky DS, Gonzales F, Lagman R. A prospective study of the pathophysiology and clinical characteristics of pain in a palliative medicine population. *Am J Hospice Palliat Med.* 2003;20:140−148.

41. Van den Beuken-van Everdingen M, De Rijke J, Kessels A, Schouten H, Van Kleef M, Patijn J. Prevalence of pain in patients with cancer: a systematic review of the past 40 years. *Ann Oncol.* 2007;18:1437−1449.

42. Green CR, Hart-Johnson T. Cancer pain: an age-based analysis. *Pain Med.* 2010;11:1525−1536.

43. Cleary JF. The pharmacologic management of cancer pain. *J Palliat Med.* 2007;10:1369−1394.

44. Marcus DA. Epidemiology of cancer pain. *Curr Pain Headache Rep.* 2011;15:231−234.

45. Donnelly S, Walsh D. The symptoms of advanced cancer. *Semin Oncol.* 1995;22:67−72.

46. Bandieri E, Romero M, Ripamonti CI, et al. Randomized trial of low-dose morphine versus weak opioids in moderate cancer pain. *J Clin Oncol.* 2016;34:436−442.

47. Davis MP, Walsh D. Epidemiology of cancer pain and factors influencing poor pain control. *Am J Hospice Palliat Med.* 2004;21:137−142.

48. Cancer Pain Guideline Panel, Agency for Health Care Policy and Research. Management of cancer pain: adults. *Am Fam Physician.* 1994;49(8):1853−1868.

49. Jadad AR, Browman GP. The WHO analgesic ladder for cancer pain management: stepping up the quality of its evaluation. *J Am Med Assoc.* 1995;274:1870−1873.

50. Smith HS. Potential analgesic mechanisms of acetaminophen. *Pain Physician*. 2009;12:269–280.
51. Larson AM, Polson J, Fontana RJ, et al. Acetaminophen-induced acute liver failure: results of a United States multicenter, prospective study. *Hepatology*. 2005;42:1364–1372.
52. Tasmacioglu B, Aydinli I, Keskinbora K, Pekel AF, Salihoglu T, Sonsuz A. Effect of intravenous administration of paracetamol on morphine consumption in cancer pain control. *Support Care Cancer*. 2009;17:1475–1481.
53. Julius D, Basbaum AI. Molecular mechanisms of nociception. *Nature*. 2001;413:203.
54. Malmberg AB, Yaksh TL. Antinociceptive actions of spinal nonsteroidal anti-inflammatory agents on the formalin test in the rat. *J Pharmacol Exp Therapeut*. 1992;263:136–146.
55. Joishy SK, Walsh D. The opioid-sparing effects of intravenous ketorolac as an adjuvant analgesic in cancer pain: application in bone metastases and the opioid bowel syndrome. *J Pain Symptom Manag*. 1998;16:334–339.
56. Miranda H, Silva E, Pinardi G. Synergy between the antinociceptive effects of morphine and NSAIDs. *Can J Physiol Pharmacol*. 2004;82:331–338.
57. Reinhart DJ. Minimising the adverse effects of ketorolac. *Drug Saf*. 2000;22:487–497.
58. Mercadante S, Fulfaro F, Casuccio A. A randomised controlled study on the use of anti-inflammatory drugs in patients with cancer pain on morphine therapy: effects on dose-escalation and a pharmacoeconomic analysis. *Eur J Cancer*. 2002;38:1358–1363.
59. Wood AJLM. Pharmacologic treatment of cancer pain. *N Engl J Med*. 1996;335(15):1124–1132.
60. Menelaou A, Hutchinson MR, Quinn I, Christensen A, Somogyi AA. Quantification of the O-and N-demethylated metabolites of hydrocodone and oxycodone in human liver microsomes using liquid chromatography with ultraviolet absorbance detection. *J Chromatogr B*. 2003;785:81–88.
61. Prommer E. Hydrocodone: does it have a role in palliative care? *J Opioid Manag*. 2010;6:295–299.
62. Reddy A, Yennurajalingam S, Desai H, et al. The opioid rotation ratio of hydrocodone to strong opioids in cancer patients. *Oncologist*. 2014;19:1186–1193.
63. Rodriguez RF, Castillo JM, Castillo MP, et al. Hydrocodone/acetaminophen and tramadol chlorhydrate combination tablets for the management of chronic cancer pain: a double-blind comparative trial. *Clin J Pain*. 2008;24:1–4.
64. Rodriguez RF, Castillo JM, del Pilar Castillo M, et al. Codeine/acetaminophen and hydrocodone/acetaminophen combination tablets for the management of chronic cancer pain in adults: a 23-day, prospective, double-blind, randomized, parallel-group study. *Clin Therapeut*. 2007;29:581–587.
65. Leppert W, Łuczak J. The role of tramadol in cancer pain treatment—a review. *Support Care Cancer*. 2005;13:5–17.
66. Prommer EE. Tramadol: does it have a role in cancer pain management? *J Opioid Manag*. 2005;1:131–138.
67. Pedersen RS, Damkier P, Brøsen K. Enantioselective pharmacokinetics of tramadol in CYP2D6 extensive and poor metabolizers. *Eur J Clin Pharmacol*. 2006;62:513–521.
68. Mejjad O, Serrie A, Ganry H. Epidemiological data, efficacy and safety of a paracetamol–tramadol fixed combination in the treatment of moderate-to-severe pain. SALZA: a post-marketing study in general practice. *Curr Med Res Opin*. 2011;27:1013–1020.
69. Wilder-Smith C, Schimke J, Osterwalder B, Senn H-J. Oral tramadol, a μ-opioid agonist and monoamine reuptake-blocker, and morphine for strong cancer-related pain. *Ann Oncol*. 1994;5:141–146.
70. Tawfik MO, Elborolossy K, Nasr F. Tramadol hydrochloride in the relief of cancer pain. A double blind comparison against sustained release morphine. *Pain*. 1990;41:S377.
71. Bono A, Cuffari S. Effectiveness and tolerance of tramadol in cancer pain. A comparative study with respect to buprenorphine. *Drugs*. 1997;53:40–49.
72. Yue Q, Hasselstrom J, Svensson J, Sawe J. Pharmacokinetics of codeine and its metabolites in Caucasian healthy volunteers: comparisons between extensive and poor hydroxylators of debrisoquine. *Br J Clin Pharmacol*. 1991;31:635–642.
73. Dean M. Opioids in renal failure and dialysis patients. *J Pain Symptom Manag*. 2004;28:497–504.
74. Dhaliwal H, Sloan P, Arkinstall WW, et al. Randomized evaluation of controlled-release codeine and placebo in chronic cancer pain. *J Pain Symptom Manag*. 1995;10:612–623.
75. Prommer EE. Pharmacological management of cancer-related pain. *Cancer Control*. 2015;22:412–425.
76. Trescot AM, Datta S, Lee M, Hansen H. Opioid pharmacology. *Pain Physician*. 2008;11:S133–S153.
77. Davis MP, McPherson ML, Mehta Z, Behm B, Fernandez C. What parenteral opioids to use in face of shortages of morphine, hydromorphone, and fentanyl. *Am J Hosp Palliat Care*. 2018;35:1118–1122.
78. Somogyi AA, Barratt DT, Coller JK. Pharmacogenetics of opioids. *Clini Pharmacol Therapeut*. 2007;81:429–444.
79. McQuay H. Opioids in pain management. *Lancet*. 1999;353:2229–2232.
80. Christrup LL. Morphine metabolites. *Acta Anaesthesiol Scand*. 1997;41:116–122.
81. de Wildt SN, Kearns GL, Leeder JS, van den Anker JN. Glucuronidation in humans. *Clin Pharmacokinet*. 1999;36:439–452.
82. Glare P, Walsh T. Clinical pharmacokinetics of morphine. *Ther Drug Monit*. 1991;13:1–23.
83. Cherny NI. Opioid analgesics. *Drugs*. 1996;51:713–737.
84. Miners J, Lillywhite K, Birkett D. In vitro evidence for the involvement of at least two forms of human liver UDP-glucuronosyltransferase in morphine 3-glucuronidation. *Biochem Pharmacol*. 1988;37:2839–2845.
85. Owen H, Plummer J, Ilsley A, Hawkins R, Arfeen Z, Tordoff K. Variable-dose patient-controlled analgesia: a preliminary report. *Anaesthesia*. 1995;50:855–857.

86. Murtagh FE, Chai M-O, Donohoe P, Edmonds PM, Higginson IJ. The use of opioid analgesia in end-stage renal disease patients managed without dialysis: recommendations for practice. *J Pain Palliat Care Pharmacother.* 2007;21:5–16.

87. Prommer EE. Methadone for cancer pain. *Palliat Care Res Treat.* 2010;4:S4847.

88. Shaiova L, Berger A, Blinderman CD, et al. Consensus guideline on parenteral methadone use in pain and palliative care. *Palliat Support Care.* 2008;6:165–176.

89. Piguet V, Desmeules J, Ehret G, Stoller R, Dayer P. QT interval prolongation in patients on methadone with concomitant drugs. *J Clin Psychopharmacol.* 2004;24:446–448.

90. McPherson ML, Walker KA, Davis MP, et al. Safe and appropriate use of methadone in hospice and palliative care: expert consensus white paper. *J Pain Symptom Manag.* 2019;57:635–645 e4.

91. Ventafridda V, Ripamonti C, Bianchi M, Sbanotto A, De Conno F. A randomized study on oral administration of morphine and methadone in the treatment of cancer pain. *J Pain Symptom Manag.* 1986;1:203–207.

92. Mercadante S, Casuccio A, Agnello A, Serretta R, Calderone L, Barresi L. Morphine versus methadone in the pain treatment of advanced-cancer patients followed up at home. *J Clin Oncol.* 1998;16:3656–3661.

93. Murray A, Hagen NA. Hydromorphone. *J Pain Symptom Manag.* 2005;29:S57–S66.

94. Nalamachu SR, Kutch M, Hale ME. Safety and tolerability of once-daily OROS® hydromorphone extended-release in opioid-tolerant adults with moderate-to-severe chronic cancer and noncancer pain: pooled analysis of 11 clinical studies. *J Pain Symptom Manag.* 2012;44:852–865.

95. Vallner J, Stewart J, Kotzan J, Kirsten E, Honigberg I. Pharmacokinetics and bioavailability of hydromorphone following intravenous and oral administration to human subjects. *J Clin Pharmacol.* 1981;21:152–156.

96. Thwaites D, McCann S, Broderick P. Hydromorphone neuroexcitation. *J Palliat Med.* 2004;7:545–550.

97. Paramanandam G, Prommer E, Schwenke DC. Adverse effects in hospice patients with chronic kidney disease receiving hydromorphone. *J Palliat Med.* 2011;14:1029–1033.

98. Q C. Hydromorphone for acute and chronic pain. *Cochrane Database Syst Rev.* 2002;1. CD003447.

99. Pigni A, Brunelli C, Caraceni A. The role of hydromorphone in cancer pain treatment: a systematic review. *Palliat Med.* 2011;25:471–477.

100. Kalso E, Vainio A. Morphine and oxycodone hydrochloride in the management of cancer pain. *Clini Pharmacol Therapeut.* 1990;47:639–646.

101. Tallgren M, Olkkola KT, Seppälä T, Höckerstedt K, Lindgren L. Pharmacokinetics and ventilatory effects of oxycodone before and after liver transplantation. *Clini Pharmacol Therapeut.* 1997;61:655–661.

102. Lauretti GR, Oliveira G, Pereira NL. Comparison of sustained-release morphine with sustained-release oxycodone in advanced cancer patients. *Br J Cancer.* 2003;89:2027.

103. Bruera E, Belzile M, Pituskin E, et al. Randomized, double-blind, cross-over trial comparing safety and efficacy of oral controlled-release oxycodone with controlled-release morphine in patients with cancer pain. *J Clin Oncol.* 1998;16:3222–3229.

104. Mucci-LoRusso P, Berman BS, Silberstein PT, et al. Controlled-release oxycodone compared with controlled-release morphine in the treatment of cancer pain: a randomized, double-blind, parallel-group study. *Eur J Pain.* 1998;2:239–249.

105. Gallego AO, Baron MG, Arranz EE. Oxycodone: a pharmacological and clinical review. *Clin Transl Oncol.* 2007;9:298–307.

106. Davis MP, Walsh D, Lagman R, LeGrand SB. Controversies in pharmacotherapy of pain management. *Lancet Oncol.* 2005;6:696–704.

107. Sloan P, Slatkin N, Ahdieh H. Effectiveness and safety of oral extended-release oxymorphone for the treatment of cancer pain: a pilot study. *Support Care Cancer.* 2005;13:57–65.

108. Adams MP, Ahdieh H. Pharmacokinetics and dose-proportionality of oxymorphone extended release and its metabolites: results of a randomized crossover study. *Pharmacotherapy.* 2004;24:468–476.

109. Kirvela M, Lindgren L, Seppala T, Olkkola KT. The pharmacokinetics of oxycodone in uremic patients undergoing renal transplantation. *J Clin Anesth.* 1996;8:13–18.

110. Prommer E. Oxymorphone: a review. *Support Care Cancer.* 2006;14:109–115.

111. Prommer E. The role of fentanyl in cancer-related pain. *J Palliat Med.* 2009;12:947–954.

112. Sathyan G, Guo C, Sivakumar K, Gidwani S, Gupta S. Evaluation of the bioequivalence of two transdermal fentanyl systems following single and repeat applications. *Curr Med Res Opin.* 2005;21:1961–1968.

113. Labroo RB, Paine MF, Thummel KE, Kharasch ED. Fentanyl metabolism by human hepatic and intestinal cytochrome P450 3A4: implications for interindividual variability in disposition, efficacy, and drug interactions. *Drug Metabol Dispos.* 1997;25:1072–1080.

114. Heiskanen T, Mätzke S, Haakana S, Gergov M, Vuori E, Kalso E. Transdermal fentanyl in cachectic cancer patients. *Pain.* 2009;144:218–222.

115. Ripamonti C, Fagnoni E, Campa T, Brunelli C, De Conno F. Is the use of transdermal fentanyl inappropriate according to the WHO guidelines and the EAPC recommendations? A study of cancer patients in Italy. *Support Care Cancer.* 2006;14:400–407.

116. Payne R, Mathias SD, Pasta DJ, Wanke LA, Williams R, Mahmoud R. Quality of life and cancer pain: satisfaction and side effects with transdermal fentanyl versus oral morphine. *J Clin Oncol.* 1998;16:1588–1593.

117. Clark A, Ahmedzai S, Allan L, et al. Efficacy and safety of transdermal fentanyl and sustained-release oral morphine in patients with cancer and chronic noncancer pain. *Curr Med Res Opin.* 2004;20:1419–1428.

118. Coluzzi PH, Schwartzberg L, Conroy Jr JD, et al. Breakthrough cancer pain: a randomized trial comparing oral transmucosal fentanyl citrate (OTFC®) and morphine sulfate immediate release (MSIR®). *Pain*. 2001;91:123—130.

119. Zeppetella G. An assessment of the safety, efficacy, and acceptability of intranasal fentanyl citrate in the management of cancer-related breakthrough pain: a pilot study. *J Pain Symptom Manag*. 2000;20:253—258.

120. Soares LGL, Martins M, Uchoa R. Intravenous fentanyl for cancer pain: a "fast titration" protocol for the emergency room. *J Pain Symptom Manag*. 2003;26:876—881.

121. Pergolizzi J, Aloisi AM, Dahan A, et al. Current knowledge of buprenorphine and its unique pharmacological profile. *Pain Pract*. 2010;10:428—450.

122. Bullingham RE, McQuay HJ, Moore A, Bennett MR. Buprenorphine kinetics. *Clini Pharmacol Therapeut*. 1980;28:667—672.

123. Kress HG. Clinical update on the pharmacology, efficacy and safety of transdermal buprenorphine. *Eur J Pain*. 2009;13:219—230.

124. Evans HC, Easthope SE. Transdermal buprenorphine. *Drugs*. 2003;63:1999—2010.

125. Davis MP. Buprenorphine in cancer pain. *Support Care Cancer*. 2005;13:878—887.

126. Picard N, Cresteil T, Djebli N, Marquet P. In vitro metabolism study of buprenorphine: evidence for new metabolic pathways. *Drug Metabol Dispos*. 2005;33:689—695.

127. Davis MP. Twelve reasons for considering buprenorphine as a frontline analgesic in the management of pain. *J Support Oncol*. 2012;10:209—219.

128. Wolff RF, Aune D, Truyers C, et al. Systematic review of efficacy and safety of buprenorphine versus fentanyl or morphine in patients with chronic moderate to severe pain. *Curr Med Res Opin*. 2012;28:833—845.

129. Sorge J, Sittl R. Transdermal buprenorphine in the treatment of chronic pain: results of a phase III, multicenter, randomized, double-blind, placebo-controlled study. *Clin Therapeut*. 2004;26:1808—1820.

130. Likar R, Lorenz V, Korak-Leiter M, Kager I, Sittl R. Transdermal buprenorphine patches applied in a 4-day regimen versus a 3-day regimen: a single-site, Phase III, randomized, open-label, crossover comparison. *Clin Therapeut*. 2007;29:1591—1606.

131. Böhme K, Likar R. Efficacy and tolerability of a new opioid analgesic formulation, buprenorphine transdermal therapeutic system (TDS), in the treatment of patients with chronic pain. A randomised, double-blind, placebo-controlled study. *Pain Clin*. 2003;15:193—202.

132. Prommer E. Levorphanol: the forgotten opioid. *Support Care Cancer*. 2007;15:259—264.

133. Zhang A, Xiong W, Bidlack JM, et al. 10-Ketomorphinan and 3-substituted-3-desoxymorphinan analogues as mixed κ and μ opioid ligands: synthesis and biological evaluation of their binding affinity at opioid receptors. *J Med Chem*. 2004;47:165—174.

134. Stringer M, Makin MK, Miles J, Morley JS. d-morphine, but not l-morphine, has low micromolar affinity for the non-competitive N-methyl-D-aspartate site in rat forebrain. Possible clinical implications for the management of neuropathic pain. *Neurosci Lett*. 2000;295:21—24.

135. Weinberg DS, Inturrisi CE, Reidenberg B, et al. Sublingual absorption of selected opioid analgesics. *Clini Pharmaco Therapeut*. 1988;44:335—342.

136. Dixon R, Crews T, Inturrisi C, Foley K. Levorphanol: pharmacokinetics and steady-state plasma concentrations in patients with pain. *Res Commun Chem Pathol Pharmacol*. 1983;41:3—17.

137. Rowbotham MC, Twilling L, Davies PS, Reisner L, Taylor K, Mohr D. Oral opioid therapy for chronic peripheral and central neuropathic pain. *N Engl J Med*. 2003;348:1223—1232.

138. Tzschentke TM, Christoph T, Kögel B, et al. (−)-(1R, 2R)-3-(3-dimethylamino-1-ethyl-2-methyl-propyl)-phenol hydrochloride (tapentadol HCl): a novel μ-opioid receptor agonist/norepinephrine reuptake inhibitor with broad-spectrum analgesic properties. *J Pharmacol Exp Therapeut*. 2007;323:265—276.

139. Prommer EE. Tapentadol: an initial analysis. *J Opioid Manag*. 2010;6:223—226.

140. Terlinden R, Ossig J, Fliegert F, Lange C, Göhler K. Absorption, metabolism, and excretion of 14 C-labeled tapentadol HCl in healthy male subjects. *Eur J Drug Metab Pharmacokinet*. 2007;32:163—169.

141. Kneip C, Terlinden R, Beier H, Chen G. Investigations into the drug-drug interaction potential of tapentadol in human liver microsomes and fresh human hepatocytes. *Drug Metabol Lett*. 2008;2:67—75.

142. Tapentadol (Nucynta)—a new analgesic. *Med Lett Drug Ther*. 2015;51(1318):61—62.

143. Kress HG, Koch ED, Kosturski H, et al. Tapentadol prolonged release for managing moderate to severe, chronic malignant tumor-related pain. *Pain Physician*. 2014;17:329—343.

144. Hartrick C, Van Hove I, Stegmann J-U, Oh C, Upmalis D. Efficacy and tolerability of tapentadol immediate release and oxycodone HCl immediate release in patients awaiting primary joint replacement surgery for end-stage joint disease: a 10-day, phase III, randomized, double-blind, active-and placebo-controlled study. *Clin Therapeut*. 2009;31:260—271.

145. Kleinert R, Lange C, Steup A, Black P, Goldberg J, Desjardins P. Single dose analgesic efficacy of tapentadol in postsurgical dental pain: the results of a randomized, double-blind, placebo-controlled study. *Anesth Analg*. 2008;107:2048—2055.

146. Oh C, Rengelshausen J, Mangold B, et al. A thorough QT/QTc study of multiple doses of tapentadol immediate release in healthy subjects. *Int J Clin Pharm Ther*. 2010;48:678—687.

147. Miguel R. Interventional treatment of cancer pain: the fourth step in the World Health Organization analgesic ladder? *Cancer Control*. 2000;7:149—156.

148. Wong GY, Schroeder DR, Carns PE, et al. Effect of neurolytic celiac plexus block on pain relief, quality of life, and survival in patients with unresectable pancreatic cancer: a

randomized controlled trial. *J Am Med Assoc.* 2004;291: 1092−1099.

149. Plancarte R, Amescua C, Patt RB, Aldrete JA. Superior hypogastric plexus block for pelvic cancer pain. *Anesthesiology.* 1990;73:236−239.

150. Whistler JL, Chuang H-h, Chu P, Jan LY, Von Zastrow M. Functional dissociation of μ opioid receptor signaling and endocytosis: implications for the biology of opiate tolerance and addiction. *Neuron.* 1999;23:737−746.

151. Finn AK, Whistler JL. Endocytosis of the mu opioid receptor reduces tolerance and a cellular hallmark of opiate withdrawal. *Neuron.* 2001;32:829−839.

152. Portenoy RK, Foley KM, Inturrisi CE. The nature of opioid responsiveness and its implications for neuropathic pain: new hypotheses derived from studies of opioid infusions. *Pain.* 1990;43:273−286.

153. Mercadante S. Opioid rotation for cancer pain: rationale and clinical aspects. *Cancer.* 1999;86:1856−1866.

154. Mercadante S, Arcuri E, Tirelli W, Casuccio A. Analgesic effect of intravenous ketamine in cancer patients on morphine therapy: a randomized, controlled, double-blind, crossover, double-dose study. *J Pain Symptom Manag.* 2000;20:246−252.

155. Bruera E, Kim HN. Cancer pain. *J Am Med Assoc.* 2003; 290:2476−2479.

156. Mercadante S, Radbruch L, Caraceni A, et al. Episodic (breakthrough) pain: consensus conference of an expert working group of the European Association for Palliative Care. *Cancer.* 2002;94:832−839.

157. Radbruch L, Trottenberg P, Elsner F, Kaasa S, Caraceni A. Systematic review of the role of alternative application routes for opioid treatment for moderate to severe cancer pain: an EPCRC opioid guidelines project. *Palliat Med.* 2011;25:578−596.

158. Muijsers RB, Wagstaff AJ. Transdermal fentanyl. *Drugs.* 2001;61:2289−2307.

159. Vasisht N, Gever LN, Tagarro I, Finn AL. Formulation selection and pharmacokinetic comparison of fentanyl buccal soluble film with oral transmucosal fentanyl citrate. *Clin Drug Invest.* 2009;29:647−654.

160. Thomas JR, von Gunten CF. Pain in terminally ill patients. *CNS Drugs.* 2003;17:621−631.

161. Collins S, Faura C, Moore RA, McQuay H. Peak plasma concentrations after oral morphine: a systematic review. *J Pain Symptom Manag.* 1998;16:388−402.

162. Stuart-Harris R, Joel S, McDonald P, Currow D, Slevin M. The pharmacokinetics of morphine and morphine glucuronide metabolites after subcutaneous bolus injection and subcutaneous infusion of morphine. *Br J Clin Pharmacol.* 2000;49:207−214.

163. Klepstad P, Kaasa S, Skauge M, Borchgrevink P. Pain intensity and side effects during titration of morphine to cancer patients using a fixed schedule dose escalation. *Acta Anaesthesiol Scand.* 2000;44:656−664.

164. De Conno F, Ripamonti C, Fagnoni E, et al. The MERITO Study: a multicentre trial of the analgesic effect and tolerability of normal-release oral morphine during 'titration phase' in patients with cancer pain. *Palliat Med.* 2008;22: 214−221.

165. Gatti A, Reale C, Occhioni R, et al. Standard therapy with opioids in chronic pain management. *Clin Drug Invest.* 2009;29:17−23.

166. McCarberg BH, Barkin RL. Long-acting opioids for chronic pain: pharmacotherapeutic opportunities to enhance compliance, quality of life, and analgesia. *Am J Therapeut.* 2001;8:181−186.

167. Network NCC. *NCCN Clinical Practice Guidelines in Oncology: Adult Cancer Pain.v2.* 2015.

168. Radbruch L, Loick G, Schulzeck S, et al. Intravenous titration with morphine for severe cancer pain: report of 28 cases. *Clin J Pain.* 1999;15:173−178.

169. Knotkova H, Fine PG, Portenoy RK. Opioid rotation: the science and the limitations of the equianalgesic dose table. *J Pain Symptom Manag.* 2009;38:426−439.

170. Mercadante S, Ferrera P, Villari P, Casuccio A, Intravaia G, Mangione S. Frequency, indications, outcomes, and predictive factors of opioid switching in an acute palliative care unit. *J Pain Symptom Manag.* 2009;37:632−641.

171. Pasternak GW. Incomplete cross tolerance and multiple mu opioid peptide receptors. *Trends Pharmacol Sci.* 2001;22:67−70.

172. McPherson ML. *Demystifying Opioid Conversion Calculations. A Guide for Effective Dosing.* 2nd ed. 2018 Chapter 1 Introduction to Opioid Conversion Calculations.

173. Cherny N, Ripamonti C, Pereira J, et al. Strategies to manage the adverse effects of oral morphine: an evidence-based report. *J Clin Oncol.* 2001;19:2542−2554.

174. Pappagallo M. Incidence, prevalence, and management of opioid bowel dysfunction. *Am J Surg.* 2001;182: S11−S18.

175. Twycross R, Sykes N, Mihalyo M, Wilcock A. Stimulant laxatives and opioid-induced constipation. *J Pain Symptom Manag.* 2012;43:306−313.

176. Mystakidou K, Befon S, Liossi C, Vlachos L. Comparison of tropisetron and chlorpromazine combinations in the control of nausea and vomiting in patients with advanced cancer. *J Pain Symptom Manag.* 1998;15: 176−184.

177. Webster L, Andrews M, Stoddard G. Modafinil treatment of opioid-induced sedation. *Pain Med.* 2003;4:135−140.

178. Peuckmann-Post V, Elsner F, Krumm N, Trottenberg P, Radbruch L. Pharmacological treatments for fatigue associated with palliative care. *Cochrane Database Syst Rev.* 2010;(12):5−10.

179. Dworkin RH, Backonja M, Rowbotham MC, et al. Advances in neuropathic pain: diagnosis, mechanisms, and treatment recommendations. *Arch Neurol.* 2003;60: 1524−1534.

180. Lussier D, Huskey AG, Portenoy RK. Adjuvant analgesics in cancer pain management. *Oncologist.* 2004;9: 571−591.

181. Tiina T. Amitriptyline effectively relieves neuropathic pain following treatment of breast cancer. *Pain.* 1996; 64:293−302.

182. Ehrnrooth CG, Zachariae R, Andersen J. Eva. Randomized trial of opioids versus tricyclic antidepressants for radiation-induced mucositis pain in head and neck cancer. *Acta Oncologica*. 2001;40:745−750.

183. Kautio A-L, Haanpää M, Saarto T, Kalso E. Amitriptyline in the treatment of chemotherapy-induced neuropathic symptoms. *J Pain Symptom Manag*. 2008;35:31−39.

184. Mercadante S, Arcuri E, Tirelli W, Villari P, Casuccio A. Amitriptyline in neuropathic cancer pain in patients on morphine therapy: a randomized placebo-controlled, double-blind crossover study. *Tumori J*. 2002;88:239−242.

185. Preskorn SH, Irwin HA. Toxicity of tricyclic antidepressants—kinetics, mechanism, intervention: a review. *J Clin Psychiatr*. 1982.

186. Derry S, Wiffen PJ, Aldington D, Moore RA. Nortriptyline for neuropathic pain in adults. *Cochrane Database Syst Rev*. 2015;(1).

187. Predictable S. Side effects of antidepressants: an overview. *Cleveland Clin J Med*. 2006;73:351.

188. Sindrup SH, Gram LF, Brøsen K, Eshøj O, Mogensen EF. The selective serotonin reuptake inhibitor paroxetine is effective in the treatment of diabetic neuropathy symptoms. *Pain*. 1990;42:135−144.

189. Sindrup SH, Bach FW, Madsen C, Gram L, Jensen T. Venlafaxine versus imipramine in painful polyneuropathy: a randomized, controlled trial. *Neurology*. 2003;60:1284−1289.

190. Smith EML, Pang H, Cirrincione C, et al. Effect of duloxetine on pain, function, and quality of life among patients with chemotherapy-induced painful peripheral neuropathy: a randomized clinical trial. *J Am Med Assoc*. 2013;309:1359−1367.

191. Tasmuth T, Härtel B, Kalso E. Venlafaxine in neuropathic pain following treatment of breast cancer. *Eur J Pain*. 2002;6:17−24.

192. Jefferson JW, Pradko JF, Muir KT. Bupropion for major depressive disorder: pharmacokinetic and formulation considerations. *Clin Therapeut*. 2005;27:1685−1695.

193. Dhillon S, Yang LP, Curran MP. Spotlight on bupropion in major depressive disorder. *CNS Drugs*. 2008;22:613−617.

194. Semenchuk MR, Davis B. Efficacy of sustained-release bupropion in neuropathic pain: an open-label study. *Clin J Pain*. 2000;16:6−11.

195. Semenchuk MR, Sherman S, Davis B. Double-blind, randomized trial of bupropion SR for the treatment of neuropathic pain. *Neurology*. 2001;57:1583−1588.

196. Leppert W, Buss T. The role of corticosteroids in the treatment of pain in cancer patients. *Curr Pain Headache Rep*. 2012;16:307−313.

197. Smith P, Bruera E. Management of malignant ureteral obstruction in the palliative care setting. *J Pain Symptom Manag*. 1995;10:481−486.

198. Yennurajalingam S, Frisbee-Hume S, Palmer JL, et al. Reduction of cancer-related fatigue with dexamethasone: a double-blind, randomized, placebo-controlled trial in patients with advanced cancer. *J Clin Oncol*. 2013;31:3076−3082.

199. Heimdal K, Hirschberg H, Slettebø H, Watne K, Nome O. High incidence of serious side effects of high-dose dexamethasone treatment in patients with epidural spinal cord compression. *J Neurooncol*. 1992;12:141−144.

200. Sørensen P, Helweg-Larsen S, Mouridsen H, Hansen H. Effect of high-dose dexamethasone in carcinomatous metastatic spinal cord compression treated with radiotherapy: a randomised trial. *Eur J Cancer*. 1994;30:22−27.

201. Vecht CJ, Hovestadt A, Verbiest H, Van Vliet J, Van Putten W. Dose-effect relationship of dexamethasone on Karnofsky performance in metastatic brain tumors: a randomized study of doses of 4, 8, and 16 mg per day. *Neurology*. 1994;44:675.

202. Loblaw DA, Wu JS, Kirkbride P, et al. Pain flare in patients with bone metastases after palliative radiotherapy—a nested randomized control trial. *Support Care Cancer*. 2007;15:451−455.

203. Jensen TS. Anticonvulsants in neuropathic pain: rationale and clinical evidence. *Eur J Pain*. 2002;6:61−68.

204. Caraceni A, Zecca E, Bonezzi C, et al. Gabapentin for neuropathic cancer pain: a randomized controlled trial from the Gabapentin Cancer Pain Study Group. *J Clin Oncol*. 2004;22:2909−2917.

205. Mishra S, Bhatnagar S, Goyal GN, Rana SPS, Upadhya SP. A comparative efficacy of amitriptyline, gabapentin, and pregabalin in neuropathic cancer pain: a prospective randomized double-blind placebo-controlled study. *Am J Hospice Palliat Med*. 2012;29:177−182.

206. Sabers A, Gram L. Newer anticonvulsants. *Drugs*. 2000;60:23−33.

207. Yajnik S, Singh GP, Singh G, Kumar M. Phenytoin as a coanalgesic in cancer pain. *J Pain Symptom Manag*. 1992;7:209−213.

208. Dunteman ED. Levetiracetam as an adjunctive analgesic in neoplastic plexopathies: case series and commentary. *J Pain Palliat Care Pharmacother*. 2005;19:35−43.

209. Rao RD, Flynn PJ, Sloan JA, et al. Efficacy of lamotrigine in the management of chemotherapy-induced peripheral neuropathy: a phase 3 randomized, double-blind, placebo-controlled trial, N01C3. *Cancer*. 2008;112:2802−2808.

210. Bruera E, Ripamonti C, Brenneis C, Macmillan K, Hanson J. A randomized double-blind crossover trial of intravenous lidocaine in the treatment of neuropathic cancer pain. *J Pain Symptom Manag*. 1992;7:138−140.

211. Lee JT, Sanderson CR, Xuan W, Agar M. Lidocaine for cancer pain in adults: a systematic review and meta-analysis. *J Palliat Med*. 2019;22:326−334.

212. Sharma S, Rajagopal M, Palat G, Singh C, Haji AG, Jain D. A phase II pilot study to evaluate use of intravenous lidocaine for opioid-refractory pain in cancer patients. *J Pain Symptom Manag*. 2009;37:85−93.

213. Reeves DJ, Foster AE. Continuous intravenous lidocaine infusion for the management of pain uncontrolled by opioid medications. *J Pain Palliat Care Pharmacother*. 2017;31:198−203.

214. Ripamonti C, Bruera E. Pain and symptom management in palliative care. *Cancer Control*. 1996;3:204−213.

215. Sloan P, Basta M, Storey P, Von Gunten C. Mexiletine as an adjuvant analgesic for the management of neuropathic cancer pain. *Anesth Analg.* 1999;89:760.

216. Wallace MS, Magnuson S, Ridgeway B. Efficacy of oral mexiletine for neuropathic pain with allodynia: a double-blind, placebo-controlled, crossover study. *Reg Anesth Pain Med.* 2000;25:459−467.

217. Garzón-Rodríguez C, Merchan MC, Calsina-Berna A, López-Rómboli E, Porta-Sales J. Lidocaine 5% patches as an effective short-term co-analgesic in cancer pain. Preliminary results. *Support Care Cancer.* 2013;21:3153−3158.

218. Cheung KWA, Chan PC, Lo SH. The use of ketamine in the management of refractory cancer pain in a palliative care unit. *Ann Palliat Med.* 2019.

219. Galer BS, Rowbotham MC, Perander J, Friedman E. Topical lidocaine patch relieves postherpetic neuralgia more effectively than a vehicle topical patch: results of an enriched enrollment study. *Pain.* 1999;80:533−538.

220. Gammaitoni AR, Davis MW. Pharmacokinetics and tolerability of lidocaine patch 5% with extended dosing. *Ann Pharmacother.* 2002;36:236−240.

221. Parsons CG. NMDA receptors as targets for drug action in neuropathic pain. *Eur J Pharmacol.* 2001;429:71−78.

222. Sikora K, Advani S, Koroltchouk V, et al. Essential drugs for cancer therapy: a World Health Organization consultation. *Ann Oncol.* 1999;10:385−390.

223. Sinner B, Graf B. Ketamine. In: *Modern Anesthetics.* Springer; 2008:313−333.

224. Hardy J, Quinn S, Fazekas B, Plummer J, Eckermann S, Agar M, Spruyt O, Rowett D, Currow DC. Randomized, double-blind, placebo-controlled study to assess the efficacy and toxicity of subcutaneous ketamine in the management of cancer pain. *J Clin Oncol.* 2012.

225. Okon T. Ketamine: an introduction for a pain and palliative medicine physician. *Pain Physician.* 2007;10:493.

226. Schmid RL, Sandler AN, Katz J. Use and efficacy of low-dose ketamine in the management of acute postoperative pain: a review of current techniques and outcomes. *Pain.* 1999;82:111−125.

227. Bell RF, Eccleston C, Kalso EA. Ketamine as an adjuvant to opioids for cancer pain. *Cochrane Database Syst Rev.* 2017;6. Cd003351.

228. Portenoy RK, Ganae-Motan ED, Allende S, et al. Nabiximols for opioid-treated cancer patients with poorly-controlled chronic pain: a randomized, placebo-controlled, graded-dose trial. *J Pain.* 2012;13:438−449.

229. Johnson JR, Burnell-Nugent M, Lossignol D, Ganae-Motan ED, Potts R, Fallon MT. Multicenter, double-blind, randomized, placebo-controlled, parallel-group study of the efficacy, safety, and tolerability of THC: CBD extract and THC extract in patients with intractable cancer-related pain. *J Pain Symptom Manag.* 2010;39:167−179.

230. Lynch ME, Cesar-Rittenberg P, Hohmann AG. A double-blind, placebo-controlled, crossover pilot trial with extension using an oral mucosal cannabinoid extract for treatment of chemotherapy-induced neuropathic pain. *J Pain Symptom Manag.* 2014;47:166−173.

231. Pérez J. Combined cannabinoid therapy via an oromucosal spray. *Drugs Today.* 2006;42:495−503.

232. Noyes Jr R, Brunk SF, Avery DH, Canter A. The analgesic properties of delta-9-tetrahydrocannabinol and codeine. *Clin Pharmacol Therapeut.* 1975;18:84−89.

233. Schreiber S, Getslev V, Backer M, Weizman R, Pick C. The atypical neuroleptics clozapine and olanzapine differ regarding their antinociceptive mechanisms and potency. *Pharmacol Biochem Behav.* 1999;64:75−80.

234. Khojainova N, Santiago-Palma J, Kornick C, Breitbart W, Gonzales GR. Olanzapine in the management of cancer pain. *J Pain Symptom Manag.* 2002;23:346−350.

235. Prommer EE. Toxicity of bisphosphonates. *J Palliat Med.* 2009;12:1061−1065.

236. Rosen LS, Gordon D, Tchekmedyian S, et al. Zoledronic acid versus placebo in the treatment of skeletal metastases in patients with lung cancer and other solid tumors: a phase III, double-blind, randomized trial—the zoledronic acid lung cancer and other Solid Tumors Study Group. *J Clin Oncol.* 2003;21:3150−3157.

237. Saad F, Gleason DM, Murray R, et al. A randomized, placebo-controlled trial of zoledronic acid in patients with hormone-refractory metastatic prostate carcinoma. *J Natl Cancer Inst.* 2002;94:1458−1468.

238. Berenson JR, Lichtenstein A, Porter L, et al. Efficacy of pamidronate in reducing skeletal events in patients with advanced multiple myeloma. *N Engl J Med.* 1996; 334:488−493.

239. Prommer E. Palliative oncology: denosumab. *Am J Hospice Palliat Med.* 2015;32:568−572.

240. Body J-J. Dosing regimens and main adverse events of bisphosphonates. *Semin Oncol.* 2001:49−53.

241. Lewington VJ, McEwan AJ, Ackery DM, et al. A prospective, randomised double-blind crossover study to examine the efficacy of strontium-89 in pain palliation in patients with advanced prostate cancer metastatic to bone. *Eur J Cancer Clin Oncol.* 1991;27:954−958.

242. Parker C, Nilsson S, Heinrich D, et al. Alpha emitter radium-223 and survival in metastatic prostate cancer. *N Engl J Med.* 2013;369:213−223.

243. Yomiya K, Matsuo N, Tomiyasu S, et al. Baclofen as an adjuvant analgesic for cancer pain. *Am J Hospice Palliat Med.* 2009;26:112−118.

244. Cohen JY, Guilbault A. Induction of psychosis by cyclobenzaprine. *Psychopharmacol Bull.* 2018;48:15−19.

245. Chou R, Clark E, Helfand M. Comparative efficacy and safety of long-acting oral opioids for chronic non-cancer pain: a systematic review. *J Pain Symptom Manag.* 2003;26:1026−1048.

246. Penn RD, Paice JA, Kroin JS. Octreotide: a potent new non-opiate analgesic for intrathecal infusion. *Pain.* 1992;49:13−19.

247. Dahaba AA, Mueller G, Mattiassich G, et al. Effect of somatostatin analogue octreotide on pain relief after major abdominal surgery. *Eur J Pain.* 2009;13:861−864.

248. Bernard SA, Bruera E. Drug interactions in palliative care. *J Clin Oncol.* 2000;18:1780−1799.

CHAPTER 8

Complementary and Integrative Health

HYUNG S. KIM, MD

OVERVIEW

Integrative healthcare is defined by the United States National Institutes of Health as a comprehensive, often interdisciplinary approach to treatment, prevention, and health promotion that brings together complementary and conventional therapies.[42] In the United States, the National Center for Complementary and Integrative Health (NCCIH) is responsible for research on promising integrative health approaches. The mission of NCCIH is to define, through rigorous scientific investigation, the usefulness and safety of complementary and integrative health approaches and their roles in improving health and healthcare.[42] Budget for NCCIH in the United States exceeded USD$146 million in 2019, testifying to interest by the public and governmental agencies in exploring efficacy and safety of many of these approaches.[43] Complementary and integrative health approaches contrast with alternative medicine, which is defined as unproven practices used in place of conventional health approaches. Some examples of complementary and integrative health approaches commonly used in the United States and other parts of the world to treat acute and chronic pain are delineated as follows. In light of the recent opioid crisis in the United States, and in search of alternatives to long-term opioid therapy to treat chronic nonmalignant pain, interest in complementary and integrative approaches has grown and adapted by many patients and clinicians alike.

ACUPUNCTURE

Acupuncture is defined as insertion of thin needles on specific points in the skin for the purposes of restoring health and promoting wellness. First known written documentation of acupuncture, *Huangdi Neijing* ("Yellow Emperor's Inner Classic"), dates back to 100 BCE.[69] Acupuncture is typically associated with Traditional Chinese Medicine (TCM) and is the form most widely adopted in the United States, although variants with different philosophies and approaches have been developed in the treatment of pain.[15] TCM approach involves belief in *qi* (life force) that courses within the body in specific channels called meridians. Disease state involves dysfunction of the *qi*, and acupuncture among other treatments is used to restore the proper flow of *qi*.[44] TCM often uses herbs as part of its treatment, along with cupping and moxibustion, which involves burning dried mugwort plant (*Artemisia vulgaris*) on different points on the body.

A typical TCM acupuncture session involves placing the patient in a comfortable position (usually supine or prone) and inserting needles for a length of time, typically 20 to 30 minutes. Needles may be stimulated with heat, pressure, manual manipulations, or electricity. Needle insertion may be associated with *de-qi*, which refers to paresthesia or deep ache as the needle is being inserted.[25] Acupuncture treatment is unique to each recipient and may be altered on subsequent treatments depending on response to prior treatments.

Practices related to acupuncture include acupressure, in which physical pressure is applied to specific points on the body for therapeutic purposes. Cupping refers to the practice of placing a suction cup on the skin for the purposes of mobilizing blood flow and promoting healing. Tui na is a method of stimulating the flow of *qi* by various techniques that do not involve needles. Electroacupuncture involves use of electrical stimulation to the acupuncture needles that are inserted in the body. Bee venom acupuncture involves injecting purified, diluted bee venom into acupuncture points.[34]

The efficacy of acupuncture for pain has been extensively studied. A meta-analysis evaluating efficacy of acupuncture for chronic pain indicated that acupuncture is effective for the treatment of chronic musculoskeletal, headache, and osteoarthritis pain.[63] Treatment effects of acupuncture persisted over time and could not be explained solely in terms of placebo effects. Authors concluded that acupuncture is a reasonable option for a patient with chronic pain.

Cochrane review for acupuncture for neck disorders concluded that there is moderate-quality evidence that suggests that acupuncture relieves pain better than sham acupuncture, as measured at completion of treatment and at short-term follow-up. Those who received acupuncture report less pain and disability at short-term follow-up than those on a waitlist. Moderate-quality evidence also indicates that acupuncture is more effective than inactive treatment for relieving pain at short-term follow-up.[62]

In a systematic review and meta-analysis, verum acupuncture was shown to be more effective than sham acupuncture for pain relief, improving sleep quality and reforming general status in fibromyalgia syndrome.[29]

While acupuncture with roots in TCM is the most widely practiced and known form of acupuncture, acupuncture from other traditions also exist. Examples include Japanese acupuncture, Korean acupuncture, French Energetic Acupuncture (French Meridian Acupuncture), scalp acupuncture, and auricular acupuncture (which includes Battlefield Acupuncture). Nonthermal, low-intensity laser to stimulate acupuncture points has been incorporated in some acupuncture treatments.[12]

Acupuncture is a relatively safe treatment, but as with any procedure involving needles, complications can be seen. In a prospective observational study of 229,230 patients who received an average of 10.2 acupuncture treatments,[71] 8.6% reported at least one adverse effect and 2.2% reported one that required treatment, with most common adverse effects being bleeding or hematoma (6.1% of patients, 58% of all adverse effects) and pain (1.7%). Two patients were found to have pneumothorax, one requiring hospital treatment and the other requiring observation only. The longest duration of a side effect was 180 days (nerve lesion of the lower limb). While relatively safe, practitioners should consider providing patients with an informed consent that reviews risks, benefits, and alternatives prior to delivery of acupuncture treatments.

TAI CHI/QIGONG

Tai Chi and Qigong are traditional Chinese exercises that integrate the body and mind. It includes breathing control, slow movements, mental relaxation, and meditation.[10] Tai Chi and Qigong are widely practiced in China and have spread internationally for their purported health benefits. As of 2017, yoga, Tai Chi, and Qigong were practiced by 14.5% of US adults, with

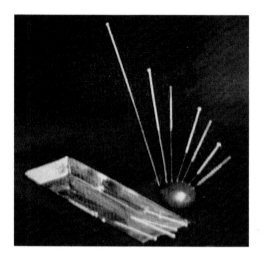

Acupuncture needles (Fig 184.1 from Chapter 184, Pfenniger and Fowler's Procedures for Primary Care (4th ed., (c) 2020), p. 1258.)

pain and arthritis as among the top medical conditions for which people used these modalities.[67]

Zou and colleagues[74] in a systematic review and meta-analysis of randomized controlled trials examining Tai Chi, Qigong, and yoga noted that these practices appear to reduce pain intensity and disability in patients with low back pain compared with control groups. Of the three, Tai Chi had a significantly superior effect on pain management irrespective of noncontrol comparison or active control comparison (conventional exercises, core training, and physical therapy programs). A systematic review by the United States Agency for Healthcare Research and Quality noted that Tai Chi and Qigong were associated with slight short-term (1–6 month) improvements in function and pain for fibromyalgia patients, although the strength of evidence was considered low.[54]

Tai Chi was shown in a systematic review and meta-analysis of 18 randomized controlled trials to have positive evidence of immediate relief of chronic pain from osteoarthritis; there were some beneficial evidence regarding the effects of Tai Chi on immediate relief of chronic pain from low back pain and osteoporosis.[30] Tai Chi has been reported to improve quality of life, functional balance, and pain in patients with multiple sclerosis.[73] Another systematic review and meta-analysis of 15 randomized controlled trials of Tai Chi for patients with chronic musculoskeletal conditions found that there is moderate-quality evidence for effectiveness of Tai Chi compared with no treatment or usual care at short term for pain and disability.[24] Additional high-quality trials with large samples sizes were recommended to assess short- and long-term benefit from Tai Chi for chronic musculoskeletal pain conditions.

AYURVEDIC MEDICINE

Ayurveda is a system of medicine originating from India and South Asia that emphasizes holistic approaches to health and a balance in lifestyle.[55] Ayurvedic medicine consists of individualized treatments consisting of multimodal components such as manual therapies, nutritional therapy, herbs, lifestyle counseling, and yoga-based exercises.[28] The term "ayurveda" is Sanskrit derived from Ayu (life) and Veda (knowledge). *Sushruta Samhita* is one of the most widely accepted Ayurvedic texts and dates back over 2000 years, although the concepts leading to the formulation of Ayurveda dates back to well before that time.

Medicinal therapy is highly individualized in Ayurveda, and pharmacy is highly developed.[55] The choice and dose of medicine are influenced not only by disease but by the individual's constitution and the environmental conditions likely to affect the individual's *Doshas*, or energy that defines every person's makeup. Ayurvedic medicine subscribes to almost 70 books containing more than 8000 recipes for the preparation of different medicines, most of which are derived from minerals and plants.

One such Ayurvedic preparation, curcumin, a yellow pigment derived from the spice turmeric and an essential component of curry powder dried from *Curcuma longa*, has been found to exert a powerful anti-inflammatory effect by blocking numerous inflammatory pathways.[1] A meta-analysis of randomized controlled trials has shown that curcumin can treat osteoarthritis patients effectively and improve Western Ontario and McMaster Universities Osteoarthritis Index Scale and Visual Analog Scale score. Side effects from the use of curcumin were not higher than that of ibuprofen.[72]

Neuropathic pain may also respond to Ayurvedic preparations.[53] Research and evaluation of effectiveness of Ayurvedic medicine are limited by wide variation and quantity of pharmacologically active substances in plants.[55] In addition, some herbs that form ingredients for Ayurvedic medicine are endangered or vulnerable plants, and cultivation in other areas are impractical, raising concerns over potential adulteration of commercially prepared drugs.[64,51]

YOGA

Yoga is a mind-body practice with origins in India. It has three main components: physical poses/posture, breathing control, and meditation/relaxation.[31] A systematic review and meta-analysis by Lauche et al.[32] found low-quality evidence for the effects of yoga on pain, physical function, and stiffness secondary to osteoarthritis. A systematic review and meta-analysis found preliminary evidence of short-term efficacy of yoga in improving headache frequency, headache duration, and pain intensity in patients suffering from tension-type headaches.[3] Agency for Healthcare Research and Quality systematic review[54] on noninvasive nonpharmacological treatment for chronic pain found that yoga was associated with slight improvements in function and pain for short- (1 to less than 6 months, strength of evidence moderate) and intermediate-term (greater than or equal to 6 months and less than 12 months, strength of evidence low).

Cochrane review on yoga for treatment of chronic nonspecific low back pain concluded that there is low-to-moderate certainty evidence that yoga compared with nonexercise controls results in small to moderate improvements in back-related function at 3 and 6 months. Yoga may also be slightly more effective for pain at 3 and 6 months. Yoga was associated with more adverse events than nonexercise controls but may have the same risk of adverse events as other back-focused exercise. Yoga was not associated with serious adverse events.[70]

A randomized trial comparing yoga, physical therapy, and education for chronic low back pain concluded that a manualized yoga program (12 weekly 75-minute classes) was noninferior to physical therapy for function (as measured by Roland Morris Disability Questionnaire) and pain (as measured by an 11-point scale), and the improvements were maintained at 1 year with no differences between maintenance strategies.[50]

In a randomized clinical trial involving military veterans with chronic low back pain, yoga improved health outcomes despite evidence that the participants had fewer resources, worse health, and more challenges attending yoga sessions than community samples studied previously; the magnitude of pain intensity decline was small, but occurred in the context of reduced opioid use.[23]

HOMEOPATHY

Homeopathy is a system of medical treatment developed by German physician Samuel Hahnemann at the end of the 18th century that utilizes highly diluted

Various yoga positions (Source: Mears SC, Wilson MR, Mannen EM, Tackett SA, Barnes CL. Position of the Hip in Yoga. *J Arthroplasty*. 2018;33(7):2306–2311.)

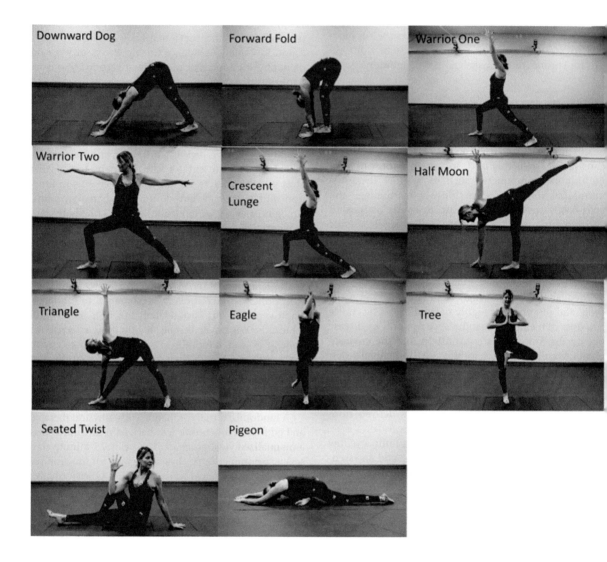

substances to promote healing.[52] Homeopathy is used by over six million people in the United States, and one of the most common uses for homeopathy includes treatments for musculoskeletal pain complaints.[13] Some conventional treatments use concepts akin to homeopathy, as evidenced by the use of minute quantities of botulinum toxin for the treatment of migraine headache.

Homeopathy has been suggested as a potential treatment option for fibromyalgia in a comprehensive literature review and meta-analysis based on 10 case reports, 3 observational studies, 1 non-randomized, and 4 randomized controlled trials, although authors acknowledged that any conclusions based on the results of the review have to be regarded as preliminary.[6] In addition, homeopathy has been suggested as a potential treatment option to treat symptoms related to low back pain, including in a randomized controlled trial by Beer et al.[5] involving 248 patients (of whom 137 completed the study) as measured by the Hannover Functional Ability Questionnaire (intent-to-treat analysis = 0.11, per-protocol analysis $p = .029$), although further studies are needed to clarify the role homeopathy may play in treatment of low back pain in the future.[40]

NATUROPATHY

Naturopathy refers to approaches to healthcare that reprioritizes the order of therapeutics, first emphasizing lifestyle-oriented self-care, preventive behaviors, nutrition, physical activity, and stress-management counseling before proceeding with medications, herbs, homeopathy, and manual therapy. There is less emphasis on the use of over-the-counter medications, prescription drug therapies, or surgical interventions.[8]

There are eight accredited schools of naturopathy in North America. In the United States, naturopathy is licensed in 22 states, the District of Columbia, and Puerto Rico and the US Virgin Islands. Third-party insurance coverage for naturopathy varies by state and range from minimal coverage (e.g., California) to legislatively mandated coverage (e.g., Washington State).[7,47]

Integrating naturopathic medicine into acute inpatient care has shown the potential to improve patient satisfaction and form a stronger relationship between care staff and patients.[49] Further research is needed to the determine effectiveness of naturopathy in the treatment of acute and chronic pain.

CHIROPRACTIC

Chiropractic approaches focus mainly but not exclusively on spinal manipulation to adjust subluxations.[16] Chiropractic was founded in the 1890s by Daniel David Palmer, a Canadian-American who proposed that most diseases of the body could be attributed to misaligned vertebrae, or spinal subluxation.[57] Existence of spinal subluxations, as defined by chiropractic practitioners, has been challenged in conventional medical literature.[39] Spinal mobilization as a treatment can also be performed by other medical providers, such as osteopaths and physical therapists, although distinctions remain between chiropractic manipulations and those employed by nonchiropractors.

A Cochrane review concluded that there is slightly improved pain and disability in the short term, and pain in the medium term, for acute/subacute low back pain when combined chiropractic interventions are utilized for low back pain.[65] In a systematic review of pragmatic studies, chiropractic care for low back pain appears to be equally effective as physical therapy.[75] Limited evidence suggests the same conclusion when chiropractic care is compared with exercise therapy and medical care, although whether chiropractic or medical care is more cost-effective could not be answered.

For the treatment of fibromyalgia, chiropractic care received a "strong against" recommendation by the European League Against Rheumatism based on studies of poor quality and lacking robust interpretable data.[36]

Risks associated with chiropractic spinal manipulation are controversial but may be not inconsiderable.[16] Existing literature indicates that benign adverse events following manual treatments to the spine are common, while serious adverse events are rare; incidence and causal relationships with serious adverse events are challenging to establish, with gaps in the literature and inherent methodological limitations of studies.[58]

OSTEOPATHY

Osteopathic medicine was founded by American A. T. Still in 1874 as a medical study of the relationship that the osseous structure and its interrelationships have on health.[66] A T. Still developed osteopathy after witnessing the death of his three children in 1864 during a meningitis outbreak and the powerlessness of the allopathic medicine of his time to treat them. He advocated abandoning all use of drugs in favor of dietary, spiritual, and mechanical functional treatment. A. T. Still found the American School of Osteopathy in Kirksville, Missouri, in 1892. American Association of College of Osteopathic Medicine was founded in 1898 to support and assist the osteopathic medical schools in the United States (https://www.aacom.org accessed Nov 30, 2019). As of 2019, there are 36 accredited colleges of osteopathic medicine in the United States, accounting for 25% of all US medical students.

Osteopathic medicine's guiding principles include the following: 1) the body is a unit; 2) structure and function are interrelated; 3) body has the innate ability to heal itself; and 4) rational practice of medicine must take these principles into account.[66] Central to its tenet is that the body is considered as a unified whole as opposed to a summation of its parts. In addition, the individual is considered an extension of his or her entire environment: social, family, environmental, nutritional, and psychospiritual. Osteopathic manipulative medicine is aimed at restoration of function. Primary structural diagnosis in osteopathic manipulative medicine is "somatic dysfunction" which is defined by the

American Osteopathic Association as "impaired or altered function of related components of the somatic (body framework) system: skeletal, arthrodial, and myofascial structures and their related vascular, lymphatic, and neural elements."[20]

Systemic reviews and meta-analysis suggest that clinically relevant effects of osteopathic manipulative treatment (OMT) were found for reducing pain and improving functional status in patients with acute and chronic nonspecific low back pain and for low back pain in pregnant and postpartum women at 3 months posttreatment.[19] Larger randomized controlled trials with robust comparison groups were felt to be needed to further validate the effects of OMT on low back pain.[60]

OMT has been proposed as a potentially effective treatment option for various types of headaches.[68] A systematic review by Orrock and Myers,[45] based on two studies, concluded that osteopathic intervention was similar in effect to a sham intervention for treatment of chronic nonspecific low back pain; and that there is similarity of effect between osteopathic intervention, exercise, and physical therapy. Further, visceral osteopathic manual therapy applications may improve results in treating patients with chronic nonspecific low back pain.[59]

MASSAGE

A Cochrane review evaluating massage therapy for nonspecific low back pain evaluated 25 trials and concluded that there was very little confidence that massage was an effective treatment for low back pain. Acute, subacute, and chronic low back pain had improvements in pain outcomes with massage, but only in the short-term follow-up. Functional improvement was observed in participants with subacute and chronic low back pain when compared with inactive controls, but again only for the short-term follow-up. Only minor adverse effects were noted with massage.[21] A systematic review of randomized controlled trials by Nelson and Churilla[41] concluded that there is low-to-moderate quality evidence that massage therapy is superior to nonactive therapies in reducing pain and improving certain functional outcomes, although it is unclear whether massage therapy is more effective than other forms of treatment.

Massage, along with warm pack and thermal manual methods, may have a role in reducing pain during labor in women in a Cochrane review.[56] The quality of evidence for studies ranged from low to very low.

AROMATHERAPY

Aromatherapy involves the use of essential oils for clinical benefit. A systematic review of randomized placebo-controlled trials concluded that there is moderate level evidence for the superiority of aromatherapy (inhalation, massage or oral use) for pain reduction over placebo in primary dysmenorrhea.[33]

MUSIC THERAPY

Music therapy has been shown in randomized controlled trials to provide statistically significant improvements in pain in critically ill patients.[61] Music therapy has been suggested as a nonpharmacologic intervention to ameliorate pain in infants undergoing painful procedures involving skin puncture as part of routine medical care.[37]

LOW-LEVEL LASER THERAPY

In a systematic review, low-level laser therapy was associated with moderate improvement in function and pain in chronic low back pain patients, with moderate strength of evidence.[54]

MINDFULNESS-BASED STRESS REDUCTION

In adults with chronic low back pain, treatment with mindfulness-based stress reduction (MBSR) or cognitive behavioral therapy (CBT), compared with usual care, resulted in greater improvement in back pain and functional limitations at 26 weeks, with no significant differences in outcomes between MBSR and CBT. These findings suggest that MBSR, as with CBT, may be an effective treatment option for patients with chronic low back pain.[11]

MBSR was evaluated in a systematic review of 7 randomized controlled trials.[2] The authors concluded that MBSR may be associated with short-term effects on pain intensity and physical functioning. Long-term randomized controlled trials that compare MBSR with active treatments were felt to be needed in order to better understand the role of MBSR in the management of low back pain.

GUIDED IMAGERY

Guided imagery may be a useful adjunct for pain management in patients undergoing orthopedic surgery,[9] nonmusculoskeletal pain,[48] arthritis, and other rheumatic diseases,[22] although additional research in this area was needed.

VIRTUAL REALITY

Virtual reality is the use of technology, such as a head-mounted display, tracking system, and sound device, to create an interactive three-dimensional experience. Augmented reality superimposes a computer-generated image on a user's visual field, thus enhancing the user's real-world view. Use of virtual reality and augmented reality has been proposed as potential treatment options for treatment of phantom limb pain[14] and pain and anxiety management in children.[4] Low-cost virtual reality headsets were shown to reduce perceived pain in healthy adults in a multicenter randomized crossover trial.[46] Virtual reality is an effective treatment for reducing acute pain and may reduce chronic pain according to a systematic review and meta-analysis by Mallari et al.[35]

REFLEXOLOGY

Reflexology proposes that the feet are representative of the body and that massaging specific points of the feet increases blood supply to mapped organs in the body.[26] Treatment uses a homunculus-like model for different points of the body as projected onto the foot. Currently research is limited on effects of reflexology in treating chronic pain.[27]

ENERGY HEALING

Energy healing for the treatment of pain may include Reiki, therapeutic touch, and healing touch.[17] There has been limited research evaluating these interventions and their effect on pain despite interest in these modalities. Evidence with a high risk of bias suggested that Reiki and prayer meditation might be associated with pain reduction.[18]

PRAYER

Active prayer, like other active coping strategies for pain, may facilitate self-management of pain and thus enhance pain outcomes.[38]

DISCUSSION

Use of integrative and complementary approaches is an evolving area with potential to improve delivery of care for patients suffering from acute and chronic pain. They are widely used in the United States and around the world, especially in areas where access to conventional Western medicine approaches may be limited. Research into effectiveness of these approaches for the treatment of pain is accelerating and suggests potential benefit for many of these approaches in the treatment of pain. A systematic review by the Agency for Healthcare Research and Quality noted that exercise, multidisciplinary rehabilitation, acupuncture, CBT, and mind-body practices are consistently associated with durable slight to moderate improvements in function and pain for specific chronic pain conditions.[54] Further research is needed to clarify their efficacy and role in the treatment of pain patient, especially with regard to comparative research on sustainability of effects beyond the immediate posttreatment period. In balance, the risk-benefit ratio appears favorable in incorporation of most of the complementary and integrative approaches to manage chronic nonmalignant pain syndromes at this time.

REFERENCES

1. Aggarwal BB. Targeting inflammation-induced obesity and metabolic diseases by curcumin and other nutraceuticals. *Annu Rev Nutr.* 2010;30:173−199.
2. Anheyer D, Haller H, Barth J, Lauch, Dobos G, Cramer H. Mindfulness-based stress reduction for treating low back pain: asystematic review and meta-analysis. *Ann Intern Med.* 2017;166(11):799−807.
3. Anheyer D, Klose P, Lauche R, Saha FJ, Cramer H. Yoga for treating headaches: a systematic review and meta-analysis. *J Gen Intern Med.* 2019;35(3):846−854. https://doi.org/10.1007/s11606-019-05413-9.
4. Arane K, Behboudi A, Goldman RD. Virtual reality for pain and anxiety management in children. *Can Fam Physician.* 2017;63(12):932−934.
5. Beer AM, Fey S, Zimmer M, Teske W, Schremmer D, Wiebelitz KR. Effectiveness and safety of a homeopathic drug combination in the treatment of chronic low back pain. A double-blind, randomized, placebo-controlled clinical trial. *MMW Fortschr Med.* 2012;154(Suppl 2):48−57.
6. Boehm K, Raak C, Cramer H, Lauche R, Ostermann T. Homeopathy in the treatment of fibromyalgia − a comprehensive literature-review and meta-analysis. *Compl Ther Med.* 2014;22(4):731−742.
7. Boon HS, Cherkin DC, Erro J, et al. Practice patterns of naturopathic physicians: results from a random survey of licensed practitioners in two US States. *BMC Compl Alternative Med.* 2004;4:14.
8. Bradley R, Harnett J, Cooley K, Mcintyre E, Goldenberg J, Adams J. Naturopathy as a model of prevention-oriented, patient-centered primary care: a disruptive innovation in health care. *Medicina.* 2019;55(9).
9. Carpenter JJ, Hines SH, Lan VM. Guided imagery for pain management in postoperative orthopedic patients: an integrative literature review. *J Holist Nurs.* 2017;35(4):342−351.
10. Cheng CA, Chiu YW, Wu D, Kuan YC, Chen SN, Tam KW. Effectiveness of Tai Chi on fibromyalgia patients: a meta-

analysis of randomized controlled trials. *Compl Ther Med.* 2019;46:1—8.

11. Cherkin DC, Sherman KJ, Balderson BH, et al. Effect of mindfulness-based stress reduction vs cognitive behavioral therapy or usual care on back pain and functional limitations in adults with chronic low back pain: a randomized clinical trial. *J Am Med Assoc.* 2016;315(12):1240—1249.

12. Chon TY, Mallory MJ, Yang J, Bublitz SE, Do A, Dorsher PT. Laser acupuncture: a concise review. *Med Acupunct.* 2019;31(3):164—168.

13. Dossett ML, Yeh GY. Homeopathy use in the United States and implications for public health: a review. *Homeopathy.* 2018;107(1):3—9.

14. Dunn J, Yeo E, Moghaddampour P, Chau B, Humbert S. Virtual and augmented reality in the treatment of phantom limb pain: a literature review. *Neurorehabilitation.* 2017; 40(4):595—601.

15. Ernst E. Acupuncture—a critical analysis. *J Intern Med.* 2006;259(2):125—137.

16. Ernst E. Chapter 43. A critical appraisal of complementary and alternative medicine. In: *Wall & Melzack's Textbook of Pain.* 6th ed. Saunders; 2013:603—608.

17. Fazzino DL, Griffin MT, Mcnulty RS, Fitzpatrick JJ. Energy healing and pain: a review of the literature. *Holist Nurs Pract.* 2010;24(2):79—88.

18. Ferraz GAR, Rodrigues MRK, Lima SAM, et al. Is reiki or prayer effective in relieving pain during hospitalization for cesarean? A systematic review and meta-analysis of randomized controlled trials. *Sao Paulo Med J.* 2017;135(2): 123—132.

19. Franke H, Franke JD, Fryer G. Osteopathic manipulative treatment for nonspecific low back pain: a systematic review and meta-analysis. *BMC Muscoskel Disord.* 2014;15:286.

20. Fryer G. Somatic dysfunction: an osteopathic conundrum. *Int J Osteopath Med.* 2016;22:52—63.

21. Furlan AD, Giraldo M, Baskwill A, Irvin E, Imamura M. Massage for low-back pain. *Cochrane Database Syst Rev.* 2015;9:CD001929.

22. Giacobbi PR, Stabler ME, Stewart J, Jaeschke AM, Siebert JL, Kelley GA. Guided imagery for arthritis and other rheumatic diseases: asystematic review of randomized controlled trials. *Pain Manag Nurs.* 2015;16(5):792—803.

23. Groessl EJ, Liu L, Chang DG, et al. Yoga for military veterans with chronic low back pain: a randomized clinical trial. *Am J Prev Med.* 2017;53(5):599—608.

24. Hall A, Copsey B, Richmond H, et al. Effectiveness of Tai chi for chronic musculoskeletal pain conditions: updated systematic review and meta-analysis. *Phys Ther.* 2017; 97(2):227—238.

25. Jang JC, Jung J, Lee H, Park YB, Kim H. Multidimensional aspects of sensations in MASS and ASQ assessment: a Pilot study. *Evid Base Compl Alternative Med.* 2017;2017: 6249329.

26. Jones J, Thomson P, Irvine K, Leslie SJ. Is there a specific hemodynamic effect in reflexology? A systematic review of randomized controlled trials. *J Alternative Compl Med.* 2013;19(4):319—328.

27. Kern C, Mccoart A, Beltranm T, Martoszek M. The benefits of reflexology for the chronic pain patient in a military pain clinic. *J Spec Oper Med.* 2018;18(4):103—105.

28. Kessler CS, Dhiman KS, Kumar A, et al. Effectiveness of an ayurveda treatemnt approach in knee osteoarthritis — a randomized controlled trial. *Osteoarthritis Cartilage.* 2018; 26(5):620—630.

29. Kim J, Kim SR, Lee H, Nam DH. Comparing verum and sham acupuncture in fibromyalgia syndrome: a systematic review and meta-analysis. *Evid Base Compl Alternative Med.* 2019:8757683.

30. Kong LJ, Lauche R, Klose P, et al. Tai chi for chronic pain conditions: a systematic review and meta-analysis of randomized controlled trials. *Sci Rep.* 2016;6:25325.

31. Lachance CC, McCormack S. *Mindfulness Training and Yoga for the Management of Chronic Non-malignant Pain: A Review of Clinical Effectiveness and Cost-Effectiveness.* CADTH Rapid Response Reports. Canadian Agency for Drugs and Technologies in Health; September 2019.

32. Lauche R, Hunter DJ, Adams J, Cramer H. Yoga for osteoarthritis: a systematic review and meta-analysis. *Curr Rheumatol Rep.* 2019;21(9):47.

33. Lee MS, Lee HW, Khalil M, Lim HS, Lim HJ. Aromatherapy for managing pain in primary dysmenorrhea: a systematic review of randomized placebo-controlled trials. *J Clin Med.* 2018;7(11).

34. Lim SM, Lee SH. Effectiveness of bee venom acupuncture in alleviating post-stroke shoulder pain: a systematic review and meta-analysis. *J Integr Med.* 2015;13(4):241—247.

35. Mallari B, Spaeth EK, Goh H, Boyd BS. Virtual reality as an analgesic for acute and chronic pain in adults: a systematic review and meta-analysis. *J Pain Res.* 2019;12:2053—2085.

36. Macfarlane GJ, Kronisch C, Dean LE, et al. EULAR revised recommendations for the management of fibromyalgia. *Ann Rheum Dis.* 2017;76(2):318—328.

37. McNair C, Yeo MC, Johnston C, Taddio A. Nonpharmacologic management of pain during common needle puncture procedures in infants: current research evidence and practical considerations: an update. *Clin Perinatol.* 2019; 46(4):709—730.

38. Meints SM, Mosher C, Rand KL, Ashburn-nardo L, Hirsh AT. An experimental investigation of the relationships among race, prayer, and pain. *Scand J Pain.* 2018; 18(3):545—553.

39. Mirtz TA, Morgan L, Wyatt LH, Greene L. An epidemiological examination of the subluxation construct using Hill's criteria of causation. *Chiropr Osteopathy.* 2009;17:13.

40. Morris M, Pellow J, Solomon EM, Tsele-tebakang T. Physiotherapy and a homeopathic complex for chronic low-back pain due to osteoarthritis: a randomized, controlled pilot study. *Alternative Ther Health Med.* 2016;22(1):48—56.

41. Nelson NL, Churilla JR. Massage therapy for pain and function in patients with arthritis: a systematic review of randomized controlled trials. *Am J Phys Med Rehabil.* 2017;96(9):665—672.

42. NIH Press Release. https://nccih.nih.gov/news/press/ 12172014. Accessed 17 June 2019.

43. NIH Press Release. https://nccih.nih.gov/about/budget/appropriations.htm. Accessed 17 June 2019.

44. Nolting MH. Chapter 31. Acupuncture. In: *Pizzorno JE and Murray MT. Textbook of Natural Medicine.* 4th ed. Churchill Livingstone; 2013:242−247.

45. Orrock PJ, Myers SP. Osteopathic intervention in chronic non-specific low back pain: a systematic review. *BMC Muscoskel Disord.* 2013;14:129.

46. Patel P, Ivanov D, Bhatt S, et al. Low-cost virtual reality headsets reduce perceived pain in healthy adults: amulticenter randomized crossover trial. *Game Health J.* 2019.

47. Physicians AAoN. *Regulated States & Regulatory Authorities;* 2019. Available online:http://www.naturopathic.org/cont ent.asp?contentid=57 . Accessed October 20, 2019.

48. Posadzki P, Lewandowski W, Terry R, Ernst E, Stearns A. Guided imagery for non-musculoskeletal pain: a systematic review of randomized clinical trials. *J Pain Symptom Manag.* 2012;44(1):95−104.

49. Romeyke T, Nohammer E, Scheuer HC, Stummer H. Integration of naturopathic medicine into acute inpatient care: an approach for patient-centred medicine under diagnosis-related groups. *Compl Ther Clin Pract.* 2017;28:9−17.

50. Saper RB, Lemaster C, Delitto A, et al. Yoga, physical therapy, or education for chronic low back pain: a randomized noninferiority trial. *Ann Intern Med.* 2017;167(2):85−94.

51. Semwal DK, Chauhan A, Kumar A, Aswal S, Semwal RB, Kumar A. Status of Indian medicinal plants in the international union for conservation of nature and the future of ayurvedic drugs: shouldn't think about ayurvedic fundamentals? *J Integr Med.* 2019;17(4):238−243.

52. Senel E. Evolution of homeopathy: a scientometric analysis of global homeopathy literature between 1975 and 2017. *Compl Ther Clin Pract.* 2019;34:165−173.

53. Singh H, Bhushan S, Arora R, Singh Buttar H, Arora S, Singh B. Alternative treatment strategies for neuropathic pain: role of Indian medicinal plants and compounds of plant origin-a review. *Biomed Pharmacother.* 2017;92:634−650.

54. Skelly AC, Chou R, Dettori JR, et al. *Noninvasive Nonpharmacological Treatment for Chronic Pain: A Systematic Review.* Rockville (MD): Agency for Healthcare Research and Quality (US); June 2018. Report No.: 18-EHC013-EF.

55. Sodhi V. Chapter 32: Ayurveda: the science of life and mother of the healing arts. In: Pizzorno JE, Murray MT, eds. *Textbook of Natural Medicine.* 4th ed. Churchill Livingstone; 2013:248−254.

56. Smith CA, Levett KM, Collins CT, Dahlen HG, Ee CC, Suganuma M. Massage, reflexology and other manual methods for pain management in labour. *Cochrane Database Syst Rev.* 2018;3:CD009290.

57. Strahinjevich B, Simpson JK. The schism in chiropractic through the eyes of a 1st year chiropractic student. *Chiropr Man Ther.* 2018;26:2.

58. Swait G, Finch R. What are the risks of manual treatment of the spine? A scoping review for clinicians. *Chiropr Man Ther.* 2017;25:37.

59. Tamer S, Öz M, Ülger Ö. The effect of visceral osteopathic manual therapy applications on pain, quality of life and function in patients with chronic nonspecific low back pain. *J Back Musculoskelet Rehabil.* 2017;30(3):419−425.

60. Task Force on the Low Back Pain Clinical Practice Guidelines. American osteopathic association guidelines for osteopathic manipulative treatment (OMT) for patients with low back pain. *J Am Osteopath Assoc.* 2016;116(8):536−549.

61. Thrane SE, Hsieh K, Donahue P, Tan A, Exline MC, Balas MC. Could complementary health approaches improve the symptom experience and outcomes of critically ill adults? A systematic review of randomized controlled trials. *Compl Ther Med.* 2019;47:102166.

62. Trinh K, Graham N, Irnich D, Cameron ID, Forget M. Acupuncture for neck disorders. *Cochrane Database Syst Rev.* 2016;5:CD004870.

63. Vickers AJ, Vertosick EA, Lewith G, et al. Acupuncture for chronic pain: update of an individual patient data meta-analysis. *J Pain.* 2018;19(5):455−474.

64. Virk JK, Gupta V, Kumar S, Singh R, Bansal P. Ashtawarga plants −suffering a triple standardization syndrome. *J Tradit Complement Med.* 2017;7(4):392−399.

65. Walker BF, French SD, Grant W, Green S. A Cochrane review of combined chiropractic interventions for low-back pain. *Spine.* 2011;36(3):230−242.

66. Walkowski S, Baker R. Chapter 18: Osteopathic manipulative medicine: afunctional approach to pain. In: *Pain Procedures in Clinical Practice.* 3rd ed. Elsevier; 2011:155−171.

67. Wang CC, Li K, Choudhury A, Gaylord S. Trends in yoga, Tai chi, and Qigong use among US adults, 2002−2017. *Am J Publ Health.* 2019;109(5):755−761.

68. Whalen J, Yao S, Leder A. A short review of the treatment of headaches using osteopathic manipulative treatment. *Curr Pain Headache Rep.* 2018;22(12):82.

69. White A, Ernst E. A brief history of acupuncture. *Rheumatology.* 2004;43(5):662−663.

70. Wieland LS, Skoetz N, Pilkington K, Vempati R, D'adamo CR, Berman BM. Yoga treatment for chronic non-specific low back pain. *Cochrane Database Syst Rev.* 2017;1:CD010671.

71. Witt CM, Pach D, Brinkhaus B, et al. Safety of acupuncture: results of a prospective observational study with 229,230 patients and introduction of a medical information and consent form. *Forsch Komplementmed.* 2009;16(2):91−97.

72. Wu J, Lv M, Zhou Y. Efficacy and side effect of curcumin for the treatment of osteoarthritis: a meta-analysis of randomized controlled trials. *Pak J Pharm Sci.* 2019;32(1):43−51.

73. Zou L, Wang H, Xiao Z, et al. Tai chi for health benefits in patients with multiple sclerosis: a systematic review. *PloS One.* 2017;12(2):e0170212.

74. Zou L, Zhang Y, Yang L, et al. Are mindful exercises safe and beneficial for treating chronic lower back pain? A systematic review and meta-analysis of randomized controlled trials. *J Clin Med.* 2019;8(5).

75. Blanchette MA, Stochkendahl MJ, et al. Effectiveness and economic evaluation of chiropractic care for the treatment of low back pain: a systematic review of pragmatic studies. *PLoS ONE.* 2016;11(8):e0160037.

CHAPTER 9

Pain and Addiction

ILENE ROBECK, BA, MD* • STEPHEN A. MUDRA, MD*

INTRODUCTION

Increased utilization of opioids for chronic pain started in the late 1990s. Although evidence of long-term benefit was never documented, opioids were recommended, often as a first-line therapy, and titrated to high doses with no upper dose limits suggested. However, opioid efficacy for pain has failed to demonstrate long-term analgesia or functional improvements. Many patients who have been managed with high dose opioid regimens were impaired by side effects including sedation, dizziness, nausea, vomiting, constipation, physical dependence, tolerance, and respiratory depression.[1] Multiple studies have shown that opioid treatment results in decreased functional outcomes.[2,3] A randomized controlled trial published in 2018 demonstrated treatment with opioids was not superior to treatment with nonopioid medications for improving pain-related function over 12 months.[4]

Currently, there is an epidemic of drug abuse and mortality associated with prescription opioid use. Prescription drug misuse is also a leading source for all-cause and unintentional death.[5,6.] In fact, there were approximately 72,000 drug overdose deaths in 2017, two-thirds (47,600) of which were related to opioids.[7] A large number of patients on long-term opioids have preexisting substance use disorders and/or psychiatric disease further complicating management.[8,9] As the opioid overdose crisis unfolds, it has become clear that the development of opioid use disorder (OUD) from prescription opioids is very common. In one study, the lifetime prevalence of OUD among patients receiving long-term opioid therapy was 41.3%. In that study the best predictors were age <65 years, current pain impairment, trouble sleeping, suicidal thoughts, anxiety disorders, illicit drug use, and history of substance abuse treatment.[10] The CDC has predicted 25% of all patients on long-term opioid therapy have OUD. The risk of developing OUD is related to dose and duration of therapy.[11]

Other addictive substances such as alcohol, marijuana, cocaine, kratom, and vaping also increase the risk of pain due to increased risk of accidents, falls, mental health complications, medical comorbidities, withdrawal symptoms, negative impact on neurotransmitters involved in the reward system (endorphins, dopamine, serotonin, and norepinephrine), sympathetic arousal, and sleep disorders. These substances on the brain interfere with sleep, decision-making, learning, and memory. Like opioids, dependence and addiction to these substances occur even if they were prescribed and/or used by patients to help with painful symptoms.[12-15]

DEFINITIONS

It is helpful to look at the current definition of addiction to understand how this impacts our ability to formulate an effective treatment approach (Table 9.1).

The American Society of Addiction Medicine (ASAM) maintains that addiction is a treatable, chronic medical disease involving complex interactions among brain circuits, genetics, the environment, and an individual's life experiences. They state that people with addiction disorders use substances or engage in behaviors that become compulsive and often continue them despite harmful consequences. Prevention efforts and treatment approaches for addiction are generally as successful as those for other chronic diseases. (ASAM)

The terms addiction and substance abuse are often used interchangeably. However, the latest version of the Diagnostic and Statistical Manual of Mental Disorders (DSM-5) released in 2013 combined "substance abuse" and "substance dependence" as "substance use disorder." This is now the preferred terminology.

- In order to be diagnosed with Substance Use Disorder, the patient must meet at least 2 of the 11 criteria for the diagnosis

---

*Board Certified in Internal Medicine and Addiction Medicine

Pain Care Essentials and Innovations. https://doi.org/10.1016/B978-0-323-72216-2.00009-0

TABLE 9.1
DSM-5 Diagnostic Criteria for OUD and Example Behaviors.

TABLE1. DSM-5 DIAGNOSTIC CRITERIA FOR OUD[A] AND EXAMPLE BEHAVIORS

DSM-5 Criteria	Example Behaviors
• Craving or strong desire or urge to use opioids	Describes constantly thinking about/needing the opioid
• Recurrent use in situations that are physically hazardous	Unwilling to cut down or discontinue opioid use despite having a job where taking an opioid is dangerous (e.g., truck driver)
• Tolerance	Needing to take more and more to achieve the same effect (asking for ↑ dose without worsened pain)
• Withdrawal (or opioids are taken to relieve or avoid withdrawal)	Feeling sick if opioid is not taken on time or exhibiting withdrawal effects (see QRD on withdrawal signs/symptoms)
• Using larger amounts of opioids or over a longer period than initially intended	Taking more than prescribed (e.g., repeated requests for early refills)
• Persisting desire or unable to cut down on or control opioid use	Has tried to reduce dose or quit opioid because of family's concerns about use but has been unable to
• Spending a lot of time to obtain, use, or recover from opioids	Driving to different doctor's offices every month to get renewals for various opioid prescriptions
• Continued opioid use despite persistent or recurrent social or interpersonal problems related to opioids	Spouse or family member worried or critical about patient's opioid use
• Continued use despite physical or psychological problems related to opioids	Unwilling to discontinue or reduce opioid use despite nonfatal accidental overdose
• Failure to fulfill obligations at work, school, or home due to use	Not finishing tasks at work due to taking frequent breaks to take opioid; getting fired from jobs

TABLE 9.1
DSM-5 Diagnostic Criteria for OUD and Example Behaviors.—cont'd

TABLE1. DSM-5 DIAGNOSTIC CRITERIA FOR OUD[A] AND EXAMPLE BEHAVIORS

DSM-5 Criteria	Example Behaviors
• Activities are given up or reduced because of use	No longer participating in weekly softball league despite no additional injury or reason for additional pain

[a] OUD DSM-5 diagnostic criteria: A problematic pattern of opioid use leading to clinically significant impairment or distress, as manifested by at least 2 of the symptoms in the table above, occurring within a 12-month period.
*VA Academic Detailing. **Tolerance and withdrawal criterion are not used for individuals taking opioids solely under appropriate medical supervision, and taking the opioid medication as directed.
Courtesy of VA PBM Academic Detailing service.

• A patient meeting 2—3 of the criteria indicates mild substance use disorder, meeting 4—5 criteria indicates moderate, and 6—7 indicates severe

The unifying features of both definitions are the individual impacted continues to use medications or substances despite significant consequences. These consequences can be related to medical (including mental health) and/or psychosocial deterioration in the ability to function. It is common that these terms are used interchangeably for the disease in which an individual exhibits an inability to stop behaviors or use of substances or medications despite significant deterioration of function. Medications or substances at high risk for users developing problems related to dependence or abuse impact the brain's reward center. Substance use problems are common medical problems; however, patients will frequently go undiagnosed and untreated. In 2017, nearly 21 million Americans needed treatment for SUD but only 4 million reported receiving any form of SUD treatment or ancillary services.[15,17]

PATHOPHYSIOLOGY

The reward center, also called the mesolimbic dopamine pathway, connects the ventral tegmental area (one of the primary dopamine producing areas in the brain) with the nucleus accumbens (the area of the brain associated with reward and motivation) and the prefrontal cortex. This system provides reward for behaviors necessary for survival of the individual and the species such as food, water, nurturing, and sex. In individuals who are addicted, the drug, substance, or behavior becomes substituted for the behaviors necessary for survival and the ability to function. One of the factors driving this change is the impact on the dopaminergic reward system.[15]

Vulnerability to developing addiction is multifactorial. This vulnerability is estimated to be 40%−60% genetic as well as associated with environmental factors related to exposure, availability, and psychosocial support. Exposure of addictive substances to the developing brain has also raised concerns over increased risk of addiction in those under 30 years of age. Medical and mental health comorbidities can also increase the risk of addiction. In addition, over the past several decades there has been increasing exposure due to medical use of opioids, benzodiazepines, and stimulants.[15,17,18]

BARRIERS TO TREATMENT

While there are many reasons for continued use despite harm, the influence of acute and protracted withdrawal has a profound impact on the development and persistence of chronic pain and addiction. Acute withdrawal usually lasts for days and produces the opposite effect of the drug or medication taken. Protracted withdrawal from drugs or medications can last months and can create or exacerbate many chronic pain problems through the development of sleeping difficulty, anxiety, depression, difficulty thinking, generalized pain, and decline in function.[13,17]

In a recent review of barriers and best practices related to SUD treatment, a key recommendation was "Co-location of SUD counseling and other services with primary care reduces the stigma of accessing a facility identified as treating SUDs, catches members in locations where they are more comfortable, and permits improved coordination between physical and behavioral health care." There are many reasons for the underdiagnosis of substance use disorders which need to be addressed, especially when evaluating chronic pain patients who may have the potential for substance use or misuse[19] Table 9.2.

ASSESSMENT

Screening questionnaires:

There are many screening tools to assess for substance use disorder. In a busy practice, it can be helpful to utilize the NIDA Quick Screening Tool available at https://www.drugabuse.gov/sites/default/files/pdf/nmassist.pdf.

This tool asks about unhealthy alcohol use, nicotine use, nonmedical use of prescription medications, and use of illicit drugs in the past year. A positive response can then be followed up with further questions about recent use of specific drugs and medications. History and physical can help determine if there has been deterioration in ability to function, medical problems related to substances or psychiatric symptoms related to substance or medication misuse.[15]

Urine Drug Testing

Urine drug testing can help understand what substances and medications a patient is taking and the potential impact on their health. It is, however, important to approach testing in a nonjudgmental manner with patients. It is also important to review with the patient that drug testing is done to improve safety and prevent future complications. Most drug screening is done through radioimmunoassay. This is less expensive and

---

TABLE 9.2
Reasons for Underdiagnosis of Substance Abuse.

1 There is a great deal of stigma associated with a substance use disorder (SUD) diagnosis on the part of patients as well as healthcare professionals

2 One of the hallmarks of this disease is denial of problems as the brain is impacted by this disease in a way that affects memory, judgement and decision-making

3 The personal and societal impact of an SUD diagnosis can be significant, leading to attempts to cover up problems and avoid diagnosing them even when apparent

4 When legal substances or medications are the cause of the problem, it can be difficult to understand when use becomes misuse

5 Treatment options can be limited for many patients leading to a therapeutic dilemma even when the diagnosis is made

faster than gas chromatography, which is typically used as a confirmatory test when there are unexplainable results or potential false positives and negatives. Whenever there is a concern about test discrepancy, it is important to discuss unexpected results with the lab.[18,20–22]

In primary care and pain clinic settings, observed urine drug screens are impractical and often unnecessary. However, when obtained, it may be helpful to check the validity of the urine sample by looking at creatinine, specific gravity, PH, and temperature (within 4 min of obtaining a specimen). A diluted specimen will have a creatinine less than 20 mg/dL and a specific gravity between 1.001 and 1.003. An adulterated specimen may have a PH less than 3 or greater than 11 or an unexplained urinary nitrate. Urinary temperatures less than 90 or over 100 can indicate an attempt to substitute a urine. It is also important to know typical detection times of the substances that are being tested. The substance with the shortest detection time is alcohol with a detection time of 7–12 h from last use. The substance with the longest detection time is chronic heavy use of cannabinoids with detection times that can last longer than 30 days.[18,20–22]

Prescription Drug Monitoring Program
Querying the prescription drug monitoring program (PDMP) available in participating states can also be an important part of an assessment for substance use disorder. It can provide helpful information such as the type and number of controlled medications that are prescribed, the number of prescribers, and the presence of overlapping prescriptions. Like urine drug screens, information obtained when checking the PDMP should be used to improve patient safety and education when seeing patients with chronic pain at risk of addiction.[17,18]

The understanding of addictive substances and medications is changing rapidly. There are a number of government websites that can help to keep clinicians up to date related to emerging drugs, impact on health, and treatment options. Table 9.3 outline the various websites available for more information.

MANAGEMENT
Treatment options for patients with pain and addiction can be highly successful when key concepts are kept in mind. As with all patients with chronic pain, effective pain care involves attention to modalities that improve movement, address cognitive behavioral approaches to pain, treat comorbidities, and address lifestyle changes.

TABLE 9.3
Additional Resources.

Organization	website
NIDA (National Institute on Drug Abuse)	www.drugabuse.gov
SAMHSA (Substance Abuse and Mental Health Services Administration)	www.samhsa.gov
CDC (Centers for Disease Control and Prevention)	www.cdc.gov
FDA (Food and Drug Administration)	www.fda.gov
Opioids.gov: US Department of Health and Human Services	www.opioids.gov
Office of the US Surgeon General	www.hhs.gov/surgeongeneral/index.html
NIAAA (National Institute of Alcohol Abuse and Alcoholism)	www.niaaa.nih.gov
US Department of Veterans Affairs	www.va.gov

These functional restoration approaches are core elements to treating both of these medical conditions. It is important to understand that treating pain and addiction in an integrated way allows for a more effective approach than treating each disorder in isolation.[13,14,23]

Addiction treatment is best individualized to meet the needs of the patient. It can also include family treatment options as well. When working with patients who have chronic pain, it is very helpful to familiarize yourself with treatment opportunities in your community and work together when pain and addiction treatment are not available in a unified clinic. Key components of behavioral approaches to addiction treatment can include strategies to modify attitudes and behaviors related to drug use, increase healthy lifestyles, setting and working toward goals to improve function, and learning coping skills related to stress and challenges that can be utilized rather than drugs.[15,17]

Behavioral Interventions
Motivational Interviewing can be a useful tool to elicit behavioral changes related to both pain and addiction. It is person-centered and allows for discussion that evokes the motivation for change. It is the engagement

in dialogue that ultimately improves involvement in and success with treatment. While there are many strategies related to this approach, key concepts include expressing empathy, avoiding arguments and confrontations, developing discrepancies between goals and current behavior, adjusting to resistance, and supporting self-efficacy. These concepts have now been shown to improve behavioral changes related to many chronic diseases.[17]

There is also increasing evidence that contingency management (CM) interventions can be effective adjuncts to care in SUD programs. CM involves providing tangible rewards for abstinence and remaining in treatment. In Voucher-Based Reinforcement treatment, vouchers are given for each urine that is negative for illicit substances or unprescribed medication. The longer the duration of negative urines, the higher the value of the voucher. Vouchers can then be exchanged for a variety of rewards. Prize Incentive CM uses the chance of winning cash prizes instead of vouchers.[15,23]

It is also important to integrate primary care into pain and addiction care as many comorbid medical conditions can also interfere with success. This can include optimizing treatment for underlying lung disease, heart disease, endocrinologic problems such as diabetes and thyroid disease, infectious diseases such as HIV disease and hepatitis C, and neurologic problems related to trauma or underlying neurologic disorders. Poor health in general will worsen chronic pain and a whole person approach is important for success.

In addition, self-help groups can be invaluable for many patients with addiction problems. While not for every patient, self-help groups can provide structure, goal-directed models for recovery, improve coping skills, and increase options for rewarding activities. They can also be an important resource for family, friends, and significant others.[17,24–26]

The most common self-help programs are 12-step groups. The programs were originally proposed by Alcoholic Anonymous (AA) as a method of recovery from alcoholism but have now been adapted to include programs for all drug and behavioral addictions (Table 9.4). The programs are organized around local groups where people meet to support each other and work through the 12 steps. Meetings are free, noncommercial, and open to anyone impacted by addiction. Some meetings are open to anyone interested in learning more such as healthcare professionals or community members. 12-step programs are available throughout the United States and internationally making meeting attendance possible during times of travel or relocation.

TABLE 9.4
The 12 Steps of Alcoholics Anonymous.

The following are the Original Twelve Steps as Published by Alcoholics Anonymous:[11]

1 We admitted we were powerless over alcohol—that our lives had become unmanageable.

2 Came to believe that a power greater than ourselves could restore us to sanity.

3 Made a decision to turn our will and our lives over to the care of God *as we understood Him.*

4 Made a searching and fearless moral inventory of ourselves.

5 Admitted to God, to us, and to another human being the exact nature of our wrongs.

6 Were entirely ready to have God remove all these defects of character.

7 Humbly asked Him to remove our shortcomings.

8 Made a list of all persons we had harmed and became willing to make amends to them all.

9 Made direct amends to such people wherever possible, except when to do so would injure them or others.

10 Continued to take personal inventory, and when we were wrong, promptly admitted it.

11 Sought through prayer and meditation to improve our conscious contact with God *as we understood Him,* praying only for knowledge of His will for us and the power to carry that out.

12 Having had a spiritual awakening as the result of these steps, we tried to carry this message to alcoholics, and to practice these principles in all our affairs.

Medication-Assisted Therapy

Treating addiction may require use of medications in some circumstances, especially when OUD is diagnosed.[27]

In addition to counseling, self-help therapy, and behavioral therapy, various medications have been used in the treatment of alcohol addiction and nicotine addiction. Common medications that are used for alcohol addiction include disulfiram, naltrexone, acamprosate, and topiramate. Those used for nicotine addiction include nicotine replacement therapy (nasal inhaler, gum, transdermal patch, etc.), varenicline, and bupropion.

While OUD can benefit from counseling and behavioral therapy, there is a high relapse rate without the use of replacement medication. OUD can be effectively treated with 3 different medications. Buprenorphine

(a partial agonist at the mu receptor), methadone (a full agonist at the mu receptor), and naltrexone (an antagonist at the mu receptor) (Table 9.5). Medication-assisted treatment (MAT) for OUD has been shown to decrease fatal overdoses, increase retention in treatment, and improve social functioning with all three agents.[28-33]

Methadone must be provided by a federally licensed methadone clinic when used for OUD. This is a highly structured, supervised setting where the patient may be required to come daily for his/her methadone dose. Methadone can be dosed once per day and is a good option if the patient has failed treatment with a partial agonist (buprenorphine) or antagonist (IM naltrexone).

Buprenorphine can be provided in an outpatient, office-based setting and has an improved safety profile compared with methadone. The outcomes of

TABLE 9.5
Opioid Use Disorder Medications in the United States[40].

Available as	Dosage (mg)	Induction Dosing (mg)	Recommended Dosing Range for Stabilization/Maintenance (mg)
METHADONE (HCL ORAL CONCENTRATE, PER ML)			
Generic	5, 10	5—10 every 4 h up to 40 in the first 24 h.	Gradual titration with close monitoring over 2 weeks to 60—120 daily; rapid metabolizers may require higher dosing
Methadone	10		
Methadone sugar-free	10		
Methadone HCL Intensol	10		
BUPRENORPHINE + NALOXONE			
Sublingual tablet			
Generic	2/0.5, 8/2	2/0.5—4/1; repeat up to 16/4 in the first 24 h.	4/1—24/6 daily
Zubsolv	1.4/0.36, 5.7/1.4	1.4/0.36—2.8/0.72; repeat up to 11.4/2.8 in the first 24 h.	2.8/0.72—17.1/4.2 daily
Suboxone Film (sublingual film)	2/0.5, 4/1, 8/2, 12/3	2/0.5—4/1; repeat up to 16/4 in the first 24 h.	4/1—24/6 daily
Bunavail (buccal film)	2.1/0.3, 4.2/0.7, 6.3/1	2.1/0.3; repeat up to 8.4/1.4 in the first 24 h	2.1/0.3—12.6/2.1 daily
BUPRENORPHINE			
Sublingual tablet (generic only)	2, 8	2—4; up to 16 in the first 24 h.	4—24 daily
NALTREXONE ER (USED IF PRETREATMENT ABSTINENCE AND NO SIGNS OF WITHDRAWAL AND WILLINGNESS TO RECEIVE MONTHLY INJECTIONS)			
Vivitrol	380	380 IM following agonist clearance; oral naltrexone 50 mg daily may precede or supplement initial induction.	380 IM every 4 weeks; oral naltrexone may be added to supplement in weeks 3—4 as needed

buprenorphine used at fixed doses above 7 mg/day were not different than methadone prescribed at 40 mg or more per day in retaining people in treatment or in suppression of illicit opioid use.[41] MAT with buprenorphine is effective with or without intensive psychosocial intervention.

The combination of buprenorphine/naloxone was developed to decrease IV misuse. There is minimal bioavailability of naloxone if used orally but the naloxone can precipitate withdrawal if injected by a current opioid user. Since concurrent use of the benzodiazepine class of medications increases risk for adverse event, efforts should be made for patients to taper off benzodiazepines prior to initiating treatment as well as abstaining from alcohol while receiving treatment with buprenorphine or methadone.[34]

Naltrexone (380 mg monthly depot injection) has no addictive potential or diversion risk and can be provided in an office-based setting. Oral naltrexone is not recommended for treatment of OUD due to the risk of nonadherence which can lead to relapse and potential overdose. Naltrexone treatment can present a challenge since patients must be off all opioids for 7–10 days before starting IM naltrexone to avoid precipitation of withdrawal.

Ongoing treatment with MAT is effective at improving retention in treatment and decreasing use of illicit opioids. In contrast, short-term treatment where MAT is tapered after a brief period of stabilization has not proven to be effective. The high relapse rate for opioid addiction, up to 90% if not treated with MAT[35], suggests that opioid maintenance therapy will play an increasing role in the future as patients are transitioned to safer medication regimens and those with OUD or opioid dependence identified.

Special Populations

There are unique needs of many special populations with substance use disorders and pain. While all care should be individualized, there can be distinctive needs that improve outcomes when addressed. While addressing the many populations that will benefit from individualizing treatment options, three special populations will be addressed in this chapter—women, veterans, and older patients.

There are a number of gender differences to consider when caring for patients with substance use disorder. Women may have different responses to many drugs and medications than men. In addition, women of childbearing age have added risks related to the impact of drugs and medications during pregnancy and postpartum on themselves, the fetus, and their children. Many women will experience difficulty with substance use more quickly and at lower doses of medications. Women are more likely to have been victims of domestic violence and often have to address childcare difficulties that may also pose barriers to treatment. In addition, early SUD research was conducted on males more than females, though there is a growing body of literature improving our understanding of the impact of drugs and medications on women.[15,17,36,37]

Veterans have increased risk of substance use disorder as well as pain-related problems compared with nonveterans. Alcohol and nicotine remain the substances most frequently misused, with marijuana the most commonly used illicit drug. In addition, mental health comorbidities such as post-traumatic stress disorder (PTSD) and depression increase the risk of suicide in veterans, especially when substance use disorder problems are not adequately addressed. Homelessness is also a problem for veterans with substance use disorder and/or mental health concerns. Fortunately, there are many programs at VA facilities to address SUD concerns requiring all who care for veterans to be knowledgeable about what is available in their community.

It is also common for clinicians to minimize the impact of substances and medications with potential for abuse in older patients. However, in a survey by SAMHSA of 2.2 million patients 50 and older, 54% had used marijuana, 28% had misused prescription drugs, and 17% had used other illicit drug(s). "Baby Boomers" had less hesitation about using substances recreationally and for coping with the aging process than older generations. Alcohol is the drug of choice for older adults but patients over 50 have lower tolerance for alcohol and an increased risk for prescription and over-the-counter medication interactions. In fact, more patients over 65 were admitted to the hospital for alcohol problems than for myocardial infarctions.[17,38.]

IMPACT OF USE, ABUSE, AND DEPENDENCE OF SPECIFIC DRUGS AND MEDICATIONS

While there are many commonalities related to pain and substance use in general, specific medications and substances have a defined impact on the development and perpetuation of chronic pain as well as treatment options.

Alcohol

Prolonged use of alcohol can cause primary painful problems related to the direct effect of alcohol. The dose needed for this impact is variable from individual to individual and related to gender (with women more susceptible at lower doses than men), genetics, and comorbidities. The pain-related problems most often associated directly to alcohol are alcohol neuropathy, myopathy, sleep disturbances, and abdominal pain (due to pancreatitis, gastritis, and/or hepatomegaly).[39,40]

In addition, patients may attempt to use alcohol to treat painful symptoms which can provide transient success but result in worsening pain over time. The dose of alcohol needed, even for transient improvement in pain symptoms, is higher than current guidelines and can result in further alcohol-related problems.[41]

Alcohol also increases risks of using other medications for pain when combined with NSAIDS, acetaminophen, and opioids as well as other sedating medications. 42% of current drinkers reported using medication that were classified as AI (Alcohol Interactive) prescription drugs. There are over 600 medications that interact with alcohol, including those needed for common chronic diseases such as hypertension, depression, and diabetes.[14]

The negative impact of even small doses of alcohol on sleep and its impact on pain cannot be overemphasized. Alcohol interferes with sleep cycles, may worsen sleep disordered breathing, and interacts with many medications utilized for sleep.[39]

Marijuana

Studies related to the benefits of marijuana and pain are varied. The current challenges of studying risk versus benefit are related to changing and inconsistent levels of tetrahydrocannabinol (THC) and cannabidiol (CBD) as well as other components of the marijuana plant, differentiating the impact of low dose versus high dose and differentiating the impact of acute, intermittent, and chronic daily use. More studies are needed to determine if long-term use of marijuana is an effective treatment for chronic pain and if so, the best dose and THC/CBD concentrations.[15,42–44]

There are marijuana receptors ubiquitously distributed throughout the brain and the periphery. Cannabinoid type 1 (CB1) receptors are concentrated in the hippocampus, amygdala, basal ganglia, cerebellum, nucleus accumbens, and cerebral cortex (anterior > posterior). Cannabinoid type 2 (CB2) receptors are primarily located in the periphery. This system is responsible for multiple functions that include learning and memory, appetite, anxiety, and fear as well as movement. There is also a well-recognized withdrawal syndrome associated with marijuana that can worsen painful symptoms. This includes irritability, depression,

anxiety, sleep difficulty, decreased appetite, restlessness, cognitive decline, abdominal pain, tremors, and sweating. This can confound treatment for patients with chronic pain.[15]

The impact of marijuana use has raised concerns due to the increasing potency of recreational and illicit marijuana which has been found to increase side effects and the risk of developing cannabis use disorder.[42,45–47] Another concern related to marijuana use, including medical marijuana, is the increasing incidence of driving while under the influence of marijuana and associated increase in motor vehicle accidents. In one study published in 2019 interviews with 790 adults with chronic pain seeking medical cannabis certification or recertification revealed that 56% of patients drove within 2 h of marijuana use, 53% reported driving while a little high, and 22% reported driving while very high.[48,49]

The current literature has not been able to document consistent results for treating chronic pain with cannabis. A 2018 Australian government study demonstrated that patients who used cannabis for pain had a greater pain severity score, pain interference score, and lower pain self-efficacy score as well as greater GAD scores. There was no evidence of an opioid sparing effect [50–52]. The more widespread use of marijuana has also raised concerns about medication interactions, interference with sleep, increased poison control calls, poor quality control, variable and changing doses, increased risks at the extremes of age with decreased perception of harm, risk of dependence, and SUD as well as unknowns about the impact of differing CBD/THC ratios and delivery methods.[53–55]

Nicotine

Nicotine use has been tied to worsening pain and poorer outcomes related to therapies for chronic pain. It has long been recognized that nicotine withdrawal symptoms can frequently make it difficult to stop using nicotine products. In addition, many symptoms of acute and protracted withdrawal can result in worsening pain. These include depressed mood, insomnia, irritability, anxiety, difficulty concentrating, and increased appetite leading to weight gain.[56,57]

A review of nicotine and pain revealed multiple epidemiologic studies demonstrating the negative impact of nicotine. Smokers with chronic pain complain of greater pain intensity and greater number of painful sites. Smokers with chronic LBP have greater long-term disability than nonsmokers. With the increasing use of nicotine in vaping products, taking a full nicotine history is important.[58]

VAPING

While many different substances are vaped, the process of vaping itself has come under scrutiny related to potential risks leading to lung disease. Further studies are underway to determine if health effects related to the process of vaping may also be a concern. A recent FDA alert raised concerns about the possibility of increased risk of seizures related to vaping.[15]

The increased use of vaped products has been related to the increased availability and perceived safety over other delivery methods for nicotine. As of October 15, 2019, 1479 lung injury cases of E-cigarette and Vaping Associated Lung disease (EVALI) have been reported to the CDC. Thirty-three deaths were confirmed in 24 states. All patients have reported a history of using e-cigarette, or vaping, products. THC was present in most, but not all of the samples tested by FDA to date.[18,59]

In addition to acute lung injury due to vaping, previous reports of lung injury due to chronic vaping have also been raised. The injury is attributed to the inhalation of heated chemicals, flavorings, and substances into the lungs. This liquid refill toxicity has been associated with cough, dry throat pneumonia, impaired lung function, and lipid pneumopathy.[60]

Of increasing concern has been the appeal of e-cigarettes to teenagers. Teenage use of addictive substances and medications has been associated with increased risk of addiction and pain-related problems. The Monitoring The Future (MTF) survey reported that between January 2017 and January 2018, the percentage of 12th graders who reported vaping nicotine during the past 30 days nearly doubled, from 11% to nearly 21%; among 10th graders, the increase was almost as great, from 8.2% to 16.1%. These were the biggest 1-year increases for any substance in the history of the MTF survey.[17]

The evidence for vaping as a replacement for nicotine use has not been substantiated, with most who vape continuing to use nicotine products. In addition, teens who vape demonstrate an increased risk of using cigarettes as well as vaping products in the future. When studied, E-cigarette users had a heavier conventional cigarette smoking history and worse respiratory health, were less likely to reduce or quit conventional cigarette smoking, had higher nicotine dependence, and were more likely to report chronic bronchitis and exacerbations of underlying lung disease. E-cigarette use was associated with worse pulmonary-related health outcomes, but not with cessation of smoking conventional cigarettes. In addition to nicotine, the most commonly vaped substance includes cannabinoids, kratom, amphetamines, and cocaine, as well as heroin and other opioids. Quality control in vaping shops has also been raised as a concern.[61,62]

Benzodiazepines

Benzodiazepines are frequently prescribed for patients with chronic pain and attempt address symptoms of sleep disorders and/or anxiety. The impact of chronic benzodiazepine can exacerbate pain care. This can include fatigue, cognitive concerns, dementia, depression, irritability, and worsening PTSD symptoms. Benzodiazepine use has also demonstrated increased risk of falls, worsening lung function, and increased risk of overdose along with other complications when combined with opioids, alcohol, or other sedating medications.[19,63−65]

Kratom

Kratom is a tree native to southeast Asia with psychotropic effects. Its use is currently legal in the United States, and it can be purchased on the Internet in many vape shops. Two compounds in kratom leaves, mitragynine and 7-α-hydroxymitragynine, interact with opioid receptors in the brain, producing sedation, pleasure, and decreased pain. Mitragynine can also interact with other receptor systems in the brain to produce stimulant effects.

A number of patients may use Kratom for the opioid-like pain relieving effect. Concerns have been raised, however, about the quality control related to Kratom products with deaths reported from Kratom related to contaminants. In addition, some patients will become addicted to Kratom with difficulty stopping use despite harms. Common side effects can include nausea, sweating, seizures, and psychotic symptoms. When mixed with other sedating medications or substances, side effects can become more severe.[15]

Cocaine

Cocaine is a highly addictive illicit substance that has been used medically in the past as a local anesthetic. Like all illicit substances, there is a significant risk of adulteration with impurities and other psychoactive substances. It is usually available as a powder which is snorted or injected. It can also be processed to a smokable form referred to as crack cocaine. The most common acute medical consequences of cocaine are cardiovascular effects, including disturbances in heart rhythm and heart attacks; neurological effects, including headaches, seizures, strokes, and coma; and gastrointestinal complications, including abdominal pain and nausea.[15,66]

Chronic cocaine use can lead to further difficulties that complicate pain care and negatively impact attention, impulse inhibition, memory, decision-making involving rewards or punishments, and performing motor tasks. Cocaine users will frequently mix cocaine and alcohol to produce coca ethylene. This further increases the risk of cardiovascular toxicity. Mixing cocaine and heroin can also be a deadly combination, leading to increased risk of overdose.[15,67]

Over-the-Counter Medications

There are three common over-the-counter medications that have been demonstrated to increase risks when mixed with other medications or drugs or taken in an unsafe way—dextromethorphan, loperamide, and pseudoephedrine.

Dextromethorphan is found in many cold and cough medications. When taken in large doses it can cause a depressant and/or hallucinogenic effect. Other symptoms reported with unsafe dextromethorphan use include hyperexcitability, poor motor control, lack of energy, stomach pain, vision changes, slurred speech, increased blood pressure, and sweating.

Loperamide is an antidiarrheal agent that can have an opioid-like effect when taken in large doses. It is sometimes used by patients with OUD to ameliorate withdrawal symptoms. Misuse of this medication can result in fainting, stomach pain, constipation, eye changes, loss of consciousness, arrhythmias, and renal disease.

Pseudoephedrine can be used to make methamphetamine. For this reason, these medications are sold behind the counter with limits on how much can be bought each month, even though it is available without a prescription. Signs and symptoms of misuse of pseudoephedrine products can include tachycardia, hypertension, anxiety, and sleeplessness.

Methamphetamines

Methamphetamine overdoses have been a cause for concern in the United States with recent increases in the number of overdoses when used alone or with opioids. In 2017, roughly 15% of all drug overdose deaths involved methamphetamine, and 50% of those deaths also involved an opioid, with half of those cases related to fentanyl. Methamphetamine can be smoked, swallowed, or injected. Long-term effects of methamphetamine include weight loss, severe dental problems, itching, anxiety, confusion, memory loss, difficulty sleeping, confusion, paranoia, hallucinations, and violent behavior.[15,18]

Opioids

Prescription opioid abuse has been the precursor for 80% of the heroin addiction.[67] The increase in heroin use is linked to patients who first become addicted to prescription opioids, then transition to heroin as their tolerance increases.[68] The increasing supplies of inexpensive heroin has made it more readily available and more cost-effective than prescription opioids.[69,70] In addition, counterfeit prescription pills made from more potent synthetic opioids such as Fentanyl and its analogs are even cheaper to manufacture than heroin.[71] Synthetic opioid overdose is now the largest driver of the overdose crisis.

Patients on opioids for years develop tolerance and dependence as central brain adaptations. The distinction between opioid dependence and opioid addiction is blurred in these patients.[72,73] OUD symptoms such as drug craving or inability to control the use of the drug often go unrecognized if patients continue to receive opioids. Opioid dependence, per ICD 10, is defined as the presence of three or more of the six features occurring simultaneously at any one time in the preceding year:

- A strong desire or sense of compulsion to take opioids (craving)
- Difficulties in controlling opioid use (onset, termination, or levels of use)
- A physiological withdrawal state
- Tolerance
- Progressive neglect of alternative interests because of opioid use
- Persisting with opioid use despite clear evidence of overtly harmful consequences

CONCLUSION

Over the past two decades, the treatment of chronic pain has led to an increase in opioid prescribing in the United States. This increase in prescribing has led to unintended and unexpected consequences, including the development of addiction disorders, such as OUD. Undoubtedly, social, cultural, genetic, and economic factors have influenced the rise of these medical complexities, but knowledge of behavioral interventions, medication-assisted therapies, substances of abuse, and the affected population may help reduce the risk. As our understanding of the impact of these drugs continues to expand, novel treatments may be developed to mitigate risk and improve outcomes.

REFERENCES

1. Benyamin, et al. Opioid complications and side effects. *Pain Physician*. 2008;11(2 Suppl):S105—S120.
2. Eriksen J, Sjsgren P, Bruera E, Ekholm O, Rasmussen NK, et al. Critical issues on opioids in chronic non-cancer pain: an epidemiological study. *Pain*. 2006.
3. Sjøgren P, Grønbæk M, Peuckmann V, Ekholm O. Population-based cohort study on chronic pain: the role of opioids. *Clin J Pain*. 2010;26:763.
4. Krebs E. *J Am Med Assoc*. 2018;319(9).
5. McHugh RK, Nielsen S, Weiss RD. Prescription drug abuse: from epidemiology to public policy. *J Subst Abuse Treat*. 2015;48(1):1—7. https://doi.org/10.1016/j.jsat.2014.08.004.
6. National Center for Health Statistics (US). *Health, United States, 2013: With Special Feature on Prescription Drugs*. Hyattsville (MD): National Center for Health Statistics (US); 2014. http://www.ncbi.nlm.nih.gov/books/NBK209224/.
7. https://www.cdc.gov.drugoverdose.datastatedeaths.
8. Seal KH, Shi Y, Cohen G, et al. Association of mental health disorders with prescription opioids and high-risk opioid use in US veterans of Iraq and Afghanistan. *J Am Med Assoc*. 2012;307(9):940—947. https://doi.org/10.1001/jama.2012.234.
9. 19992016. NCHS Data Brief.2017;(294):1—8 Edlund MJ, Martin BC, Devries A, Fan MY, Braden JB, Sullivan MD. Trends in use of opioids for chronic noncancer pain among individuals with mental health and substance use disorders: the TROUP study. *Clin J Pain*. 2010;26(1):1—8. https://doi.org/10.1097/AJP.0b013e3181b99f35.
10. Boscarino JA, Hoffman SN, John J. Han Substance abuse and rehabilitation 2015 Opioid-use disorder among patients on long-term opioid therapy: impact of final DSM-5 diagnostic criteria on prevalence and correlates. *Subst Abuse Rehabil*. 2015;6.
11. Edlund. *Clin J Pain*. 2014;30(7):557—564.
12. Modesto-Lowe V, Brooks D, Freedman K, Hargus E. Addiction and chronic pain: diagnostic and treatment dilemmas. *Conn Med*. 2007;71(3):139—144.
13. Larson MJ, Paasche-Orlow M, Cheng DM, et al. Persistent pain is associated with substance use after detoxification: a prospective cohort analysis. *Addiction*. 2007;102(5):752—760.
14. Manhapra, Becker. Pain and addiction an integrative therapeutic approach. *Med Clin N Am*. 2018;102:745—763.
15. National Institute on Drug Abuse, National Institutes of Health,U.S. Department of Health and Human Services.
16. VA PBM Academic Detailing Service.
17. SAMHSA — Substance Abuse Mental Health Services Administration.
18. CDC — Centers for Disease Control.
19. Tannenbaum. *J Psychiatr Neurosci*. 2015;40(3):E27—E28.
20. Raouf, et al. A practical guide to urine drug monitoring. *Fed Prac*. 2018:38—44.
21. Moeller KE, Lee KC, Kissack JC. Urine drug screening: practical guide for clinicians. *Mayo Clin Proc*. 2008;83(1):66—76.
22. Gourlay DL, Heit HA, Caplan YH. *Urine Drug Testing in Clinical Practice*. 6th ed. The Art and Science of Patient Care; August 31, 2015. https://www.remitigate.com/wp-content/up-loads/2015/11/Urine-Drug-Testing-in-Clinical-Practice-Ed6_2015-08.pdf.
23. Prendergast M, Podus D, Finney J, Greenwell L, Roll J. Contingency management for treatment of substance use disorders: a meta-analysis. *Addiction*. 2006;101(11):1546—1560.
24. Vederhus, Christensen. High effectiveness of self-help programs after drug addiction therapy. *BMC Psychiatr*. 2006;6:35.
25. Galanter M. Spirituality, evidence-based medicine, and alcoholics anonymous. *Am J Psychiatr*. 2008;165(12):1514—1517.
26. Laudet AB. The impact of alcoholics anonymous on other substance abuse-related twelve- step programs. *Recent Dev Alcohol*. 2008;18:71—89.
27. Douaihy, et al. Medications for substance use disorders. *Soc Work Publ Health*. 2013;28(0):264—278.
28. Kakko J, Svanborg KD, Kreek MJ, Heilig M. 1-year retention and social function after buprenorphine-assisted relapse prevention treatment for heroin dependence in Sweden: a randomised, placebo-controlled trial. *Lancet*. 2003;361:662—668.
29. Dupouy J, Palmaro A, Fatséas M, et al. Mortality associated with time in and out of buprenorphine treatment in French office-based general practice: a 7-year cohort study. *Ann Fam Med*. 2017;15(4):355—358.
30. Evans E, Li L, Min J, et al. Mortality among individuals accessing pharmacological treatment for opioid dependence in California, 2006—2010. *Addiction*. 2015;110(6):996—1005.
31. Hunt WA, Barnett LW, Branch LG. Relapse rates in addiction programs. *J Clin Psychol*. 1971;27(4):455—456.
32. Lee JD, Nunes Jr EV, Novo P, et al. Comparative effectiveness of extended release naltrexone versus buprenorphine-naloxone for opioid relapse prevention (X: BOT): a multicentre, open-label, randomised controlled trial. *Lancet*. 2018;391:309—318.
33. Hser Y, Saxon AJ, Huang D, et al. Treatment retention among patients randomized to buprenorphine/naloxone compared to methadone in a multi-site trial. *Addiction*. 2014;109(1):79—87.
34. Häkkinen M, Launiainen T, Vuori E, Ojanperä I. Benzodiazepines and alcohol are associated with cases of fatal buprenorphine poisoning. *Eur J Clin Pharmacol*. 2012;68(3):301—309.
35. Kakko, Svanborg, Kreek, Helig. 1 year retention and social function after Buprenorphine-assisted relapse prevention treatment for heroin dependence in Sweden: a randomized, placebo controlled trial. *Lancet*. 2003;361:662—668.

36. Hecksher, Hesse. Women and substance use disorders. *Mens Sana Monogr.* 2009;7(1):50–62.

37. American College of Obstetricians and Gynecologists (ACOG) Committee Opinion. *Opioid Use and Opioid Use Disorder in Pregnancy.*

38. Han B, Gfroerer JC, Colliver JD, Penne MA. Substance use disorder among older adults in the United States in 2020. *Addiction.* 2009;104(1):88–96. https://doi.org/10.1111/j.1360-0443.2008.

39. Obermeyer WH, Benca RM. Effects of drugs on sleep. Neurol Clin.14;827-841

40. Brower JK, Perron BE. Sleep disturbance as a universal risk factor for relapse in addictions to psychoactive substances. *Med Hypothesis.* 2010;74:928–933.

41. Brennan PL, Schutte KK, Moos RH. Pain and use of alcohol to manage pain: prevalence and 3-year outcomes among older problem and non-problem drinkers. *Addiction.* 2005;100:777–786.

42. Mehmedic Z, Chandra S, Slade D, Denham H, Foster S, Patel AS, Ross SA, Khan IA, ElSohly MA. Potency trends of Δ9-THC and other cannabinoids in confiscated cannabis preparations from 1993 to 2008. *J Forensic Sci.* 2010;55(5):1209–1217.

43. National Academies of SciencesE. *The Health Effects of Cannabis and Cannabinoids: The Current State of Evidence and Recommendations for Research;* 2017. Available from: https://www.nap.edu/catalog/24625/the-health-effects-of-cannabis-and-cannabinoids-the-current-state.

44. Ware MA, Wang T, Shapiro S, Robinson A, Ducruet T, Huynh T, Gamsa A, Bennett GJ, Collet J-P. Smoked cannabis for chronic neuropathic pain: a randomized controlled trial. *Can Med Assoc J.* 2010;182(14): E694–E701. PMCID: PMC2950205.

45. Tucker JS, Rodriguez A, Pedersen ER, Seelam R, Shih RA, D'Amico EJ. Greater risk for frequent marijuana uses and problems among young adult marijuana users with a medicalmarijuana card. *Drug Alcohol Depend.* 2019;194: 178–183.

46. Boehnke, et al. High frequency medical cannabis use is associated with worse pain among individuals with chronic pain. *J Pain.* 2019;(19):30814. pii: S1526-5900.

47. Arterberry BJ, et al. Higher national cannabis potency is associated with progression to cannabis use disorder symptoms. *Drug Alcohol Depend.* 2019;195:186–192.

48. Salomonsen-Sautel S, Min S-J, Sakai JT, Thurstone C, Hopfer C. Trends in fatal motor vehicle crashes before and after marijuana commercialization in Colorado. *Drug Alcohol Depend.* July 1, 2014;140:137–144.

49. Bonar EE, et al. Drivingunder the influence of medical cannabis. *Drug Alcohol Depend.* 2019;195:193–197.

50. Whiting PF, Wolff RF, Deshpande S, Di Nisio M, Duffy S, Hernandez AV, Keurentjes JC, Lang S, Misso K, Ryder S, Schmidlkofer S, Westwood M, Kleijnen J. Cannabinoids for medical use: asystematic review and meta-analysis. *J Am Med Assoc.* 2015;313(24):2456–2473. PMID: 26103030.

51. *Madras Update of Cannabis and its Medical Use.* Commissioned by Secretariat of the Expert Committee on Drug Dependence, Department of Essential Medicines and HealthProducts, World Health Organization.

52. Campbell, et al. Effect of cannabis use in people with chronic non-cancer pain prescribed opioids: findings from a 4-year prospective cohort study National Health and Medical Research Council and the Australian Government. *Lancet Publ Health.* 2018;3:e341–e350.

53. Atkinson, Fudin. Interactions between pain medications and illicit street drugs. *Pract Pain Manag.* 2014;14.

54. Babson, et al. Cannabis, cannabinoids, and sleep: a review of the literature. *Curr Psychiatr Rep.* 2017;19:23.

55. Whitehill, et al. Incidence of pediatric cannabis exposure among children and teenagers aged 0 to 19 years before and after medical marijuana legalization in Massachusetts. *JAMA Netw Open.* 2019;2(8):e199456.

56. Shi, et al. Smoking and pain: pathophysiology and clinical implications. *Anesthesiology.* 2010;113:977–992.

57. Mclaughlin. Nicotine withdrawal. *Curr Top BehavNeurosci.* 2015;24:99–123.

58. Ditre, et al. Pain, nicotine, and smoking: research findings and mechanistic considerations. *Psychol Bull.* 2011;137(6): 1065–1093.

59. Christiani. Vaping induced lung injury. *N Engl J Med.* 2019;382.

60. Flower, et al. Respiratory bronchiolitis-associated interstitial lung disease secondary to electronic nicotine delivery system use confirmed with open lung biopsy. *Respirol Case Rep.* 2017;5(3).

61. *Surgeon General's Report: E-Cigarette Use Among Youth and Young Adults.* 2016.

62. Kalkhoran, Glantz. E-cigarettes and smoking cessation in real-world and clinical settings: a systematic review and meta-analysis. *Lancet Respir Med.* 2016;4(2):116–128.

63. Cunningham, et al. Benzodiazepine use in patients with chronic pain in an interdisciplinary pain rehabilitation program. *J Pain Res.* 2017;10:311–317.

64. Golombok S, Moodley P, Lader M. Cognitive impairment in long-term benzodiazepine users. *Psychol Med.* 1988;18: 365–374.

65. Bachhuber MA, Hennessy S, Cunningham CO, Starrels JL. Increasing benzodiazepine prescriptions and overdose mortality in the United States, 1996–2013. *Am J Publ Health.* 2016;106(4):686–688.

66. O'Brien et al. Best Practices and Barriers to Engaging People with SUD in Treatment.

67. Spronk DB, van Wel JHP, Ramaekers JG, Verkes RJ. Characterizing the cognitive effects of cocaine: a comprehensive review. *Neurosci Biobehav Rev.* 2013;37(8):1838–1859.

68. kolodny A, Courtwright DT, Hwang CS, Kreiner P, Eadie JL, Clark TW, Alexander GC. The prescription opioid and heroin crisis: apublic health approach to an epidemic of Addiction. *Annu Rev Publ Health*. 2015;36: 559–574.

69. Taite R. *Prescription Opioid Abuse: AGateway to Heroin and Overdose Psychology Today*. November 2014.

70. Dreamland. *The True Tale of America's Opiate Epidemic*. Sam Quinones; 2015.

71. Compton WM, Jones CM. Relationship between nonmedical prescription-opioid use and heroin use. *N Engl J Med*. 2016:154–163.

72. Frank Richard G, Pollack HA. Addressing the fentanyl threat to public health. *N Engl J Med*. 2017;376: 605–607. https://doi.org/10.1056/NEJMp1615145.

73. Ballantyne JC, Sullivan MD, Kolodny A. Opioid dependence vs addiction: a distinction without a difference? *Arch Intern Med*. 2012;172(17):1342–1343.

CHAPTER 10

Geriatric Pain Management

DIXIE ARAGAKI, MD • CHRISTOPHER BROPHY, MD

INTRODUCTION

In 2018, for the first time in history the number of persons aged 65 years or above exceeded the number of children under the age of 5 years on the planet. By 2050, it is predicted that one in four persons living in North America or Europe will be over the age of 65 years.[1,2] Health conditions and comorbidities, such as persistent pain, rise in prevalence within an aging population. Therefore it is vital to be aware of the nuances in geriatric pain assessment and management to meet the unique demands of this growing sect of the world population.

The differences in pain experience for older adults compared to their younger counterparts are related to higher prevalence of chronic illnesses, physiologic changes, polypharmacy, cognitive or communication deficits, frailty, and socioeconomic or psychosocial stressors. Despite these challenges, the approach to pain management for older persons is similar to the effective strategies used in younger cohorts.[3] The multimodal approach includes accurate and thoughtful assessment and diagnosis, focus on optimal function and quality of life, individualized application of pharmacologic and nonpharmacologic interventions, continued monitoring of response and adherence, and adjustments to patient and caregiver needs.

EPIDEMIOLOGY

The prevalence of pain in older persons is difficult to estimate and reports differ greatly among countries, living settings (e.g., community vs. long-term care vs. hospital), pain duration (e.g., acute, chronic, intermittent), and type or site of pain. Pain prevalence estimates in community-dwelling older adults vary from 20% to 76% and long-term nursing care setting pain estimates vary from 28% to 93% (higher end of ranges reflect chronic pain).[3] Despite this variability, several studies agree that approximately half of older adults report pain that interferes with their normal function.[4-6] The overall prevalence of bothersome pain in the past month was 52.9% and the inability to do some activities of daily living (ADLs) was 70%−80% more common in American older adults with pain than in those who denied pain. These functional impacts are even more pronounced in those with pain in multiple sites.[4]

Role of Aging in Types/Sites of Pain

Older adults may process pain differently, with decreased endogenous inhibition of noxious stimuli (particularly with the dopaminergic neurons in the basal ganglia)[7] that could lead to greater bodily chronic pain.[8] However, there is also evidence that older individuals are less sensitive to pain, which could indicate that the pain they feel is due to a more severe underlying pathologic condition. In the peripheral nervous system, the density of unmyelinated fibers can decrease considerably and be associated with nerve conduction slowing. However, mixed research study findings regarding pain perception in older adults underscore that their pain experience cannot be summarized as a simple "increase" or "decrease" in pain sensitivity.[9]

Multisite and widespread pain are significantly more common in older adults, which likely reflects multiple underlying pain-associated conditions and physiologic mechanisms leading to their pain. Up to 75% of older adults report pain at three or more locations, which is associated with more severe disability and a higher risk of falls.[10,11] A sample of American adults aged 65−90+ years showed nearly a third of older adults reported back pain, while a quarter had knee pain. Shoulder, hip, foot, hand, and neck were the next most common set of pain sites; stomach and arm were the least common. The prevalence of neck pain actually decreased with advancing age.[4] Curiously, some other common sources of pain such as myocardial infarction-related pain, migraine and severe headaches, and cancer pain appear to peak in the fifth and sixth decades of life but tend to decrease beyond the seventh decade.[3]

Pain Care Essentials and Innovations. https://doi.org/10.1016/B978-0-323-72216-2.00010-7

Community-dwelling older adults with chronic pain who reported a combination of sensory pain (aching, throbbing, stiff, sore), cognitive/affective pain (troublesome, nagging, tiring, miserable), and neuropathic pain (sharp, penetrating, numb, shooting) had more severe pain and more interference with daily activities. Neuropathic pain, although least common, was associated with the widest variety of pathologic conditions.[12]

Risk Factors Associated With Chronic Pain in Older Adults

Chronic pain is frequently associated with depressive symptoms; those with persistent pain have a higher risk of developing depression and those with depression are, interestingly, at higher risk of developing chronic pain.[13] Older adults with both chronic musculoskeletal pain and depressive symptoms are at a significantly higher risk of developing disability than older persons with either condition alone.[14]

Chronic pain is also associated with frailty (increased vulnerability to adverse health outcomes) leading to deterioration of physical and psychologic function.[15,16] The association appears to be bidirectional. In longitudinal studies, those with chronic pain had twice the risk of eventually developing frailty.[17] In the surgical setting, those with preoperative frailty prior to elective noncardiac surgery had significantly more intrusive postsurgical pain than those who were not frail.[18]

Some other risk factors associated with higher risk of chronic pain in the older population include female gender, osteoporosis, and obesity. Central abdominal obesity is a metabolic syndrome component shown to have a strong independent association with pain and is associated with nearly doubling the risk of chronic pain in the elderly.[19]

According to numerous studies, race/ethnicity is another risk factor, with reports of higher pain intensity/prevalence and poorer pain management in minority adults aged over 60 years.[3] In a study of more than 1.3 million US nursing home long-stay residents between 2011 and 2012, racial/ethnic minorities (non-Hispanic blacks vs. whites) and severely cognitively impaired residents had an increased prevalence of untreated and undertreated pain.[20] Older adults with lower levels of education were more likely to report pain than those with higher levels of education. This may reflect the cumulative effects of social disadvantage on disease burden and the persistent effects of occupational, work-related injury.[4]

GERIATRIC PAIN ASSESSMENT
Barriers to Accurate Assessment

Older adults can exhibit several unique attitudes about health and function relevant to their perception of pain. They may downplay specific symptoms with stoicism because of the belief that pain and disability are normal and expected with age when in fact it is important for them to seek evaluation and relief whenever possible. They may avoid medical evaluation for pain and harbor fears of an unfavorable diagnosis; treatments with side effects or high-cost, ineffective treatment options; medication addiction; loss of independence; becoming a burden on others; or being labeled a "hypochondriac" or "bad patient."[9,21]

Patients who display high levels of pain catastrophizing have poorer pain outcomes, but there is evidence that optimism/hope can lessen pain perception via reduced catastrophizing. Therefore psychologic service referrals are prudent if negative attitudes and beliefs are detected.[3]

Other barriers to geriatric pain assessment and management include communication and cognitive deficits, especially in the memory and language domains. This could potentially limit the reliability of self-reports of pain, but self-report scales for pain have still been shown to be meaningful for patients with mild-moderate dementia.[3,9]

Tools to Evaluate and Diagnose Geriatric Pain

Self-report pain assessment methods are typically appropriate for older adults but are often inadequate for those with advanced stages of dementia. There are multiple alternative tools available to assess pain in patients with dementia, or who are otherwise unable to communicate their needs. These tools rely on assessment of nonverbal behavior, such as facial expressions and vocalizations. The Pain Assessment in Advanced Dementia (PAINAD)[22] has been thoroughly validated and has good interrater reliability; conveniently, it also takes little time to complete (see Fig. 10.1). Other more thorough scales include the Pain Assessment Checklist for Seniors with Limited Ability to Communicate (PACSLAC) and Pain Assessment in Impaired Cognition (PAIC15), which may be more sensitive in detecting pain but have the disadvantage of requiring more time to administer.[23–25]

	0	1	2	Score
Breathing, independent of vocalization	Normal	▪Occasional labored breathing ▪Short period of hyperventilation	▪Noisy labored breathing ▪Long period of hyperventilation ▪Cheyne-Stokes respirations	
Negative vocalization	None	▪Occasional moan or groan ▪Low-level speech with a negative or disapproving quality	▪Repeated troubled calling out ▪Loud moaning or groaning ▪Crying	
Facial expression	Smiling or inexpressive	▪Sad, frightened ▪Frown	▪Facial grimacing	
Body language	Relaxed	▪Tense ▪Distressed pacing ▪Fidgeting	▪Rigid, fists clenched ▪Knees pulled up ▪Pulling or pushing away ▪Striking out	
Consolability	No need to console	▪Distracted or reassured by voice or touch	▪Unable to console, distract, or reassure	
			TOTAL	

FIG. 10.1 Pain Assessment in Advanced Dementia (PAINAD). (Adapted from Warden V, Hurley AC, Volicer L. Development and psychometric evaluation of the Pain Assessment in Advanced Dementia (PAINAD) scale. *J Am Med Dir Assoc.* 2003; with permission received from Elsevier "Copyright Clearance Center's RightsLink Service.")

GERIATRIC PAIN MANAGEMENT AND SPECIAL CONSIDERATIONS

General Principles

Safe and effective pain management in the older population requires an understanding of individual patient-centered factors such as comorbidities, risks of polypharmacy, potential drug-disease interactions, motivation for treatment adherence, financial burden, and expectations. An optimal treatment plan aims to reduce pain and disability and improve function and quality of life but should be based on realistic goals set in collaboration with the patient (and primary caregivers when indicated).

When nonpharmacologic treatments are considered, it is helpful to explore the biopsychosocial model of interdisciplinary pain management options using a heuristic approach.[26] Treating the "whole" person is more important than focusing narrowly on a disease state. Providers can employ psychosocial support tools (e.g., psychologic counseling/coaching, cognitive behavior therapy, spiritual/religious guidance, meditation/mindfulness, community integration), physical interventions (e.g., therapy, modalities, bracing, assistive devices, massage), and procedural interventional strategies (e.g., epidural steroid injections and other spine interventions). Many of these approaches will be described later in this chapter.

If medications are initiated, the general wisdom is to "start low and go slow" because of pharmacokinetic factors, but it is vital to monitor response and adjust the regimen when appropriate in a timely manner. Despite the risks associated with polypharmacy, it may be advantageous to use more than a single medication to achieve a synergistic effect or reduce adverse event risks associated with monotherapy dose escalation. The route of drug administration is also important because although the oral route is the most convenient, sometimes swallowing difficulties or cognitive/behavior issues in older adults warrant transdermal, rectal, transmucosal, intravenous, or other invasive alternative medication delivery methods.[27] Intramuscular injections should be avoided when possible due to discomfort. The decisions to give immediate-release or modified-release formulations or provide scheduled medications versus on-request administration may rely on the nature of episodic or continuous pain or the older person's level of awareness and cognition, respectively. Owing to the unpredictable age-related alterations in drug absorption, metabolism, or clearance, sometimes short-acting analgesics perform more like long-acting agents. Some important age-related physiologic changes and their associated clinical pharmacologic impacts are outlined in Table 10.1.

Age-Related Physiologic Impacts on Drug Handling (Pharmacokinetics)

See Table 10.1 for a brief list of age-related physiologic changes that can impact pharmacokinetics.

Nonpharmacologic Treatments
Therapies (physical therapy, occupational therapy, others)

Broadly speaking, increased physical activity is associated with decreased pain due to endogenous pain modulation. Individuals with chronic pain tend to have higher sensitivity to painful stimuli and decreased capacity to endogenously inhibit pain. A similarly dysregulated modulation system is seen in older adults. Each level of physical activity (light and moderate to vigorous) affects a different mode of pain inhibition in older adults.[28] This suggests that any degree of physical activity may have a unique impact on pain modulation. Physical activity and exercise are often prescribed for older adults with chronic pain with goals to prevent disuse muscle atrophy, to improve strength and joint range of motion, and to maintain or improve functional mobility.[27] Additional benefits of attending various types of therapies include socialization, establishment of new social support networks, and empowerment through active symptom self-management. Low dose of moderate-vigorous activity was also shown to reduce mortality by 22% in adults aged over 60 years, and higher doses of activity improved all-cause mortality in a linear fashion.[29] The 2018 Physical Activity Guidelines for Americans[30] recommends multicomponent physical activities to include balance training and aerobic and muscle-strengthening exercises for older adults. However, caution regarding fall risk or cardiopulmonary adverse events is advised and appropriate precautions should be considered when prescribing therapy.

Alternative movement-based activities such as yoga or tai chi may also be appropriate options to enhance balance and flexibility, but the evidence base for people aged over 65 years is not very well established. One study of the efficacy of hatha yoga compared to aerobic/strengthening exercises showed equal if not superior benefits for function and knee osteoarthritis symptoms in older adults aged over 60 years.[31] Another

TABLE 10.1
Physiologic Changes in Older People and Pharmacokinetic Impacts.

Physiologic Domain	Age-Related Change	Clinical Pharmacologic Impact
Volume of distribution	Decreased body water	Reduced distribution of water-soluble drugs
	Increased body fat	Prolonged elimination and half-life of lipid-soluble drugs
	Lower plasma protein	Increased free fraction of drugs that are usually protein-bound with the potential for drug-drug interactions
Hepatic function	Reduced hepatic blood flow Reduced liver mass and functioning cells	Decreased first pass metabolism Drug metabolism via conjugation is usually preserved, but half-life of drugs metabolized by oxidative enzyme reaction is prolonged
Renal function	Reduced renal blood flow	Increased half-life of renal eliminated drugs and accumulation of the drug or metabolites
Gastrointestinal function	Delayed gastric emptying and reduced peristalsis	Increased risk of bowel dysmotility (e.g., constipation from opioids)
Skin/integumentary function	Reduced hydration, tissue thickness, surface lipids	Decreased predictability of transdermal penetration and drug distribution/retention

promising pilot randomized controlled trial of the effects of chair yoga on pain and function among community-dwelling older adults aged over 65 years and with lower limb osteoarthritis showed association with reduction in pain for up to 3 months after an 8-week "Sit 'N' Fit Chair Yoga" program compared to a standard Health Education program.[32] The efficacy of tai chi in treating chronic pain conditions specifically in older adults remains unclear, but a systematic review and meta-analysis of 18 randomized controlled trials revealed some positive support regarding tai chi as a viable low-risk complementary and alternative medicine tool for immediate benefits for chronic osteoarthritis, lower back pain, and osteoporosis.[33]

Modalities (kinesiotaping, heat, ice, vibration, massage, electrotherapy)

For knee osteoarthritis in older adults, kinesiotaping may have at least short-term beneficial effects on gait, balance, and knee pain, which may in turn facilitate exercise and other more long-term beneficial effects for pain.[34,35] Physical modalities such as superficial heat, vibration, therapeutic massage, and transcutaneous electric nerve stimulation are intended to reduce pain intensity. Most of these modalities have limited evidence and are not practical for persistent pain relief but can provide relatively brief periods of comfort.

Superficial heat is generally well tolerated by older adults but has risk of burns if used in patients with impaired sensation or communicative/cognitive deficits. Product information and instructions should be closely followed to prevent thermal damage. Heat modalities should generally be avoided in acute injuries because they may promote edema or hyperalgesia.

Superficial cooling modalities may provide temporary pain relief via reduction in local inflammation. However, older adults may be less tolerant to cold-based treatments than to heat-based treatments. Vibration, massage, and electrotherapy modalities have mixed evidence supporting utilization but should be avoided over areas of broken skin, local malignancies, infections, or local trauma. Transcutaneous electric nerve stimulation (TENS) electrodes should not be positioned over the carotid sinuses or near metallic implants or cardiac devices.[27]

Massage therapy has been shown to have positive effects on musculoskeletal and general chronic pain through a proposed mechanism of increased serotonin and dopamine levels, enhanced local blood flow, and acting through the gate control theory. Studies in older adults have shown slow-stroke back massage to reduce shoulder pain and anxiety in senior stroke survivors, with benefits observed up to 3 days after the massage.[36] Another form of massage known as "Tender Touch" (gentle comfort massage) has improved pain and anxiety in older adults living in a long-term care facility and can improve patient-staff communication.[37]

Psychologic and behavior therapies

Psychologic therapies have been shown to be well received by older adults, with improvements in self-reported pain.[3] Cognitive behavior therapy in older adults living in the community and in nursing home settings has been shown to improve pain severity, self-rated disability, mood disturbance, coping skills, social engagement, and quality of life.[27] Self-management strategies for pain control include relaxation, coping skills, exercise, adapted activities, assistive device use, and education. There is mixed evidence for the efficacy of self-management practices in the older adult population, but they are generally safe options to be offered in conjunction with other methods of pain management. Specifically, there is some evidence that assistive devices can reduce functional decline, care costs, and pain intensity and help older adults maintain community living.[36]

Procedural (injections, manipulation, surgery)

Acupressure is a noninvasive technique that can be taught to laypeople without professional training. In frail older adults, acupressure resulted in decreased pain and increased quality of life compared with waitlisted controls, when applied continuously, almost daily, for 12 weeks.[38]

For uncomplicated low-back pain, there is some retrospective evidence that chiropractic care may buffer against ADL and instrumental ADL decline, as well as increase self-rated health when compared with routine medical care.[39] When comparing spinal manipulative therapy to exercise and physical therapy, both groups demonstrated improvements in pain and function over time, without significant differences between groups.[40] However, when compared against sham therapy, spinal manipulative therapy does not consistently demonstrate improved pain outcomes, suggesting that there may be a nonspecific therapeutic effect of patient interaction itself.[41]

Spinal stenosis due to degenerative changes narrowing the vertebral canal and/or neural foramina is a common cause of axial or radicular pain and limited functional mobility in older persons. There is some evidence to support the use of epidural steroid injections via fluoroscopic guidance, preferentially using the transforaminal approach, for short-term basis symptom

TABLE 10.2
Pain Management Medications With Dosing Considerations for Older Adults.

Medication	Indications	Starting Dose	Maximum Dose	Renal Adjust	Hepatic Adjust	Comments
Acetaminophen	Mild-moderate pain Nociceptive pain Tension headache	325 mg q4–8h	3 g per day	CrCl 10–50: q6h CrCl <10: q8h	2 g per day max	First line, but minimal effect on knee/hip OA, no effect on chronic low-back pain. Avoid with alcohol. Monitor OTC use. Low therapeutic index → overdose.
NSAIDs	Inflammatory pain Nociceptive pain					Risk of GI bleed, kidney damage, and cardiovascular adverse events in susceptible patients.
Ibuprofen	Mild-moderate pain	200 mg q6–q8h	2400 mg per day	Avoid in CKD or AKI	None	Short-term trial. Give with food. Consider GI PPx (H$_2$ blocker or PPI) to prevent GI ulcer. Caution with antiplatelet or anticoagulation therapy. Avoid in cardiovascular disease.
Naproxen	Mild-moderate pain	250 mg q12h	500 mg q12h	CrCl <30: avoid	Avoid in liver disease	Similar profile to ibuprofen but easier to take because of bid dosing.
Celecoxib	Mild-moderate pain	100 mg qd	200 mg bid	Avoid in CKD or AKI	Avoid in liver disease	Reduced risk of gastroduodenal toxicity and minimal platelet inhibition (can take with aspirin). Equivalent cardiovascular risk as other NSAIDs.
Meloxicam	Osteoarthritis	7.5 mg qd	15 mg qd	Hemodialysis 7.5 mg qd	Unknown	Low risk of gastroduodenal toxicity at 7.5mg (mostly COX-2), higher risk at 15 mg (mostly COX-1). Increased risk of hemorrhagic stroke.
Salsalate	Mild-moderate pain	500 mg bid	3 g per day	Avoid in CKD or AKI	Avoid in liver disease	Minimal GI side effects and minimal effect on platelet function. Old drug, but few studies in geriatric population.

Drug	Indication	Starting dose	Max dose	Renal	Hepatic	Comments
Anticonvulsants	Central/peripheral neuropathic pain					
Gabapentin	Postherpetic neuralgia Diabetic peripheral neuropathy Fibromyalgia	300 mg qd ×1d, then bid ×1d, then tid	1200 mg tid	CrCl <60: reduce dose proportionately to CrCl, administer bid	No adjustment	Titrate up dose as tolerated. To discontinue drug taper over 7 days. Increased risk of falls due to common side effects: dizziness and somnolence. Consider qhs dosing.
Pregabalin	Postherpetic neuralgia Diabetic peripheral neuropathy Fibromyalgia	150 mg/day divided bid or tid	300 mg/day, divided bid or tid	CrCl <60: reduce dose proportionately to CrCl	No adjustment	Titrate up dose as tolerated. To discontinue drug taper over 7 days.
Antidepressants	Neuropathic pain Off-label: chronic pain					
Duloxetine	Chronic MSK pain Diabetic peripheral neuropathy Fibromyalgia	30 mg qd	120 mg/day	CrCl <30: avoid	Avoid in liver disease	Preferred SNRI in older adults. Tolerable side effect profile. Caution for hyponatremia. To discontinue drug taper gradually.
Venlafaxine ER	Off-label: same as duloxetine	37.5 mg qd, increase by 75 mg qwk	225 mg qd	CrCl 10–70: decrease dose by 25%–50%	Mild-moderate impairment: decrease dose by 50%	Second-line SNRI. Recommend trial of duloxetine first. Side effects: hypertension, anxiety, insomnia, and hyponatremia. Can impair platelets → bruising and bleeding. To discontinue drug taper over 2 weeks.
Nortriptyline	Off-label: diabetic peripheral neuropathy Fibromyalgia	10 mg qhs, increase by 10 mg q5d	160 mg qhs	No adjustment	Caution	Preferred over amitriptyline because of fewer anticholinergic side effects, but still must monitor. On Beers list.
Amitriptyline	Off-label: diabetic peripheral neuropathy Fibromyalgia	10 mg qhs, increase by 10–25 mg qwk	75 mg qhs	No adjustment	Caution	Recommend avoiding because of anticholinergic side effects in older adults. On Beers list.

Continued

	Pain type	Dose	Max dose	Renal	Hepatic	Comments
Muscle relaxants						
Baclofen	Nociceptive pain Chronic spasticity off-label: MSK pain	5 mg bid/tid	80 mg/day	No adjustment	No adjustment	Can use long term. Risk of withdrawal. To discontinue drug taper gradually.
Dantrolene	Chronic spasticity off-label: MSK pain	25 mg qd, dose/frequency q7days	100 mg qid	Not defined	Contraindicated in liver disease	Monitor hepatic function because of risk of hepatotoxicity. Can cause sun sensitivity.
Cyclobenzaprine	MSK pain Fibromyalgia	5 mg qd (IR tablet only)	10 mg tid 3 weeks max	Not defined	Avoid in moderate-severe impairment	Avoid extended release in older adults. Almost identical structure to amitriptyline; caution for anticholinergic side effects. Short-term use only.
Methocarbamol	MSK pain	500 mg qid	1000 mg qid (max 4 g/day)	Not defined	Not defined	Very short half-life. Also has IM/IV formulation. Can change urine color to brown/black/green.
Carisoprodol	MSK pain	250 mg qhs	350 mg tid 3 weeks max	Caution	Caution	Avoid in older adults. Increases risk of fall. Risk of withdrawal. Monitor for orthostatic hypotension. To discontinue long-term use taper gradually.
Topical analgesics	Nociceptive pain Inflammatory pain Neuropathic pain					Consider as first line in older adults because of the superior side effect profile compared with oral medications.
Diclofenac 1% gel	OA off-label: MSK pain	2 g Upper Extremity joints 4 g Lower Extremity joints	8 g/joint 32 g/day	Caution, monitor	Caution	Minimal (~7%) systemic absorption, low incidence of typical NSAID adverse reactions. Enhanced tissue penetration with ultrasonography/iontophoresis. Efficacy may subside after 6–12 weeks.

Drug	Indication				Comments
Lidocaine 5% patch	Peripheral neuropathic pain off-label: MSK pain	1 patch	3 patches	Not defined	Not defined	Apply patch 12 h on and 12 h off. Monitor for skin reaction. Can also consider lidocaine gel for short duration. Minimal systemic absorption, minimal penetration into soft tissue.
Capsaicin <1% cream	Peripheral neuropathic pain Fibromyalgia	Apply tid to qid	Apply tid to qid	Not defined	Not defined	Works by exhausting peripheral nerve substance P. Takes multiple applications (up to 3 weeks) before achieving analgesic benefit. Transient burning pain, erythema, itch.
Capsaicin 8% patch	Peripheral neuropathic pain	1–4 patches for 30 min (feet) or 60 min (other)	1 treatment every 3 months	Not defined	Not defined	High concentration 8% patch more effective in peripheral neuropathy, with only 1 application every 3 months.
Opioids						Adjunctive therapy for severe pain refractory to nonopioid analgesics and nonpharmacologic modalities.
Tramadol	Moderate-severe pain	25 mg bid	50 mg q6h	CrCl <30: q12h, max 200 mg/day	Cirrhosis: 50 mg q12h, max 100 mg/day	Lowest effective dose for shortest duration. Avoid extended release in older adults. If long-term use taper gradually to discontinue. Dose-dependent QT prolongation.
Oxycodone	Severe pain	2.5 mg q6h	10 mg q6h	CrCl <60: titrate slowly	Impairment: 50% starting dose	Lowest effective dose for shortest duration. Consider extended release for maintenance of chronic pain.

AKI, acute kidney injury; *bid*, twice a day; *CKD*, chronic kidney disease; *COX-1*, cyclooxygenase 1; *GI*, gastrointestinal; *H₂*, histamine receptor 2; *IM*, intramuscular; *IR*, immediate-release; *IV*, intravenous; *MSK*, musculoskeletal; *NSAIDs*, nonsteroidal antiinflammatory drugs; *OA*, osteoarthritis; *OTC*, over-the-counter; *PPI*, proton pump inhibitor; *PPx*, prophylaxis; *qd*, every day; *qhs*, every bedtime; *qid*, four times a day; *SNRI*, serotonin–norepinephrine reuptake inhibitor; *tid*, three times a day.

benefit, but literature is mixed and limited in the older population.[42] If conservative management fails or if neurologic deficits arise, surgical spinal decompression may be indicated.

Pharmacologic Treatments (see Table 10.2)
Older adults with moderate and severe pain are more likely to use daily oral analgesics, often multiple medications concomitantly, and are more likely to feel they need a stronger pain medication.[43] Owing to age-related pharmacokinetics, oral analgesic medication recommendations can differ for older people.

Acetaminophen
Acetaminophen (paracetamol or APAP) has long been considered the first-line therapy for pain (especially musculoskeletal pain) because of its efficacy and safety profile, but more recent studies have created some controversy. In a large prospective study of nursing home residents older than 80 years, acetaminophen dosages of approximately 2000 mg per day were not found to increase the risk of mortality or myocardial infarction but did increase the risk of stroke in diabetic subjects.[44] Another case series reported acute liver failure in malnourished patients (weight <50 kg). In general, the risk of renal, central nervous system, cardiovascular, and hepatic adverse effects is low if patients are educated to not exceed the dose of 3 g per 24-h period (or maximum of 2 g/24 h in malnourished patients) and avoid use in the setting of chronic alcohol abuse/dependence.[36]

Nonsteroidal antiinflammatory drugs and cyclooxygenase 2 inhibitors
Nonsteroidal antiinflammatory drugs (NSAIDs) are widely prescribed for pain and inflammation and have been particularly useful and more effective than acetaminophen for persistent musculoskeletal inflammatory pain.[45] Despite their good efficacy, they must be used with great caution in older adults because of the higher risk of hematologic (bleeding), gastrointestinal (ulceration), renal (fluid retention, worsening of chronic renal failure), hepatic, and cardiovascular (hypertension, thromboembolic) adverse events. NSAIDs have been associated with up to a quarter of hospital admissions attributed to drug adverse reactions in older people.[45] Cyclooxygenase 2 (COX-2) inhibitors have also demonstrated cardiovascular risks and are contraindicated in patients with known ischemic heart disease and cerebrovascular disease. They should also be used with caution in patients with hypertension, hyperlipidemia, tobacco smoking, or diabetes mellitus. Because of their side effect profiles, NSAIDs are not recommended in older adults. But if considered necessary, the lowest dose should be used for the shortest duration with education on possible adverse effects and strong consideration of proton pump inhibitor or misoprostol co-prescription.

Topical agents
Age-related skin changes include reduced hydration, tissue thickness, and surface lipids, which make it more difficult to predict the transdermal penetration in older adults. Dry, thin, or broken skin without a good subcutaneous layer can lead to overtreatment or undertreatment effects. This can make dose response variable so closer monitoring is necessary in older patients than in younger patients.[46]

Topical NSAIDs are generally considered safer than oral formulations because of their minimal (~7%) systemic absorption and risk of harmful effects. There is limited data in older adults with baseline renal insufficiency and use of anticoagulants so initial careful monitoring is advised.[46] A 2015 Cochrane review reported that diclofenac, ibuprofen, and ketoprofen gel formulations, as well as some diclofenac patches, provided relatively favorable benefit for acute conditions such as sprains, strains, and overuse injuries with minimal adverse events (1 in 20 people experienced a mild temporary redness at the application site).[47] Menthol and methyl salicylate combinations (e.g., Bengay, Icy Hot, Salonpas) are available over the counter or by prescription but care should be taken to avoid applying them over damaged skin or leaving a patch on for >8 h (maximum two patches in 24 h).

Topical lidocaine 5% can be effective for postherpetic neuralgia, and because of its low side effect profile and ease of application, it has been used in many types of localized neuropathic and nonneuropathic pain with low-moderate quality of evidence.[27] It is recommended to use the lowest effective amount of product to reduce systemic absorption and the risk of central nervous system or cardiac effects.

Topical capsaicin cream can be used for osteoarthritis or neuropathic pain, but many older patients are unable to tolerate the intense burning sensation with application (or they can suffer if the cream accidently contacts sensitive skin). Because it works by exhausting peripheral nerve substance P, multiple tedious applications for weeks are necessary for an optimal effect. A potent 8% capsaicin patch has been approved for more convenient use as a 1-h application that is effective for several months for postherpetic neuralgia.[36]

Tramadol

Tramadol is not well studied or supported for use in older people. It has two mechanisms of action: a weak opioid agonist activity and inhibition of monoamine uptake. It reduces the seizure threshold and should be used with caution in patients taking other serotonergic drugs. Despite it possibly having less effect on respiratory and gastrointestinal function than other opioids, it has been more associated with delirium in older adults.[48] Avoiding delirium may be particularly important in the postoperative setting, as there is evidence that postoperative delirium is associated with increased mortality, as well as a significant decline in both ADLs and cognition up to 3 years after the surgery.[49,50]

Genetic polymorphisms of the cytochrome P450 enzyme CYP2D6 largely explain individual difference in tramadol metabolism.[51] Combined with reduced renal clearance, there can be marked variability in the pharmacokinetics of tramadol in older individuals. The concentration of tramadol's primary metabolite, which induces both the opioid analgesic and the opioid side effects, is significantly increased in healthy older patients, which may explain the increased risk of delirium and sedation.[52]

Neuropathic adjuvants

Adjuvants such as antidepressants and anticonvulsants can be useful, particularly for neuropathic pain. However, attention to adverse and drug-drug reactions is important. Tricyclic antidepressants (such as amitriptyline or imipramine) may have considerable anticholinergic effects of urinary retention, confusion, dry mouth, and sedation, but a second-generation tricyclic (such as nortriptyline) may have less side effects while still reducing neuropathic pain from postherpetic neuralgia or peripheral diabetic neuropathy. Selective serotonin reuptake inhibitors are better tolerated by older adults, but they are not considered effective for pain relief.

Although there is mounting evidence that serotonin-noradrenaline reuptake inhibitors such as duloxetine or venlafaxine can improve both neuropathic pain and depression, a subgroup analysis in older patients demonstrated that concurrent use of an opioid diminished the analgesic effects of venlafaxine, while preserving its antidepressant effects.[53] Venlafaxine may also cause hypertensive episodes, whereas duloxetine has not been shown to elevate blood pressure.[46] The UK National Institute for Health and Care Excellence (NICE) guidelines recommend duloxetine as an option for initial management of painful diabetic peripheral neuropathy.[36]

Antiepileptic drugs have not been very well studied in older people, but gabapentin and pregabalin have been considered effective for neuropathic pain and are well tolerated if titrated slowly and carefully from the lowest dose possible with monitoring for response and side effects (sedation, confusion, edema). Dose adjustment of gabapentin and pregabalin is required in renal impairment. Older antiepileptic agents such as carbamazepine, sodium valproate, and phenytoin carry a higher risk of central nervous system adverse effects and require blood laboratory testing for potential drug-drug or drug-disease interactions,[36] making them less safe and practical.

Muscle relaxants

Skeletal muscle relaxants (baclofen, dantrolene, tizanidine, methocarbamol, cyclobenzaprine, metaxalone, carisoprodol) used for antispastic or antispasmodic effects in older adults are associated with sedation, confusion, and weakness leading to risk of falls and injuries. Carisoprodol should not be used because of additional risk of addiction and abuse. According to the 2015 Beers Criteria, some muscle relaxants including cyclobenzaprine, carisoprodol, methocarbamol, and metaxalone are high-risk medications because of their anticholinergic and sedating effects. Use of methocarbamol or cyclobenzaprine in veterans over the age of 65 years was associated with increased emergency department visits and hospitalizations.[54] Dantrolene can cause hepatotoxicity with chronic use, but it is relatively less sedating because it works peripherally. Tizanidine use is limited by dose-dependent adverse drug events, drug-drug interactions, and the possibility of prolonged QT intervals with chronic use.

Baclofen, not included in the Beers Criteria, is a centrally acting skeletal muscle relaxant with an FDA indication to treat spasticity related to central nervous system lesions. Baclofen is generally well tolerated in older adults and can be used chronically if the patient is monitored for sedation and educated to avoid abrupt cessation due to the risk of withdrawal.[54]

Opioids

In general, long-term use of opioids in older people should be considered only when other pain treatment avenues have been exhausted or there are significant negative impacts on the function or quality of life. Opioids are a particularly sensitive subject in the United States, given their unprecedented common use as an analgesic, followed by mounting evidence of adverse outcomes and questionable efficacy in widespread conditions such as osteoarthritis. Older individuals are particularly susceptible to their side effects such as constipation and sedation, both due to underlying physiologic changes associated with aging and common drug-drug interactions. As a result, the culture of opioid prescribing has changed significantly. In 2013, the Veterans Health Administration implemented the Opioid Safety Initiative. An analysis of prescribing trends to older veterans demonstrated an abrupt shift from steadily increasing to suddenly decreasing opioid prescriptions, with a corresponding rise in acetaminophen prescription. Interestingly, there was a small increase in the number of veterans reporting pain but no overall change in pain intensity.[55]

Older individuals are more sensitive not only to the analgesic effects but also to the sedative and respiratory depressant effects of opioids.[56–58] Even though older patients with dementia are just as likely to receive opioids for pain, there are few studies on the safety of opioids in this vulnerable population; instead, they are often excluded from studies. Because the randomized controlled trials are of small size and there is a lack of long-term cohort studies, the evidence does not indicate whether opioids are safe in this population.[59]

Older patients with continuous moderate to severe pain can be treated with a low-dose short-acting opioid (such as oxycodone or liquid morphine 2.5 mg every 6–8 h) for a trial, especially if not previously exposed to an opioid medication. Due to age-related pharmacokinetic changes, a short-acting opioid may have a longer half-life than anticipated, so it is not necessary to use a modified-release long-acting opioid unless the response to treatment justifies a change. Care should be taken to avoid inadvertent overdose of acetaminophen if included in hydrocodone or oxycodone combination formulations. If the opioid trial is tolerated well but the pain is not adequately reduced at the low starting dose, then a careful stepwise titration (using the "start low, go slow" strategy) can be performed while continuing to monitor for sedation, nausea/vomiting, constipation, or respiratory depression. Appropriate laxative therapy should be provided throughout opioid treatment. If the opioid dose is effective but wears off prematurely, then the provider can consider modified-release oral or transdermal opioid formulations with a goal of more constant plasma concentration. However, transdermal fentanyl patches should be used only in patients who are not opioid-naïve and at the lowest anticipated effective dose because of the unpredictable skin absorption, drug release and retention, and long-acting risk in older adults.

Some opioids are associated with particularly higher adverse effect risk-to-benefit ratios and are therefore not recommended for use in older patients. Meperidine (primarily due to its metabolite, normeperidine) is associated with an increased risk of delirium, seizures, anxiety, and hallucinations.[48,60] Meperidine is also a Beers list medication strongly associated with unplanned hospitalizations.[61] Propoxyphene is similarly dangerous in older patients because of the neurotoxic effects of its metabolite norpropoxyphene. Because of the age-related reduced renal clearance and accumulation of active and toxic metabolites, morphine is also a higher risk medication in older individuals.[58] However, liquid morphine has the advantage of being available in concentrations as low as 1 mg/mL, whereas the lowest dose of morphine tablet is 5 mg. Therefore a starting trial of liquid morphine 1–3 mg/mL three times a day has been shown to safely improve pain while minimizing potential risks.[62] Codeine is not recommended, especially in patients with hepatic insufficiency, because of its lower relative potency yet comparable risk of opioid adverse effects such as constipation. Methadone is safe for patients with renal insufficiency but should be prescribed only by clinicians with knowledge and experience due to its very long half-life and risk of accumulation in patients with liver disease. Hydromorphone should be used with caution in patients with hepatic or renal insufficiency because its metabolite can cause central nervous system toxicity (do not use if glomerular filtration rate is <30 mL/min).[63]

SUMMARY/CONCLUSION

Comprehensive pain management in older adults is a defining issue in this age of overwhelming information, technology, and change. Epidemiologic data harken a call to focus our attention, research, and resources on the growing number of aging individuals. The approach to successful pain mitigation in older persons relies heavily on navigating age-related factors and the judicious application of age-appropriate interventions. Biopsychosocial pain management tools give us more power and opportunity to optimize comfort, function, and quality of life for the senior members of our society.

REFERENCES

1. Vespa J. *The Graying of America: More Older Adults Than Kids by 2035*. United States Census Bureau; 2019. https://www.census.gov/library/stories/2018/03/graying-america.html.

2. United Nations, Department of Economic and Social Affairs, Population Division. *World Population Prospects 2019: Highlights*. 2019.

3. Savvas SM, Gibson SJ. Overview of pain management in older adults. *Clin Geriatr Med*. 2016;32(4):635−650.

4. Patel KV, Guralnik JM, Dansie EJ, Turk DC. Prevalence and impact of pain among older adults in the United States: findings from the 2011 National Health and Aging Trends Study. *Pain*. 2013;154(12):2649−2657.

5. Rao A, Cohen HJ. Symptom management in the elderly cancer patient: fatigue, pain, and depression. *J Natl Cancer Inst Monogr*. 2004;(32):150−157.

6. Tsang A, Von Korff M, Lee S, et al. Common chronic pain conditions in developed and developing countries: gender and age differences and comorbidity with depression-anxiety disorders. *J Pain*. 2008;9(10):883−891.

7. Cole LJ, Farrell MJ, Gibson SJ, Egan GF. Age-related differences in pain sensitivity and regional brain activity evoked by noxious pressure. *Neurobiol Aging*. 2010;31(3):494−503.

8. Naugle KM, Cruz-Almeida Y, Fillingim RB, Riley 3rd JL. Loss of temporal inhibition of nociceptive information is associated with aging and bodily pain. *J Pain*. 2017;18(12):1496−1504.

9. Molton IR, Terrill AL. Overview of persistent pain in older adults. *Am Psychol*. 2014;69(2):197−207.

10. Eggermont LH, Bean JF, Guralnik JM, Leveille SG. Comparing pain severity versus pain location in the MOBILIZE Boston study: chronic pain and lower extremity function. *J Gerontol A Biol Sci Med Sci*. 2009;64(7):763−770.

11. Eggermont LH, Leveille SG, Shi L, et al. Pain characteristics associated with the onset of disability in older adults: the maintenance of balance, independent living, intellect, and zest in the Elderly Boston Study. *J Am Geriatr Soc*. 2014;62(6):1007−1016.

12. Thakral M, Shi L, Foust JB, et al. Pain quality descriptors in community-dwelling older adults with nonmalignant pain. *Pain*. 2016;157(12):2834−2842.

13. Kroenke K, Wu J, Bair MJ, Krebs EE, Damush TM, Tu W. Reciprocal relationship between pain and depression: a 12-month longitudinal analysis in primary care. *J Pain*. 2011;12(9):964−973.

14. Murata S, Ono R, Omata J, Endo T, Otani K. Coexistence of chronic musculoskeletal pain and depressive symptoms and their combined and individual effects on onset of disability in older adults: a cohort study. *J Am Med Dir Assoc*. 2019;20(10), 1263−1267 e1263.

15. Wade KF, Lee DM, McBeth J, et al. Chronic widespread pain is associated with worsening frailty in European men. *Age Ageing*. 2016;45(2):268−274.

16. Hirase T, Kataoka H, Nakano J, Inokuchi S, Sakamoto J, Okita M. Impact of frailty on chronic pain, activities of daily living and physical activity in community-dwelling older adults: a cross-sectional study. *Geriatr Gerontol Int*. 2018;18(7):1079−1084.

17. Saraiva MD, Suzuki GS, Lin SM, de Andrade DC, Jacob-Filho W, Suemoto CK. Persistent pain is a risk factor for frailty: a systematic review and meta-analysis from prospective longitudinal studies. *Age Ageing*. 2018;47(6):785−793.

18. Esses GJ, Liu X, Lin HM, Khelemsky Y, Deiner S. Preoperative frailty and its association with postsurgical pain in an older patient cohort. *Reg Anesth Pain Med*. 2019;44:695−699.

19. Ray L, Lipton RB, Zimmerman ME, Katz MJ, Derby CA. Mechanisms of association between obesity and chronic pain in the elderly. *Pain*. 2011;152(1):53−59.

20. Hunnicutt JN, Ulbricht CM, Tjia J, Lapane KL. Pain and pharmacologic pain management in long-stay nursing home residents. *Pain*. 2017;158(6):1091−1099.

21. Brown D. A literature review exploring how healthcare professionals contribute to the assessment and control of postoperative pain in older people. *J Clin Nurs*. 2004;13(6B):74−90.

22. Warden V, Hurley AC, Volicer L. Development and psychometric evaluation of the Pain Assessment In Advanced Dementia (PAINAD) scale. *J Am Med Dir Assoc*. 2003;4(1):9−15.

23. Lukas A, Hagg-Grun U, Mayer B, Fischer T, Schuler M. Pain assessment in advanced dementia. Validity of the German PAINAD-a prospective double-blind randomised placebo-controlled trial. *Pain*. 2019;160(3):742−753.

24. Ruest M, Bourque M, Laroche S, et al. Can we quickly and thoroughly assess pain with the PACSLAC-II? A convergent validity study in long-term care residents suffering from dementia. *Pain Manag Nurs*. 2017;18(6):410−417.

25. de Waal MWM, van Dalen-Kok AH, de Vet HCW, et al. Observational pain assessment in older persons with dementia in four countries: observer agreement of items and factor structure of the pain assessment in impaired cognition. *Eur J Pain*. 2019.

26. Gatchel RJ, Okifuji A. Evidence-based scientific data documenting the treatment and cost-effectiveness of comprehensive pain programs for chronic nonmalignant pain. *J Pain*. 2006;7(11):779−793.

27. Christo PJ, Li S, Gibson SJ, Fine P, Hameed H. Effective treatments for pain in the older patient. *Curr Pain Headache Rep*. 2011;15(1):22−34.

28. Naugle KM, Ohlman T, Naugle KE, Riley ZA, Keith NR. Physical activity behavior predicts endogenous pain modulation in older adults. *Pain*. 2017;158(3):383−390.

29. Hupin D, Roche F, Gremeaux V, et al. Even a low-dose of moderate-to-vigorous physical activity reduces mortality by 22% in adults aged >/=60 years: a systematic review and meta-analysis. *Br J Sports Med*. 2015;49(19):1262−1267.

30. Piercy KL, Troiano RP, Ballard RM, et al. The physical activity guidelines for Americans. *J Am Med Assoc*. 2018;320(19):2020−2028.

31. Cheung C, Wyman JF, Bronas U, McCarthy T, Rudser K, Mathiason MA. Managing knee osteoarthritis with yoga or aerobic/strengthening exercise programs in older adults:

a pilot randomized controlled trial. *Rheumatol Int.* 2017; 37(3):389–398.

32. Park J, McCaffrey R, Newman D, Liehr P, Ouslander JG. A pilot randomized controlled trial of the effects of Chair yoga on pain and physical function among community-dwelling older adults with lower extremity osteoarthritis. *J Am Geriatr Soc.* 2017;65(3):592–597.

33. Kong LJ, Lauche R, Klose P, et al. Tai chi for chronic pain conditions: a systematic review and meta-analysis of randomized controlled trials. *Sci Rep.* 2016;6:25325.

34. Park JS, Yoon T, Lee SH, et al. Immediate effects of kinesiology tape on the pain and gait function in older adults with knee osteoarthritis. *Medicine.* 2019;98(45):e17880.

35. Park KN, Kim SH. Effects of knee taping during functional activities in older people with knee osteoarthritis: a randomized controlled clinical trial. *Geriatr Gerontol Int.* 2018;18(8):1206–1210.

36. Abdulla A, Adams N, Bone M, et al. Guidance on the management of pain in older people. *Age Ageing.* 2013; 42(Suppl 1):i1–57.

37. Sansone P, Schmitt L. Providing tender touch massage to elderly nursing home residents: a demonstration project. *Geriatr Nurs.* 2000;21(6):303–308.

38. Chan CWC, Chau PH, Leung AYM, et al. Acupressure for frail older people in community dwellings-a randomised controlled trial. *Age Ageing.* 2017;46(6):957–964.

39. Weigel PA, Hockenberry J, Bentler SE, Wolinsky FD. The comparative effect of episodes of chiropractic and medical treatment on the health of older adults. *J Manip Physiol Ther.* 2014;37(3):143–154.

40. de Luca KE, Fang SH, Ong J, Shin KS, Woods S, Tuchin PJ. The effectiveness and safety of manual therapy on pain and disability in older persons with chronic low back pain: a systematic review. *J Manip Physiol Ther.* 2017;40(7):527–534.

41. Dougherty PE, Karuza J, Dunn AS, Savino D, Katz P. Spinal manipulative therapy for chronic lower back pain in older veterans: a prospective, randomized, placebo-controlled trial. *Geriatr Orthop Surg Rehabil.* 2014;5(4):154–164.

42. Botwin KP, Gruber RD, Bouchlas CG, et al. Fluoroscopically guided lumbar transformational epidural steroid injections in degenerative lumbar stenosis: an outcome study. *Am J Phys Med Rehabil.* 2002;81(12):898–905.

43. Nawai A, Leveille SG, Shmerling RH, van der Leeuw G, Bean JF. Pain severity and pharmacologic pain management among community-living older adults: the MOBILIZE Boston study. *Aging Clin Exp Res.* 2017;29(6):1139–1147.

44. Girard P, Sourdet S, Cantet C, de Souto Barreto P, Rolland Y. Acetaminophen safety: risk of mortality and cardiovascular events in nursing home residents, a prospective study. *J Am Geriatr Soc.* 2019;67(6):1240–1247.

45. American Geriatrics Society Panel on Pharmacological Management of Persistent Pain in Older Persons. Pharmacological management of persistent pain in older persons. *J Am Geriatr Soc.* 2009;57(8):1331–1346.

46. Marcum ZA, Duncan NA, Makris UE. Pharmacotherapies in geriatric chronic pain management. *Clin Geriatr Med.* 2016;32(4):705–724.

47. Derry S, Moore RA, Gaskell H, McIntyre M, Wiffen PJ. Topical NSAIDs for acute musculoskeletal pain in adults. *Cochrane Database Syst Rev.* 2015;6:CD007402.

48. Swart LM, van der Zanden V, Spies PE, de Rooij SE, van Munster BC. The comparative risk of delirium with different opioids: a systematic review. *Drugs Aging.* 2017; 34(6):437–443.

49. Shi Z, Mei X, Li C, et al. Postoperative delirium is associated with long-term decline in activities of daily living. *Anesthesiology.* 2019;131(3):492–500.

50. Inouye SK, Marcantonio ER, Kosar CM, et al. The short-term and long-term relationship between delirium and cognitive trajectory in older surgical patients. *Alzheimers Dement.* 2016;12(7):766–775.

51. Seripa D, Latina P, Fontana A, et al. Role of CYP2D6 polymorphisms in the outcome of postoperative pain treatment. *Pain Med.* 2015;16(10):2012–2023.

52. Skinner-Robertson S, Fradette C, Bouchard S, Mouksassi MS, Varin F. Pharmacokinetics of tramadol and O-desmethyltramadol enantiomers following administration of extended-release tablets to elderly and young subjects. *Drugs Aging.* 2015;32(12):1029–1043.

53. Stahl ST, Jung C, Weiner DK, Pecina M, Karp JF. Opioid exposure negatively affects antidepressant response to venlafaxine in older adults with chronic low back pain and depression. *Pain Med.* 2019.

54. Makris UE, Pugh MJ, Alvarez CA, et al. Exposure to high-risk medications is associated with worse outcomes in older veterans with chronic pain. *Am J Med Sci.* 2015; 350(4):279–285.

55. Trentalange M, Runels T, Bean A, et al. Analgesic prescribing trends in a national sample of older veterans with osteoarthritis: 2012–2017. *Pain.* 2019;160(6):1319–1326.

56. Macintyre PE, Jarvis DA. Age is the best predictor of postoperative morphine requirements. *Pain.* 1996;64(2):357–364.

57. Shafer SL. The pharmacology of anesthetic drugs in elderly patients. *Anesthesiol Clin N Am.* 2000;18(1):1–29 (v).

58. Andres TM, McGrane T, McEvoy MD, Allen BFS. Geriatric pharmacology: an update. *Anesthesiol Clin.* 2019;37(3): 475–492.

59. Erdal A, Ballard C, Vahia IV, Husebo BS. Analgesic treatments in people with dementia – how safe are they? A systematic review. *Expet Opin Drug Saf.* 2019;18(6):511–522.

60. Friesen KJ, Falk J, Bugden S. The safety of meperidine prescribing in older adults: a longitudinal population-based study. *BMC Geriatr.* 2016;16:100.

61. Price SD, Holman CD, Sanfilippo FM, Emery JD. Association between potentially inappropriate medications from the Beers criteria and the risk of unplanned hospitalization in elderly patients. *Ann Pharmacother.* 2014; 48(1):6–16.

62. Lee J, Lakha SF, Mailis A. Efficacy of low-dose oral liquid morphine for elderly patients with chronic non-cancer pain: retrospective chart review. *Drugs Real World Outcomes.* 2015;2(4):369–376.

63. Wu A. Special considerations for opioid use in elderly patients with chronic pain. *US Pharm.* 2018;43(3):26–30.

CHAPTER 11

Cannabis in Pain

KENNETH FINN, MD

CANNABINOIDS: INTRODUCTION

Cannabinoids are the chemical constituents of the *Cannabis* plant. There are three general categories of cannabinoids present, including phytocannabinoids, endocannabinoids, and synthetic cannabinoids. Phytocannabinoids are cannabinoids found in the plant and are structurally related to delta-9-tetrahydrocannabinol (THC). Endocannabinoids are found in human and animal tissue and exert effects typically on the nervous and immune system. Synthetic cannabinoids are commercially produced substances that attach to cannabinoid receptors and exert an effect on the body. The highest concentration of phytocannabinoids is found in flowers of the *Cannabis* plant but leaves and stems are also used to produce medicinal products, such as edibles, oils, tinctures, resins, and plant extracts (Table 11.1).

Depending on the form of Cannabis product used, the route of administration changes from oral to smoking, vaporization, and topical applications. Although smoking and vaporization produce rapid drug onset and peak levels, vaporization results in a substantially higher blood concentration level of THC. This may lead to increased adverse effects in novice users compared with smoking. Cannabis can also be added to foods such as brownies, cookies, and other common items commonly referred to as edibles. Ingesting edibles results in a slower drug onset and longer duration of action, making dose titration difficult. After ingestion, THC is metabolized to 11-OH-Δ9-tetrahydrocannabinol (11-OH-THC), a more potent psychoactive form. The presence of 11-OH-THC metabolites increases the risk of overdose in novice users (Table 11.2).

CANNABINOID AND OPIOID RECEPTORS: THE EVIDENCE

In this chapter, cannabis and marijuana will be used interchangeably. There is scientific evidence as to how and why cannabinoids may be potentially useful in pain. It is also important to note there are different neurobiological mechanisms in acute and chronic pain. Pain, generically, is a broad diagnosis and there are many different types of pain. Generally speaking, there are somatic, visceral, neuropathic, and psychogenic pain disorders and pain of different origins may respond differently to different types of medications. Under each of those generic types of pain, there may be several other subtypes of pain. For example, neuropathic pain may be due to an organic cause, such as diabetes mellitus, or may be related to underlying central nervous system trauma or disease, such as spinal cord injury. Visceral pain may be related to gastrointestinal disease or space occupying lesions. The management of each of these conditions will likely be different, with some potential overlap.

The two most studied cannabinoids used for medicinal purposes are THC and cannabidiol (CBD) depicted in Fig. 11.1. Both THC and CBD have the same molecular formula ($C_{21}H_{30}O_2$) and interact with cannabinoid receptors. However, they have different molecular configurations, receptor activities, and physiological effects. CBD is a nonpsychoactive cannabinoid with some analgesic, antiinflammatory, antineoplastic, and chemopreventive activities.[51] THC is the primary psychoactive component with effects on euphoria, mood, and cognition.[52]

THC was initially identified in the 1960s[3] and has since been more thoroughly described, with the discovery of the primary molecules anandamide (AEA), 2-arachidonoylglycerol (2-AG), and fatty acid amide hydrolase.[4] Subsequently, mechanisms on how those molecules work have been identified, particularly as it related to its interaction with pain modulation pathways.[5] THC exerts its physiologic effects in the endocannabinoid (endogenous cannabinoid) system, interacting primarily with receptors CB_1 and to lesser degree CB_2.[6] CB_1 receptors are primarily localized in the central nervous system, but may also be found in the periphery, while CB_2 receptors are found in tissues of the immune system but may also be found in the

Pain Care Essentials and Innovations. https://doi.org/10.1016/B978-0-323-72216-2.00011-9

TABLE 11.1

Form	Other Terms	Development	Route of Administration
Plant	Flower, bud	The highest concentration of cannabinoids is found in the flower, not the lead, of the female plant; topical preparation and rectal suppositories can be made with dried flower or plant extract	Smoking Vaporization Topical Rectal
Edibles	Brownies, cookies, candy	Typically butter or oil used to extract cannabinoids and put into a variety of edible products	Oral
Tincture	Golden dragon Green dragon	Alcohol or glycerin used to extract active ingredients	Oral Sublingual Oromucosal
Oil	Rick Simpson oil	Alcohol use to make highly viscous concentrated extract	Oral Topical
Resin	Hash, dry sift, kief	Concentrate made by mechanically separating trichomes (hair-like protrusion on flower with high concentration of cannabinoids) from the plant	Oral mucosal
Nabiximols	Sativex™	Pharmaceutically prepared whole plant extract in spray form; 1:1 THC:CBD concentration; approved for prescription use in many countries outside of United States	Oromucosal
Dab	Wax, shatter	Ultraconcentrated extract made with solvents such as butane; very high levels of THC; risk of overdose and acute psychosis	Dabbing (concentrate placed on very hot metal rod and inhaled)
Pharmaceutical cannabinoids	Dronabinol™ Nabilone™ Epidiolex™	Dronabinol™ and Nabilone™ are FDA-approved synthetic THC (used for chemotherapy-induced nausea, vomiting; AIDS-related cachexia); Epidiolex™ is a highly purified CBD plant extract and is FDA approved for the treatment of two rare epilepsy syndromes	Oral

Adapted from Kansagara, D, MD, Cannabis Provider Education Packet; Portland Evidence Synthesis Program, Department of Veterans Affairs, VA HSRD ESP #05-225We, February 2020.

brain[7] (Fig. 11.2). Cannabinoid and opioid receptors belong to the same rhodopsin subfamily of G protein-coupled receptors, which when activated inhibit adenylyl cyclase, leading to decreases in cellular levels of cyclic adenosine monophosphate.

Opioid and cannabinoid receptors are also localized primarily at the presynaptic nerve terminals, and when activated via cellular mechanisms, inhibit release of multiple neurotransmitters which may modulate pain pathways. They also colocalize in GABA-ergic neurons

TABLE 11.2

Route	Smoking	Vaporization ("Vaping")	Oral/Edibles	Topical
Notes	Combustion of dried cannabis flower using several methods: cigarettes (joints, spliffs), pipes, water pipes (bongs)	Vaporizer is used to heat dried flower or concentrated extract (oil, resin) and the resultant vapor is inhaled	Variety of edibles is available; often dose/single serving is a fraction of the product (i.e., one part of a cookie or brownie)	Many forms are available: creams, ointments, patches, poultices, oils
Pharmacology	Rapid onset and peak	Rapid onset and peak similar to smoking	No inhalation; broad range of products; slower onset and longer duration of action	None of the pulmonary effects associated with inhalation; probably much less intoxicating
Cautions	Bronchial irritation; cough, sputum; production contains carcinogens; potential for adverse effects on lungs function with heavy use over many years	Substantially higher blood THC concentrations achieved at a given dose than with smoking; higher risk of adverse effects in novice users; long-term lung safety is unknown; need for potentially costly equipment; potentially fatal vaping-related pulmonary illness	Onset and peak are delayed, and effects can last many hours which make it more difficult to titrate dose; oral metabolite of THC (11-OH-THC) may have fourfold more powerful psychoactive effect; risk of overdose; caution especially in novice users	Very little is known about topical preparations; unknown systemic absorption

At this time, providers should caution patients against vaping given the lack of certainty regarding the cause and scope of the recently described series of severe vaping-related pulmonary illness cases.
Adapted from Kansagara, D, MD, Cannabis Provider Education Packet; Portland Evidence Synthesis Program, Department of Veterans Affairs, VA HSRD ESP #05-225We, February 2020.

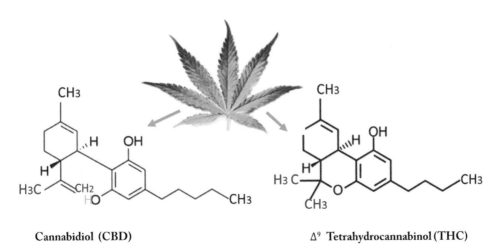

Cannabidiol (CBD) Δ^9 **Tetrahydrocannabinol (THC)**

FIG. 11.1 Cannabidiol (CBD) and delta-9-tetrahydrocannabinol (THC) are both found in the *Cannabis sativa* plant. Note that although they have the same chemical formula ($C_{21}H_{30}O_2$), their configurations and properties are different.

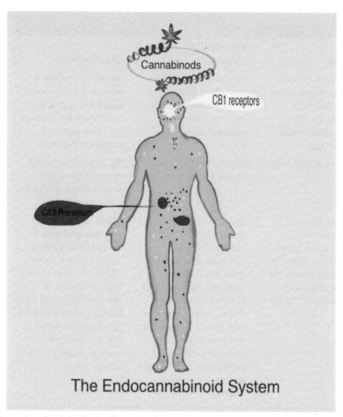

FIG. 11.2 THC exerts physiological effects in the endocannabinoid system through the CB_1 and CB_2 receptors. CB_1 receptors are primarily localized in the central nervous system, but may also be found in the periphery, while CB_2 receptors are found in tissues of the immune system but may also be found in the brain.

the primary inhibitory neurons in the central nervous system. Activation of both opioid and cannabinoid receptors effects the permeability of calcium, potassium, and sodium channels, which may also explain how they may modulate pain pathways.[5,8,9] Inhibition of glutamate release from nociceptive neurons and pain-associated regions is felt to be one of the primary antinociceptive mechanisms.[10] Norepinephrine, 5-hydrotryptamine, glycine, and dopamine are other neurotransmitters, both opioids and cannabinoids may modulate and may have an impact on pain modulation. Opioids and cannabinoids have similar pharmacologic profiles which may cause hypothermia, hypotension, hypoventilation, sedation, and antinociception.[5,8] Naloxone is a mu-opioid inverse agonist as well as kappa- and gamma-receptor antagonist which has been shown to have effects on the cannabinoid system in multiple animal model studies.[11–14] There have been case reports of treating cannabinoid overdose with naloxone infusion.[15]

CBD has been receiving more attention recently due to its nonpsychoactive properties and its potential benefit for a narrow spectrum of pediatric seizures.[16] Its benefits in pain have also been touted due to its possible impacts in inflammatory processes.[17] Due to its molecular makeup, it does not bind well to the CB_1 or CB_2 receptors, although some of its analogs may have low binding affinity for that receptor. Some of the evidence supporting its antiinflammatory properties are its affinity to adenosine A2A, and GPR55 (G protein receptor 55) receptors which may modulate cellular calcium (Ca^{++}) and potassium (K^+) channels. Other signaling events in inflammatory processes identified in animal models include stimulating arachidonic acid release and phospholipid hydrolysis, stimulation of cyclo-oxygenase-2 (COX-2), reduction of prostaglandin E_2 (PGE_2), reduction of nitrous oxide (NO), and other oxygen-derived free radicals. In addition, signaling events may be related to CBD's effect on cytokine production. The effects or benefit of purified CBD use in human inflammatory processes have not been rigorously evaluated.

A serious concern regarding the use of artisanal CBD products for medicinal purposes has much to do with "product integrity." Currently, there is only one FDA-approved and purified CBD: Epidiolex.[18] It is approved for Dravet and Lennox-Gastaut syndromes, effecting a very small percent of the pediatric population. It has been claimed that CBD is federally legal in all 50 states and can be purchased CBD online. It has been reported that medical CBD products purchased in regulated markets failed to meet basic label accuracy standards for pharmaceuticals.[19] In those products, only 59% had detectable levels of CBD, only 17% were accurately labeled with respect to THC content, and only 17% had CBD content labeled. It has been further reported that CBD products purchased online, only 31% were accurately labeled and THC was detected in 21% of the samples,[20] which is federally illegal to be mailed through the postal service.

With the expansion of multiple marijuana markets over the past several years, there appears to be an increasing inability to test and regulate marijuana products which are used for both medical and recreational purposes. In January 2019, the Oregon Secretary of State published an audit of their marijuana programs.[21] They reported that the state was only able to inspect 3% of retailers and 32% of growers due to a variety of issues. There was a significant lack of testing for pesticides and solvents, as well as heavy metals and microbiological contaminants which could pose a consumer risk. They concluded that Oregon's marijuana testing program could not ensure that test results were reliable or that products were safe.

CANNABINOIDS AND PAIN: LITERATURE REVIEW

Despite general restrictions on the study of cannabis from federal levels, there has been ongoing research on cannabis for decades since the discovery of its primary psychoactive component, THC, and subsequently identification of the many other components of the plant which may have potential physiologic activity. Reviews of the medical use of cannabinoids in several conditions have evaluated the evidence at the time.[2,22,32] Currently, many countries are in the midst of an opioid epidemic and there are thoughts that cannabis may be a good opioid substitute and could potentially impact such epidemic.

In 2014, Bachhuber reviewed opioid overdose deaths in medical marijuana states and concluded that medical cannabis laws are associated with a significantly lower state-level opioid overdose mortality rates, however also felt more research was needed to evaluate the interaction between medical cannabis laws and opioid analgesic overdose deaths.[23] In 2016, this was followed by Bradford's research[24] which suggested that medical marijuana laws are associated with lower Medicare D prescriptions and may have influenced opioid prescribing patterns and spending in Medicare Part D. In this day and age of health insurance, cost savings are important to take into consideration. They noted limitations of their study, which included the fact that Medicare D population comprised a very small percentage (13%–27%) of people who use medical marijuana, and physician prescribing behavior is difficult to quantify.

In 2017, Livingston looked at opioid-related deaths in Colorado between 2000 and 2015,[25] utilizing the Centers for Disease Control and Prevention WONDER (Wide-Ranging Online Data for Epidemiologic Research) system. They found a statistically significant reduction of 6% in opioid-related deaths following recreational cannabis legalization in Colorado. A potential confounder they noted was Colorado's prescription drug monitoring program registration mandate in 2014. In 2019, the Colorado Medical Society issued a report[26] showing that PDMP utilization increased by 650% since marijuana legalization in 2014 and the rate of retail-filled opioid prescriptions had decreased to the lowest in 5 years, dropping almost 30% from 2013 to 2018. In that period of time, there has also been an increased physician and public awareness of the opioid epidemic, a significant increase in utilization of naloxone, the reversal agent for opioid overdose, development of atypical opioids, and abuse-deterrent formulations which have less abuse potential, and there may be an increase reluctance for physicians to prescribe, or patients to receive, an opioid prescription.

Despite those efforts and available data, Colorado had a record number of prescription opioid overdose deaths in 2017, with 2018 having the second highest number of deaths (Fig. 11.3). It is important to understand that Colorado has had a medical marijuana program since 2001, and consistently over time, more than 90% of the marijuana recommendations were for a pain condition.[27] Similar data have occurred in other marijuana states, such as Illinois, where their Department of Public Health has been tracking such data. Despite a steady decline in the number of opioid prescriptions, the number of opioid overdose deaths has continued to climb (Fig. 11.4 and 11.5). Interestingly, in Colorado, since legalization for medical and

Number of Drug Overdose Deaths by Substances Mentioned, Colorado, 2000-2018

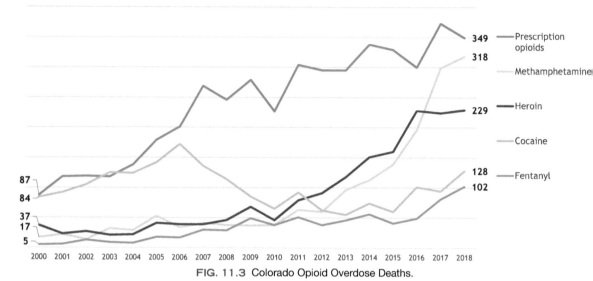

FIG. 11.3 Colorado Opioid Overdose Deaths.

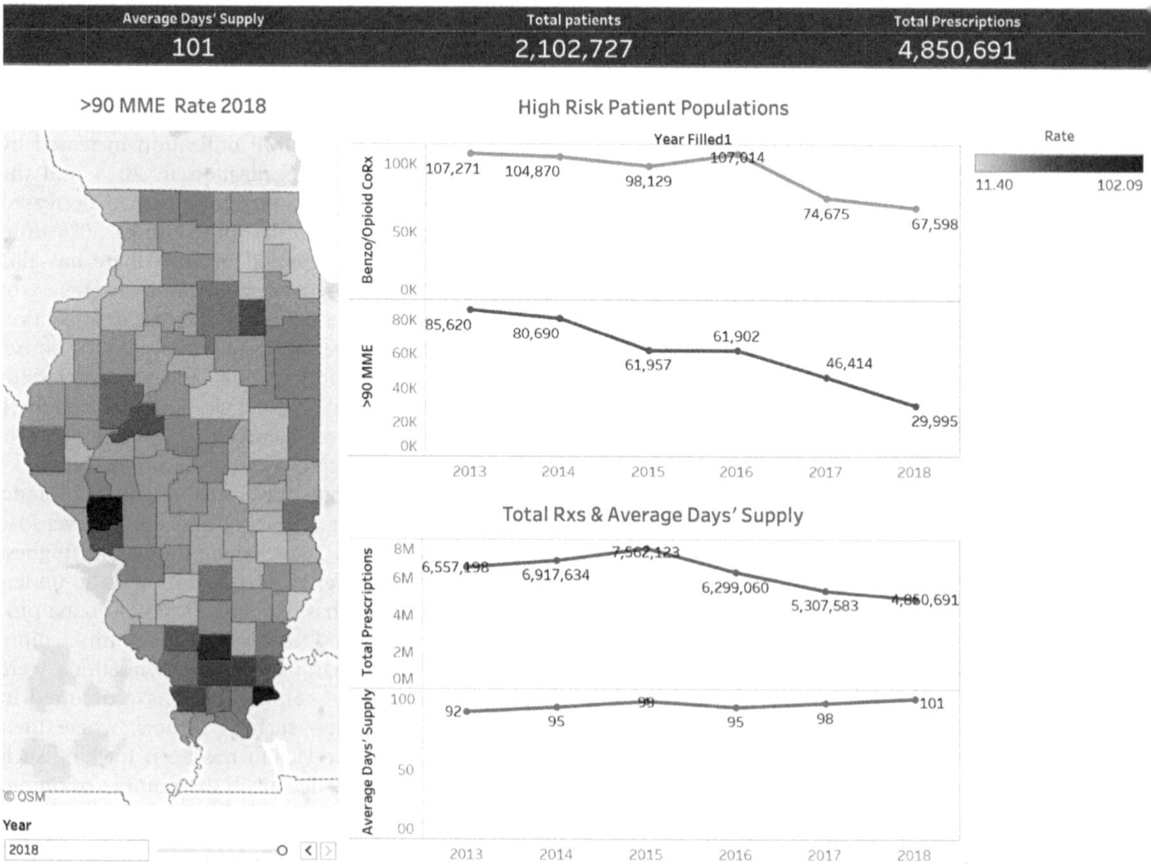

Average Days' Supply	Total patients	Total Prescriptions
101	2,102,727	4,850,691

>90 MME Rate 2018

High Risk Patient Populations

Total Rxs & Average Days' Supply

FIG. 11.4 Illinois Prescription Data.

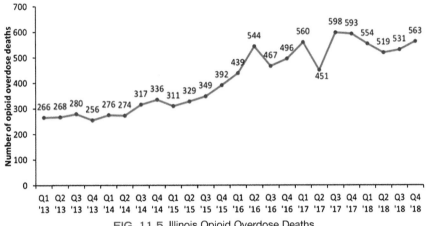

FIG. 11.5 Illinois Opioid Overdose Deaths.

subsequently for recreational use, the number of overdose deaths related to other drugs also increased, including cocaine, methamphetamine, heroin, and fentanyl. In 2018, they noted 16 overdose deaths mentioning marijuana, the highest ever. It is unclear as to the nature or circumstances of those deaths, including an incidental finding or possibly synthetic cannabinoid present.

In 2018, Bradford again looked at the association between US state medical cannabis laws and opioid prescribing in the Medicare Part D population.[28] They determined that medical cannabis laws are associated with significant reductions in opioid prescribing in the Medicare Part D population. Again, a select subset of patients was evaluated, comprising a small percentage of people who may be using cannabis or may be using opioids. The authors were unable to demonstrate a direct relationship between less opioid use and substitution with cannabis.

In September 2019, Bleyer and Barnes looked at opioid mortality data from the US Centers for Disease Control from each marijuana-legalizing state and D.C. before and after legalization implementation. They concluded that legalizing marijuana appears to have contributed to the nation's opioid mortality epidemic.[29]

Furthermore, in 2018, Caputi and Humphries subsequently investigated medical marijuana patients and their use of other prescription medications.[30] Utilizing 2015 data from the National Survey on Drug Use and Health, it was determined that medical marijuana users were significantly more likely to report medical use of prescription drugs in the past 12 months. Those using medical marijuana were also significantly likely to report nonmedical use in the past 12 months of any

prescription drug, with elevated risks for pain relievers, stimulants, and tranquilizers.

In 2017, Olfson published a paper surveyed 43,000 adults in 2001–02 with follow-up of 34,000 adults in 2004–05[31] to determine whether individual patients who use cannabis have a lower or higher risk of developing opioid use disorder. They evaluated the population in 2 waves, establishing baseline data a wave 1 and follow-up data at wave 2, assessing possible associations between cannabis use (at wave 1) and nonmedical prescription opioid use and opioid use disorder (at wave 2). Utilizing the Epidemiologic Survey on Alcohol and Related Conditions and logistic regression models, they concluded that cannabis use increases, rather than decreases the risk of developing nonmedical prescription opioid use and opioid use disorder. Marijuana potency was significantly less at that time compared with potencies of 2019, with some products now reaching close to 99% THC.

In 2017, the National Academies of Science, Engineering and Medicine[32] published a review of the literature for the use of cannabis in several medical conditions. Regarding pain, they concluded that there is substantial evidence that cannabis is an effective treatment for chronic pain in adults. They relied heavily on previous analyses of the literature[22] and were not clear in stating the fact that the majority of studies up to that time supporting use of cannabinoids were with Nabiximols, which are not commercially available in the United States, or with synthetic cannabinoid-based medications, and in less common pain conditions, neuropathic pain and cancer pain. They did note that only a handful of studies evaluated the use of cannabis in the United States and all of those evaluated cannabis in flower form provided by the National Institute on Drug Abuse that was either vaporized or smoked. In addition, they noted that cannabis products sold in state-regulated markets bear little resemblance to products available for research at the federal level and did not include edible or topical artisanal products, which are more widely available in those markets. They also concluded that there is very little known about routes of administration, side effects, and most importantly, efficacy, of commonly used and commercially available products in the United States and supported the need for ongoing research along these lines. They failed to note that Sativex, a natural, purified cannabinoid with a nearly 1:1, THC:CBD ratio, failed two Phase III clinical trials in patients with cancer pain that had maximized opioid therapy.[33] A comparison and contrast of routes of administration is provided in Table 11.2.

Shortly thereafter, Nugent, who reviewed the same literature, came to different conclusions.[34] They wanted to review the benefits of plant-based cannabis preparations for treating chronic pain in adults and the harms of cannabis use in chronic pain and general adult populations. They felt there was low strength evidence that cannabis alleviates neuropathic pain but insufficient evidence in other pain populations. Harms in general patient populations included psychotic symptoms, short-term cognitive impairment, and increased risk for motor vehicle accidents. Review of the literature was limited by few methodologically rigorous trials, cannabis formulations studied may not reflect commercially available products, and there may be limited application to older or chronically ill populations and heavy cannabis users. In 2018, Finn[35] also reached similar conclusions, and highlighted that studies to date were with natural cannabis-based medications not available in the United States or with synthetic or semisynthetic cannabis-based medications, and in less common pain conditions, and importantly, not with dispensary cannabis, which is frequently contaminated.

A 4-year prospective, national, observational cohort of people with chronic noncancer pain prescribed opioids were followed in Australia[36] to evaluate the effect of cannabis use in people with chronic noncancer pain prescribed opioids from August 2012 to April 2014. They noted that cannabis use was common in people with chronic noncancer pain who had been prescribed opioids, but there was no evidence that cannabis use improved patient outcomes. They found participants who used cannabis had a greater pain severity score, greater pain interference score, and greater generalized anxiety disorder severity scores.

There was also no evidence that cannabis use reduced prescribed opioid use or increased rates of opioid discontinuation.

Rogers[37] et al. demonstrated similar findings in 2019. With the passage of medical cannabis laws, by nature there will likely be an increase of cannabis use. Given that opioids are commonly prescribed in chronic pain states, couse of opioids and cannabis is becoming more common. Their results suggest that, compared with opioid use alone, opioid and cannabis couse was associated with elevated anxiety and depression symptoms, as well as tobacco, alcohol, cocaine, and sedative use problems, but not with pain experience. These findings are consistent with experimental pain models[38] that showed that there is a significant, yet small, association between cannabinoid administration and pain threshold but not between pain intensity. Cannabinoids may make experimental pain feel less unpleasant and more tolerable, suggesting there is an affective component. Importantly, cannabis-induced improvements in pain-related negative affect may be the mechanism by which cannabis relieves pain, rather than changes in pain threshold.

Another study[39] evaluated the relationship between cannabis use and aberrant behaviors during chronic opioid therapy for noncancer pain. Higher risk of opioid misuse was found in patients using cannabis and opioids for chronic pain; therefore, closer monitoring for opioid-related aberrancy was recommended for that group of patients.

It was noted that most evidence to date was associated with less common pain conditions, such as cancer pain or neuropathic pain. Chronic lower back pain is one of the most common pain conditions effecting the general population. It has been reported that about 80% of adults will experience low back pain at some point in their lives and about 20% of people affected by low back pain will become chronic.[40] Given that, does the use of inhaled cannabis reduce overall opioid use? Early literature reviews showed that persons who used cannabis for pain had a higher oral morphine equivalent dose than those who did not use cannabis for pain and persons using cannabis for pain were more likely to meet criteria for substance abuse disorders and were more likely to be nonadherent with their prescription opioids.[41] Patients with chronic pain using cannabis may be at higher risk for substance-related outcomes.[42]

Currently, there is little evidence that cannabinoids are effective for acute pain.[43] Authors concluded that in most studies reviewed, cannabinoids were found to provide equivalent analgesia to placebo and there were no synergistic or additive analgesic effect observed when cannabinoids were used in combination with opioids. The authors felt there was no role for the use of cannabinoids in acute pain. There is also no evidence that cannabis is an opioid substitute.[44] Using data on 627,000 individuals aged 12 years and older from the 2004−14 National Survey on Drug Use and Health, the association between state-level medical marijuana law enactment with individual-level nonmedical prescription opioid use and prescription opioid use disorder among prescription opioid users was investigated. The authors determined that medical marijuana law enactment was not associated with a reduction in individual-level nonmedical prescription opioid use, contradicting the hypothesis that people would substitute marijuana for opioids.

In 2018, Salottolo and colleagues looked at marijuana use and acute pain management following traumatic injury. In that retrospective, multiinstitutional pilot study, the effect of posttrauma analgesic pain management was reviewed in chronic and episodic marijuana use and nonuse. They concluded that marijuana use, particularly chronic use, may affect response to injury by requiring greater use of opioid analgesia, and the results were less pronounced in patients who used other drugs, were episodic marijuana users, or nonusers.[45] In May 2019, Twardowski and colleagues published an article in the Journal of the American Osteopathic Society evaluating on the effects of cannabis use on sedation requirements during endoscopic procedures. They found that compared with

Growing medical cannabis (Photo credit: Tilray; Epilepsy & Behavior Special Issue: Cannabinoids and EpilepsyTable of Contents and articles at www.epilepsybehavior.com/issue/S1525-5050(17)X0007-3)

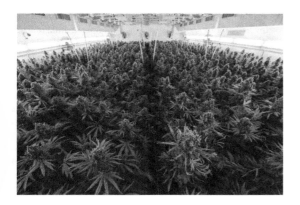

people who did not regularly use cannabis, people who regularly used cannabis required an amount of sedation for endoscopic procedures that was significantly higher ($P = 0.05$). The statistical significance persisted when adjusted for age, sex, and use of alcohol, benzodiazepines, and opiates.[46]

More recently, in September 2019, Liu and colleagues examined the impact of preoperative cannabis use on postop pain scores and pain-related outcomes in patients undergoing major orthopedic surgery. They found that patients who were on preoperative cannabinoids had a higher numerical rating score at rest and with movement and a higher incidence of moderate-to-severe pain at rest and with movement in the early postoperative period compared with patients who were not on cannabinoids. There was also a higher incidence of sleep interruption in the early postoperative period for patients who used cannabinoids.[47]

Large pain organizations have also developed positions on cannabis use as medicine. The British Pain Society (BPS) acknowledges that the use of cannabis may have a place in pain management for a small number of carefully selected people.[48] They also felt that based on metaanalysis on cannabinoids for the management of pain concluded, there is no positive evidence to support routing use in pain management, which include neuropathic, chronic nonmalignant pain, and cancer pain. The BPS considers there may be a role for medical cannabis in pain management, but more reliable evidence is warranted following robust clinical evaluation.

The European Pain Federation published their position paper on appropriate use of cannabis-based medicines and medical cannabis for chronic pain management in the European Journal of Pain in 2018.[49] They made the important distinction between cannabis-based medicines and medical cannabis. They defined "medical cannabis" or "medical marijuana" as cannabis plants and plant material, for example, flowers, marijuana, hashish, buds, leaves, or full plant extracts used for medical reasons. On the other hand, registered medicinal cannabis extracts with defined and standardized THC and THC/CBD content should be classified as "cannabis-derived" or "cannabis-based" medicines. Some of their key points included do not prescribe cannabis flowers with a high (>12.5%) THC content. A dose of no more than one inhalation four times per day to avoid cannabis intoxication and cognitive impairment is recommended. They also recommended screening for anxiety and depression, screening for substance abuse, utilization of treatment agreements, and discouraged smoking.

CONCLUSION

There is evidence that cannabinoids may have antinociceptive properties based on animal, preclinical, and some clinical evidence. Many of the studies to date have demonstrated some improvements with two less common pain diagnoses: neuropathic and cancer pain with products that are not commercially available in the United States or with synthetic cannabinoids. There should be serious concern that current commercially available products are not regulated as expected, or to the degree required, to ensure public health and safety and there should be mechanisms in place to inform consumers on contaminated products.

There are multiple additional negative societal effects associated with marijuana expansion programs which are outside the prevue of this chapter, yet should be taken into consideration in the realm of medicine and include driving impairment, youth use and addiction, pregnancy, in utero exposure, mental health and psychiatric concerns, as well as environment impacts, to name only a few. More recently, severe pulmonary effects, including death,[50] have been associated with use of marijuana products and should raise further concern for medical providers supervising patients using cannabis products. Informed consent and agreements should be utilized similar to those by providers prescribing opioids.

The endocannabinoid system has been well studied and outlined, and there is likely much more understanding needed with the expansion of marijuana markets, both for medicinal and recreational use, in order to determine what role, if any, cannabinoids have in the management of pain. Currently, there is a paucity of evidence that dispensary cannabis, which may be contaminated and poorly regulated,[21] is beneficial with more common pain conditions. FDA drug development protocols and products which are free of contaminants and proven to be effective for pain conditions should be supported.

Cannabis-based medications should be able to be prescribed under the supervision of a qualified medical provider and dispensed through a pharmacy. Dispensary cannabis is not medication and due to the significant variability and potency of products, any intended effect may not be readily achieved. The use of cannabis-based medications in conjunction with opioids and/or benzodiazepines should be avoided until patient safety data are more widely studied, accumulated, and available, as they are all centrally acting substances and may have potential additive effects, which may lead to impairment. Close patient monitoring is recommended for evidence of addiction, other medication misuse or diversion, or other adverse health effects.

Provider education is paramount in order to be better equipped to recognize such effects. Science, not public opinion or industry interests, should direct public policy on the use of cannabinoids as medicine or for personal use.

REFERENCES

1. National Institute of Health, US National Library of Medicine. ClinicalTrials.gov.
2. The National Academies of Sciences, Engineering, and Medicine. *The Health Effects of Cannabis and Cannabinoids: The Current State of Evidence and Recommendations for Research*. The National Academies Press; 2017.
3. Mechoulam R, Gaoni Y. The absolute configuration of delta-1-tetrahydrocannabinol, the major active constituent of hashish. *Tetrahedron Lett*. 1967;12:1109−1111.
4. Devane WA, Hanus L, Breuer A, et al. Isolation and structure of a brain constituent that binds to the cannabinoid receptor. *Science*. 1992;258(5090):1946−1949.
5. Robledo P, Berrendero F, Ozaita A, Maldonado R. Advances in the Field of Cannabinoid−Opioid Crosstalk. *Addict Biol*. 2008;13.
6. Bjorn J, Chen J, Furnish T, Wallace M. Medical marijuana and chronic pain: areview of basic science and clinical evidence. *Curr Pain Headache Rep*. 2015;19:50.
7. Pertwee RG. Pharmacological actions of cannabinoids. In: Pertwee RG, ed. *Handbook of Experimental Pharmacology*. Berlin Heidelberg: Springer-Verlag; 2005:1−51.
8. Scavone JL, Sterling RC, Van Bockstaele EJ. Cannabinoid and opioid interactions: implications for opiate dependence and withdrawal. *Neuroscience*. 2013;248:637−654.
9. Pickel VM, Chan J, Kash TL, Rodriguez JJ, MacKie R. Compartment-specific localization of cannabinoid 1 (CB1) and μ-opioid receptors in rat nucleus accumbens. *Neuroscience*. 2004;127(1):101−112.
10. Lotsch J, Weyer-Menkhoff I, Tegeder I. Current evidence of cannabinoid-based analgesia obtained in preclinical and human experimental settings. *Eur J Pain*. 2018;22:471−484.
11. Sirohi S, Dighe SV, Madia PA, et al. The relative potency of inverse opioid agonists and a neutral opioid antagonist in precipitated withdrawal and antagonism of analgesia and toxicity. *J Pharmacol Exp Therapeut*. 2009;330:513−519.
12. Chen JP, Paredes W, Li J, et al. Delta 9-tetrahydrocannabinol produces naloxone blockable enhancement of presynaptic basal dopamine efflux in nucleus accumbens of conscious, freely moving rats as measured by intracerebral microdialysis. *Psychopharmacology*. 1990;102:156−162.
13. Justinova Z, Tanda G, Munzar P, et al. The opioid antagonist naltrexone reduces the reinforcing effects of Delta 9 tetrahydrocannabinol (THC) in squirrel monkeys. *Psychopharmacology*. 2004;173:186−194.
14. Navarro M, Carrera MR, Fratta W, et al. Functional interaction between opioid and cannabinoid receptors in drug self-administration. *J Neurosci*. 2001;21:5344−5350.

15. Richards JR, Shandera V, Elder JW. Treatment of acute cannabinoid overdose with naloxone infusion. *Toxicol Commun.* 2017;(1):29−33.
16. Welty TE, Luebke A, Gidal BE. Cannabidiol: promise and pitfalls. *Epilepsy Current.* 2014;14(5):250−252.
17. Burstein S. 1377−1385 Cannabidiol (CBD) and its analogs: a review of their effects on inflammation. *Bioorg Med Chem.* 2015;23.
18. *Will Need to Know How to Reference Related to FDA Process.* epidiolex.com:
19. Vandrey R. *J Am Med Assoc.* 2015;313(24).
20. Bonn-Miller MO, Loflin MJE, Thomas BF, et al. *J Am Med Assoc.* 2017;318(17).
21. Secretary of State, Oregon Audits Division. *Oregon's Framework for Regulating Marijuana Should Be Strengthened to Better Mitigate Diversion Risk and Improve Laboratory Testing.* January 2019.
22. Whiting PF, Wolff RF, Deshpande S, et al. Cannabinoids for medical use a systematic review and meta-analysis. *J Am Med Assoc.* 2015;313(24):2456−2473.
23. Bachuber MA, Saloner B, Cunningham CO. Medical cannabis laws and opioid analgesic overdose mortality in the United States. *JAMA Intern Med.* 2014;174(10):1668−1673.
24. Bradford WD, Bradford AC. Medical Marijuana state laws associated with reduced medicare prescriptions. *Health Aff.* 2016;35:1230−1236.
25. Livingston MD, Barnett TE, Delcher C, Wagenaar AC. Recreational cannabis legalization and opioid-related deaths in Colorado, 2000−2015. *Am J Publ Health.* 2017;107(11):1827−1829.
26. Colorado Medical Society. *Physicians Taking Steps to Reverse Opioid Epidemic Nationally and in Colorado;* June 7, 2019. https://www.cms.org/articles/physicians-taking-steps- to-reverse-opioid-epidemic-nationally-and-in-colora.
27. Colorado Department of Public Health and Environment, Medical Marijuana Registry. *Medical Marijuana Statistics and Data.* https://www.colorado.gov.
28. Bradford AC, Bradford WD, Abraham A, Adams GB. Association between US state medical cannabis laws and opioid prescribing in the medicare part D population. *JAMA Intern Med.* 2018;178(5):667−673.
29. Bleyer A, Barnes B. *Contribution of Marijuana Legalization to the U.S. Opioid Mortality Epidemic: Individual and Combined Experience of 27 States and District of Columbia;* medRxiv, Preprinted and Online: https://www.medrxiv.org/content/10.1101/19007393v1. Accessed 2 October 2019.
30. Caputi TL, Humphries K. Medical Marijuana users are more likely to use prescription drugs medically and nonmedically. *J Addiction Med.* 2018;12(4):295−299.
31. Cannabis use and risk of prescription opioid use disorder in the United States; Olfson, M, Wall, MM, Liu, S, Blanco, C;Am J Psychiatr175(1): 47-53.
32. *The Health Effects of Cannabis and Cannabinoids: The Current State of Evidence and Recommendations for Research.* National Academies Press; 2017.
33. Fallon MT, Wolff RF, Deshpande S, et al. Sativex oromucosal spray as adjunctive therapy in advanced cancer patients with chronic pain unalleviated by optimized opioid therapy: two double-blind, randomized, placebo-controlled phase 3 studies. *Br J Pain.* 2017;11(3):119−133.
34. Nugent SM, Morasco BJ, O'Neil ME. The effects of cannabis among adults with chronic pain and an overview of general harms. *Ann Intern Med.* 2017;167(5):319−331.
35. Finn K. Why marijuana will not fix the opioid epidemic. *Missouri Med.* 2018;115(3):191−193.
36. Campbell G, Hall WD, Peacock A, et al. Effect of cannabis use in people with chronic non-cancer pain prescribed opioids: findings from a 4-year prospective cohort study. *Lancet Publ Health.* 2018;3:341−350.
37. Rogers H, et al. Opioid and cannabis co-use among adults with chronic pain: relations to substance misuse, mental health, and pain experience. *J Addiction Med.* 2019;13(4):287−294.
38. De Vita MJ, Moskal D, Maisto SA, Ansell E. Association of cannabinoid administration with experimental pain in healthy adults a systematic review and meta-analysis. *JAMA Psychiatry.* 2018;75(11):1118−1127.
39. DiBenedetto DJ, Weed VF. The association between cannabis use and aberrant behaviors during chronic opioid therapy for chronic pain. *Pain Med.* 2018;19:1997−2008.
40. National Institute of Neurological Disorders and Stroke. *Low Back Pain Fact Sheet.* www.nids.nih.gov.
41. Smaga S, Gharib A. In adults with chronic low back pain, does the use of inhaled cannabis reduce overall opioid use? *Evidence Based Pract.* 2017;20(1):E10−E11.
42. Shah A, Craner J, Cunningham J. Medical cannabis use among patients with chronic pain in an interdisciplinary pain rehabilitation program: characterization and treatment outcomes. *J Subst Abuse Treat.* 2017;77:95−100.
43. Stevens AJ, Higgins MD. A systematic review of the analgesic efficacy of cannabinoid medications in the management of acute pain. *Acta Anaesthesiol Scand.* 2017;61:268−280.
44. Segura LE, Mauro CM, Levy N. Association of US medical marijuana laws with nonmedical prescription opioid use and prescription opioid use disorder. *JAMA Netw Open.* 2019;2(7). e197216.
45. Salottolo, et al. The grass is not always greener: a multiinstitutional pilot study of marijuana uses and acute pain management following traumatic injury. *Patient Saf Surg.* 2018;12:16.
46. Mark A, Twardowski DO, Margaret M, et al. BS effects of cannabis use on sedation requirements for endoscopic procedures. *J Am Osteopath Assoc.* 2019;119(5):307−311.
47. Liu CW, et al. Weeding out the problem: the impact of preoperative cannabinoid use on pain in the perioperative period. *Anesth Analg.* 2019;129(3):874−881.
48. *British Pain Society Position Statement on the Medicinal Use of Cannabinoids in Pain Management, British Pain Society.* britishpainsociety.org. Accessed 26 September 2019.

49. Hauser W, et al. European Pain Federation (EFIC) position paper on appropriate use of cannabis-based medicines and medical cannabis for chronic pain management. *Eur J Pain*. 2018;22:1547–1564.

50. https://learnaboutsam.org/wp-content/uploads/2019/09/VapeTP.pdf.

51. National Center for Biotechnology Information. PubChem Database. Cannabidiol, CID=644019. https://pubchem.ncbi.nlm.nih.gov/compound/Cannabidiol. Accessed 3 March 2020.

52. Gaoni Y, Mechoulam R. Isolation, structure and partial synthesis of an active constituent of hashish. *J Am Chem Soc*. 1964;86:1646.

CHAPTER 12

Inpatient Pain

REBECCA OVSIOWITZ, MD

INTRODUCTION

Inpatient pain management is a critical component of hospital care. Patients followed by an acute pain service are typically those who have undergone surgery, were involved in trauma, have a chronic medical condition that causes pain, such as pancreatitis, or are being managed for cancer pain. Traditional inpatient pain services have focused on postsurgical care. Warfield et al. (Anesthesiology, Oct 31, 1995, 83(5): 1090–1094) noted that as many as 57% of adult patients reported pain was their primary fear before surgery and 77% reported experiencing pain after surgery. Enhanced Recovery After Surgery (ERAS) programs were introduced to allay these concerns and improve postsurgical outcomes. These programs are common in Europe and expanding in the United States to ensure patients have reasonable expectations for postoperative pain control, which may reduce the incidence of chronic postsurgical pain.

PAIN EVALUATION AND ASSESSMENT

For patients admitted to the hospital, assessment for the source of pain should be undertaken. This may be obvious in postsurgical cases but challenging for acute and chronic pain conditions. A comprehensive chart review and careful history and physical examination can illuminate influencing factors contributing to an individual's pain complaint. Other important information includes presence of allergies to pain medications, previous trials of pain medications (including prescriptions, herbal supplements, and over-the-counter medications), current medical status, mental health, and current or prior substance abuse.

Pain is a subjective phenomenon, characterized by individual experiences and variable expressions. Regular and routine pain assessment is essential to optimal pain management. There are many available scales that can be used for patients to communicate their symptoms. The most commonly used are the numeric rating scale in which patients rate their pain from 0 to 10, and the verbal quantitative scale, when a description (no pain, moderate pain, severe pain, etc.) is given. The visual analog scale (Fig. 12.1) requires patients to rate their pain on a horizontal line from no *pain* to *worst possible pain*. Other measures are also available, including the Simple Descriptive Pain Intensity Scale, the Numeric Pain Intensity Scale, and the faces scales, which include the Wong-Baker scale and the Oucher scale (Fig. 12.1). The faces scales consisting of drawings (Wong-Baker) or photographs (Oucher) of young faces in certain pain states can be used to assess pain in children who lack the language or number sophistication to describe their pain. Currently, activity and function scales are becoming more common. These include the PEG: three-item brief screening scale (Fig. 12.2) and the DVPRS (Defense and Veterans Pain Rating Scale).

Pain assessment in patients who are unable or lack the capacity to communicate verbally can be challenging. The Pain Assessment in Advance Dementia tool was developed to assist in pain assessment in patients with dementia, using observation of facial expression, vocalization, and physiologic indicators to create a pain scale score (Fig. 12.3). Patients in intensive care units can be assessed with CPOT (Critical Care Pain Observation Tool),[1-3] which considers compliance with ventilation, body movement, facial expressions, and vocalization (Fig. 12.4). New metrics are being designed and tested to improve pain assessment, including the Clinically Aligned Pain Assessment (CAPA) developed by Donaldson and Chapman. The CAPA promotes patient conversations that incorporate comfort, sleep, function, changes in pain, and pain control.[2] (Fig. 12.5)

SPECIAL POPULATIONS

Certain populations, including geriatric, pediatric, mentally disabled, physically disabled, and the opioid dependent, will require adjustments in the assessment

Pain Care Essentials and Innovations. https://doi.org/10.1016/B978-0-323-72216-2.00012-0

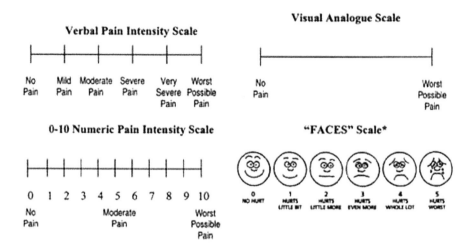

FIG. 12.1 Pain Scales. (Adapted from Analgesic agents: Pharmacology and Application in Critical Care Lisa G. Hall PharmD Lance J.Oyen PharmD, BCPS[a] Michael J.Murray MD, PhD.

1. What number best describes your <u>pain on average</u> in the past week:

0   1   2   3   4   5   6   7   8   9   10

No pain   Pain as bad as
                                                                       you can imagine

2. What number best describes how, during the past week, pain has interfered with your <u>enjoyment of life</u>?

0   1   2   3   4   5   6   7   8   9   10

Does not   Completely
interfere   interferes

3. What number best describes how, during the past week, pain has interfered with your <u>general activity</u>?

0   1   2   3   4   5   6   7   8   9   10

Does not   Completely
interfere   interferes

FIG. 12.2 The PEG three-item scale. (The PEG three-item scale * Items from the Brief Pain Inventory adapted from Krebs EE, Lorenz KA, Bair MJ, et al. *J Gen Intern Med.* 2009;24:733.

and management of their pain complaints. Polypharmacy and impaired organ function are common in the geriatric population, requiring judicious prescribing. Assessment of pain is also challenging in the elderly due to dementia, delirium, or stoicism, which may contribute to undertreatment of pain. In physically or cognitively impaired patients, it can be difficult to assess pain and address pain complaints due to the potentially limited ability to communicate. An example where special precaution should be taken is when prescribing a controlled analgesia pump for a patient who is visually or physically impaired, as they may not be able to use the pump as directed. Patients in the intensive care unit setting may be physically impaired by endotracheal tubes, or cognitively impaired due to sedation, making adequate pain assessment more challenging. Those with mental health comorbidities, such as anxiety or depression, may be at higher risk for overdose due to drug-drug interactions as well as increased sensitivity to pain medications. Pain management in patients with a history of substance use disorder may also be challenging due to tolerance, drug-seeking behavior, and behavioral difficulties.

	0	1	2	Score
Breathing Independent of vocalization	Normal	Occasional labored breathing. Short period of hyperventilation	Noisy labored breathing. Long period of hyperventilation. Cheyne-Stokes respirations.	
Negative vocalization	None	Occasional moan or groan. Low-level speech with a negative or disapproving quality.	Repeated troubled calling out. Loud moaning or groaning. Crying.	
Facial expression	Smiling, or inexpressive	Sad. Frightened. Frown	Facial grimacing	
Body language	Relaxed	Tense. Distressed pacing. Fidgeting.	Rigid. Fists clenched. Knees pulled up. Pulling or pushing away. Striking out.	
Consolability	No need to console	Distracted or reassured by voice or touch.	Unable to console, distract or reassure.	
			TOTAL	

FIG. 12.3 Pain Assessment advanced Dementia (PAINAD). (Adapted from Development and Psychometric Evaluation of the Pain Assessment in Advanced Dementia (PAINAD) Scale.)

PAIN MANAGEMENT
Route of Administration

In general, the least invasive route of drug administration is preferred. Typically, the least invasive route is the oral route; however, other minimally invasive methods include intranasal and transdermal routes. The transmucosal route is also available, but drug bioavailability is variable. More invasive and less preferred routes for medication administration include intramuscular and rectum administration. If immediate pain relief is needed, intravenous (IV), (PCA), patient-controlled epidural analgesia (PCEA), and regional anesthesia can be considered. It is important to reassess pain control after medication administration or intervention to assess for treatment effectiveness and adverse effects.

Medication Selection

Appropriate implementation of pharmacologic interventions can enhance pain control on the inpatient pain service. Providers should consider a multimodal approach to pain control including nonpharmacologic and pharmacologic interventions.

Acetaminophen

Acetaminophen is widely used for its antipyretic and analgesic effects. The exact mechanism of action of acetaminophen is unclear, but it[4] weakly inhibits prostaglandin (PG) synthesis in vitro and may have antiinflammatory activity, earning the classification as a

nonsteroidal antiinflammatory drug (NSAID). It is typically felt to work through a central mechanism with predominant effects on analgesia and fever control with limited antiinflammatory effects. Acetaminophen is commercially available as an IV solution, rectal suppository, and a variety of oral products. Acetaminophen is also available in oral formulations in combination with opioids (codeine, hydrocodone, oxycodone, etc.), that may provide synergy. The Federal Drug Administration set a daily dose limit of 4 g for acetaminophen, but caution should be exercised above 3 g, and less for patient with impaired liver function. The recommended oral dose is 500–1000 mg twice or three times daily.

NSAIDS

NSAIDs act peripherally to inhibit PG synthesis and provide antiinflammatory, antipyretic, and analgesic effects. NSAIDs are used for mild to moderate pain, and when combined with opioids, can be used for severe pain. With the growing concern for opioid use in the United States, NSAIDs are more prevalent in inpatient and outpatient settings. NSAIDs can assist in managing postoperative pain, leading to reductions in opioid use, time to first ambulation, and time to first bowel movement.[5,6] However, NSAIDs carry a black box warning for increased risk of serious cardiovascular thrombotic events and gastrointestinal adverse events, including bleeding, ulceration, and perforation. NSAIDs can cause kidney injury and reduced renal blood flow, may affect bone healing,

Indicator	Score		Operational Definition
Facial Expressions	Relaxed, neutral	0	No muscle tension observed
	Tense	1	Presence of frowning, brow lowering, orbit tightening, and levator contraction or any other change (e.g., opening eyes or tearing during nociceptive procedures)
	Grimacing	2	All previous facial movements plus eyelid tightly closed (the patient may present with mouth open or biting the endotracheal tube)
Body Movements	Absence of movements or normal position	0	Does not move at all (doesn't necessarily mean absence of pain) or normal position (movements not aimed toward the pain site or not made for the purpose of protection)
	Protection	1	Slow, cautious movements, touching or rubbing the pain site, seeking attention through movements
	Restlessness	2	Pulling tube, attempting to sit up, moving limbs/thrashing, not following commands, striking at staff, trying to climb out of bed
Compliance with the ventilator (intubated patients)	Tolerating ventilator or movement	0	Alarms not activated, easy ventilation
	Coughing but tolerating	1	Coughing, alarms may be activated but stop spontaneously
	Fighting ventilator	2	Asynchrony: blocking ventilation, alarms frequently activated
Or			
Vocalization (extubated patients)	Talking in normal tone or no sound	0	Talking in normal tone or no sound
	Sighing, moaning	1	Sighing, moaning
	Crying out, sobbing	2	Crying out, sobbing
Muscle tension: Evaluation by passive flexion and extension of upper limbs when patient is at rest or evaluation when patient is being turned	Relaxed	0	No resistance to passive movements
	Tense, rigid	1	Resistance to passive movements
	Very tense or rigid	2	Strong resistance to passive movements, incapacity to complete them
Total		/8	

FIG. 12.4 Description and Directives to use the Critical Care Pain Observation Tool (CPOT). (Adapted from Céline Gélinas RN, PhD. Nurses' evaluations of the feasibility and the clinical utility of the critical-care pain observation tool. *Pain Manag Nurs*. 2010;11(2):115–125, Copyright © 2010 American Society for Pain Management Nursing.)

Question	Response
Comfort	• Intolerable • Tolerable with discomfort • Comfortably manageable • Negligible pain
Change in Pain	• Getting worse • About the same • Getting better
Pain Control	• Inadequate pain control • Partially effective • Fully effective *Would like to reduce medication (why?)*
Functioning	• Can't do anything because of pain • Pain keeps me from doing most of what I need to do • Can do most things, but pain gets in the way of some • Can do everything I need to
Sleep	• A wake with pain most of night • Awake with occasional pain • Normal Sleep

FIG. 12.5 CAPA tool. (Adapted from Donaldson G, Chapman. *Pain is More Than Just a Number*. 2013: University of Utah Health Care/Department of Anesthesiology.)

and are contraindicated for perioperative use in coronary artery bypass surgery. There are several NSAID classes that vary in selectivity, potency, and formulation (Fig. 12.6). The classes of NSAIDs include carboxylic acids (which include salicylic acid), propionic and acetic acids, anthranilic acid derivatives, and cyclooxygenase-2 selective (COX-2). Unlike other NSAIDs, aspirin specifically inhibits platelet aggregation and irreversibly blocks cyclooxygenase. Because each NSAID class has unique efficacy and side effect profiles, patients who did not respond to one class may respond to a drug in another class. NSAIDs are most commonly prescribed in oral formulations. Topical formulations of NSAIDs, including diclofenac and ketoprofen, show promising results when used for musculoskeletal conditions.[7] An IV NSAID formulation, such as ketorolac, has been shown to have an equivalent analgesic effect to morphine in major abdominal surgery and reduce the use of opioid medications.[8–11] Both ibuprofen and diclofenac are also available in an IV formulation for use in postsurgical pain.

Opioids

Opioids act on central receptors in the brain and spinal cord to mediate pain. Among the opioid receptors (mu (μ), kappa (κ), and sigma (σ)), mu receptors contribute significantly to analgesia and respiratory depression. A short-term trial of opioids in the acute postoperative period may be used along with a plan to reduce the medication as pain improves with healing. Often, the type and amount of opioid prescribed after common surgical procedures varies greatly, resulting in more medication prescribed than necessary after discharge.[12–14] The incidence of persistent opioid use after minor or major surgical procedures is noted to be significantly higher (approximately 6%) than in the nonoperative group (0.4%) and associated with behavioral and pain disorders.[15] In an attempt to offer guidelines to provide appropriate pain treatment, Overton et al. described utilizing a modified Delphi procedure to determine the maximum number of opioid tablets required at discharge for various surgical procedures.[14] Furthermore, after the CDC guidelines for opioid prescribing was published, 31 states (as of March 2016) have implemented a 7-day limit for initial or postoperative prescriptions.[16]

Short-acting opioids. Short-acting opioids are used for fast reduction of pain. Opioid regimens vary widely, but short-term judicious management with a sliding scale can assist in determining the opioid requirements. An example of sliding scale includes use of morphine sulfate-immediate release (IR) 5 mg po for mild pain (1–3/10), 10 mg po for moderate pain

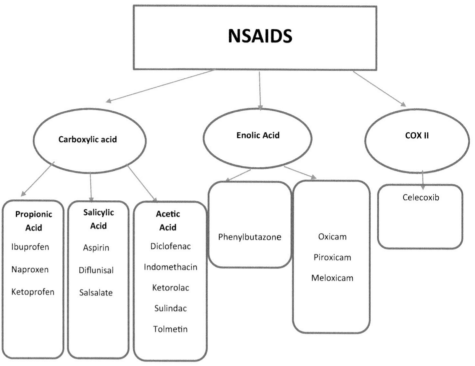

FIG. 12.6 NSAID classification by chemical structures.

(4−6/10), or 15 mg for severe pain 7−10/10, given every 4−6 h. Similarly, oxycodone sliding scale can be used from 5 to 15 mg every 4−6 h using the same scale for mild, moderate, and severe pain in opioid naïve patients. Concurrent use of more than one short-acting opioid should be avoided due to an increase in adverse effects. If adequate pain control is not achieved despite dose increase, or side effects are intolerable, opioid rotation to another short-acting opioid should be considered. Medication regimens should also consider formulations that include acetaminophen, as acetaminophen is limited by the total 24-hour total amount (i.e., > 4 g/daily.). Clinician should be extra cautious when using opioids in older individuals per the Beers Criteria.[17,18] The Beers Criteria was first published in the American Journal of Geriatric Society in 1991 and last updated in 2019. It includes a list of medications that may be used with caution in older adults due to safety, drug-drug interactions, side effects, etc.

Patient-controlled analgesia and patient-controlled epidural analgesia. Patient controlled analgesia (PCA) and PCEA offers patients immediate pain relief and is considered the gold standard for postoperative pain control after major surgery. PCA and PCEA treatment allows self-administration of IV or epidural opioids, respectively, to provide individuals continuous (basal rate) and/or on-demand dosing with triggered bolus. The PCA and PCEA drug delivery units have built-in safety features such as time lock, maximum dose limits, and capnography. The delivery units also document medication use, including bolus frequency. Basal rate infusions should be avoided in opioid naïve patients due to increased risk of adverse effects, such as sedation and respiratory depression, but can be used with caution in patients on chronic opioids. Standard PCA often utilizes morphine but hydromorphone and fentanyl are options for patients with renal impairment. PCEA uses opioids or opioids in combination with anesthetics (i.e., bupivacaine). In complex abdominal, thoracic, and major gynecological cancer surgeries, PCEA is preferred due to improved postsurgical outcomes[19] and superior pain relief with less sedative effects.[20] During transition from IV opioids to oral formulations, it is recommended to allow approximately 90 min of overlap time for oral medication to reach steady state.[21] The conversion ratio of opioids depends on the drug's molecular weight, lipophilicity, and membrane permeability. The general conversion between different formulations is noted below and can be adjusted based on a patient's tolerance and cross-reacting medications(Table 12.1).

Long-acting opiates. The use of long-acting opioid formulations is generally not supported for acute pain management. In individuals with chronic pain with identified pathology that warrants long-term regimens, appropriate use of long-acting or sustained released opioids may offer improved steady-state pain control. For individuals maintained on a long-acting opioid regimen, weaning to a lowest possible oral medication equivalent preoperatively may improve postoperative pain control. During the acute postsurgical period, individuals may require higher doses of short-acting opioids to cover baseline requirements and once tolerating orals, patients may resume their home regimen with additional oral breakthrough dosing. The goal for opioid use in the perioperative period is to use the lowest amount of medication necessary for pain control and then taper off medications as healing occurs.

Synthetic opioids and medication-assisted treatment. Synthetic opioids such as methadone and fentanyl are potent analgesics. Methadone and fentanyl can be used in the postoperative period for select patients that are opioid tolerant or have renal and/or hepatic dysfunction. Individuals with organ impairment require careful consideration when choosing opioids to address new/acute postsurgical pain or flares/exacerbations that contribute to acute hospitalizations.[22–24]

Equally challenging is pain management for patients admitted to the hospital who are on medication-assisted treatment (MAT) for substance use disorder. Individuals on the partial agonist buprenorphine undergoing elective surgery can hold the medication 3 days prior to surgery to minimize side effects of poor pain control related to mu-opioid receptor binding and potential for increased respiratory depression once buprenorphine is fully eliminated from the body.[15] Individuals on chronic MAT, who require emergency surgery or those admitted with acute pain, can continue buprenorphine with nonopioid adjuvants, if postsurgical pain is expected to be mild to moderate. In the case of severe pain, the recommendation is to discontinue buprenorphine and carefully titrate a short-acting opioid while monitoring for respiratory depression, as higher doses of pure mu agonists will typically be needed for analgesic effect.[25–27]

Opioid-induced constipation. Constipation is a common side effect of opioids, affecting 40%–60% of patients on opioids for noncancer pain. Opioids inhibit gastric emptying and peristalsis in the GI tract as well as increase anal sphincter tone, resulting in hardened infrequent stool, incomplete emptying, and constipation. Patients who are older, female, and unemployed are more likely to be affected. A review of different opioids showed no difference in rates of opioid-induced constipation (OIC) between morphine, hydrocodone, and hydromorphone.[28] However, the rates of OIC for transdermal opioids (fentanyl and buprenorphine) are numerically lower than for oral opioids.[29]

Prophylaxis agents should be initiated at the same time that opioids are started. In addition, patients should be encouraged to increase dietary fiber, fluid intake, and increase physical activities to promote healthy bowel motility. If medication is needed, stimulant laxatives (i.e., bisacodyl, sodium picosulfate, sennoside, polyethylene glycol), macrogol, and synthetic sugars (i.e., lactulose, sorbitol) have shown effectiveness in relieving OIC.[29] Bulk laxatives such as psyllium should be avoided as they may cause bowel distention, leading to possible bowel obstruction.[30]

Newer formulations such as prucalopride (a potent and highly selective agonist of $5\text{-}HT_4$ serotonin receptors) and lubiprostone (a chloride [Cl$^-$] channel activator derived from PG E1) are now available. In addition, peripherally acting μ-opioid receptor antagonists (PAMORAs) have been shown to improve OIC. This class of medication includes naloxone, methylnaltrexone, naloxegol, and alvimopan.[30]

TABLE 12.1
IV and Epidural Opioid Conversion

	Properties	Ratio	Oral	IV	Epidural	Intrathecal
Morphine	Hydrophilic	1/10	30 mg	10 mg	1.0 mg	0.10 mg
Hydromorphone	Intermediate	1/5	5 mg	1 mg	0.2 mg	0.04 mg
Fentanyl	Lipophilic	1/3 to 1/5	N/a	100 μg	33 μg	6–10 μg

Adjuvants

Selective serotonin reuptake inhibitors/Serotonin norepinephrine reuptake inhibitors. Selective serotonin reuptake inhibitor antidepressants block serotonin reuptake in the central nervous system and increase serotonin availability in the synaptic cleft. Similarly, serotonin norepinephrine reuptake inhibitors (SNRIs) increase time and availability of serotonin and norepinephrine in the synaptic cleft. These inhibitory neuromodulators are effective antidepressants which may diminish the affective components of pain. SNRIs also appear to play an additional role in the pain cascade (targeting among others, the mu-opioid receptors and chloride channels).[31,32] SNRIs can improve symptoms of pain, with or without concurrent depression. Currently, there are two SNRIs that are approved by the Food and Drug Administration (FDA) for the treatment of pain, duloxetine and milnacipran. Duloxetine is approved for the treatment of fibromyalgia, chronic musculoskeletal pain, and diabetic peripheral polyneuropathy. A trial of duloxetine 30–60 mg daily may be helpful for these conditions, but caution is advised in patients with hepatic impairment or renal impairment (creatinine clearance < 30 mL/min). Milnacipran if FDA approved for fibromyalgia, typically prescribed 12.5 –200mg daily with caution in end-staged renal disease (ESRD)/severe renal impairment.[33,34] Another SNRI, venlafaxine (approved for migraine prophylaxis) is also used for management of neuropathic pain. SNRIs should be used with caution in patients who are concurrently taking tricyclic antidepressants (TCAs), monoamine oxidase inhibitors, triptans, and antiemetics due to increased risk for serotonin syndrome. Serotonin syndrome is a condition caused by serotonin toxicity presenting with mental status changes (confusion, agitation, anxiety, etc.), autonomic manifestation (diaphoresis, hypertension, tachycardia, etc.), and neuromuscular hyperactivity (clonus, increased muscle tone and deep tendon reflexes, etc.). In addition to serotonin syndrome, the seizure threshold can be lowered in patients taking SNRIs if tramadol (a weak μ agonist with serotoninergic and norepinergic properties) is concurrently used.[35,36]

Tricyclics. TCAs block catecholamines which allow serotonin and norepinephrine more time and exposure in the synaptic cleft. Low dose TCAs can offer analgesic action and improve sleep, although TCAs have significant anticholinergic side effects and caution is advised for use in the geriatric population (>65; Beers Criteria). TCAs can prolong the QTc interval and an electrocardiogram (EKG) should be obtained prior to initiation. In addition, abrupt discontinuation can precipitate withdrawal symptoms and should be avoided. Tertiary amine TCAs, such as amitriptyline, may lead to intolerable dry mouth and monitoring should be done for neurologic, cardiovascular, and hematologic effects. Secondary amine TCAs, like nortriptyline and desipramine, may be better tolerated with fewer anticholinergic side effects.[33,36]

Anticonvulsants. The anticonvulsant class of medications was initially developed to treat seizure disorders, but the gabapentinoid class was shown to improve nerve pain. The gabapentinoids (gabapentin, pregabalin) are membrane stabilizers that play a role in neuropathic pain, postherpetic neuralgia, and migraines by antagonizing the alpha-2-delta Ca++ channels =.[33,37] The gabapentinoids also have efficacy in treating central pain.[38,39] Gabapentin is often initiated at 300 mg q.h.s (100 mg for older/frail individuals) and titrated by 300 mg every 3 days (i.e., 300 mg BID, then TID) to a maximum dose of 3600 mg daily (renal dose is max 1200–1400 mg). More recently, there has been concern for sedation with concurrent use of gabapentinoids with opioids, increasing the risk for respiratory depression.[33]

Muscle relaxants. Muscle relaxants are used to reduce skeletal muscle tone or spasticity associated with pain. With the exception of dantrolene sodium, which works directly on the muscle by inhibiting Ca^{2+} ions release from sarcoplasmic reticulum, most muscle relaxants work at the level of the central nervous system. For example, cyclobenzaprine exerts its action at the brain stem to reduce tonic somatic motor activity. Baclofen, an agonist of presynaptic GABA-B receptors works at the level of the spinal cord to block transmission of monosynaptic and polysynaptic reflexes and reduce the release of excitatory transmitters, including glutamic and aspartic acids. Tizanidine, an alpa-2 adrenergic agonist, acts as an antinociceptive agent, increasing presynaptic inhibition of motor neurons thereby reducing release of excitatory amino acids blocking caeruleospinal pathways. Other muscle relaxants like carisoprodol block intraneuronal activity in the descending reticular formation and spinal cord, but there is concern that carisoprodol has addiction/abuse potential. Diazepam is a benzodiazepine that enhances gamma-amino butyric acid and allows increased chloride ion permeability across membrane channels, which may facilitate spasticity management in spinal cord injury.[33] However, side effects and the habit-forming nature of benzodiazepines limit their long-term use.

Topicals agents. Topical analgesics like lidocaine, capsaicin, and topical diclofenac can provide local pain relief. Lidocaine blocks sodium ion channels required for initiation and conduction of neuronal impulses, and topical application may provide analgesic effects to intact integument. Topical capsaicin acts by depleting substance P in the peripheral nerve endings thereby interrupting pain signal transmission to the brain. The patch formulation of capsaicin affects heat detection and sharp sensations by stimulating transient receptor potential vanilloid-1 receptors (TRPV1), resulting in reduction in pain signal transmission from nerve endings. Topical diclofenac is an NSAID pain reliever that is FDA approved for knee osteoarthritis. Topical diclofenac carries a black box warning for increased risk of serious cardiovascular thrombotic events and gastrointestinal side effects. Topical menthol/salicylate may offer cooling effects and act as a pain distractor.[33,40]

N-methyl-D-aspartate receptor antagonists. N-methyl-D-aspartate receptor antagonists may reduce central sensitization, hyperalgesia, and opioid tolerance; however, many are limited by their side effect profile. In 1956, the Parke-Davis lab discovered a process to synthesize phencyclidine (PCP). Shortly thereafter, ketamine was formulated with similar properties. Ketamine was described to have cataleptic, analgesic, and anesthetic actions without hypnotic properties and the first studies performed on prisoners elucidated dissociative anesthetic effects. Ketamine was utilized as a field anesthetic during the Vietnam War, but abuse and psychedelic properties pushed it out of favor. Ketamine is experiencing a resurgence, especially in treatment-resistant depression and pain. Indications for ketamine use include those undergoing surgical procedures with expected severe postoperative pain such as abdominal or thoracic surgeries, and individuals who are opioid tolerant and/or dependent undergoing surgery or experiencing a flare of chronic pain (sickle cell disease, pancreatitis pain, Ehlers-Danlos syndrome).[41,42] Ketamine IV infusion dosing is individualized but typically the maximum dosing is 0.9 mg/kg/h and with a total of 600 mg.[43–50]

Neural blockade
Perioperative regional, local, or percutaneous anesthetic blocks may offer improved postoperative pain control.

IV ketamine, lidocaine, magnesium, and esmolol (beta blocker) are available and may improve perioperative pain control. In addition, alpha-2 agonists can facilitate analgesia with effects on anxiolysis, sedation, and hypnosis.[51] New technologies allow for placement of percutaneous pumps and catheters to deliver postoperative treatment.[19]

Interdisciplinary pain management
Pain is a conscious experience and is greatly affected by stress and mood, specifically depression and anxiety. The aforementioned factors are common in hospitalized patients and a comprehensive treatment plan should incorporate supportive psychology, addiction, and/or psychiatry assistance if a patient is not progressing as expected. MAT may be necessary for those with current or prior substance use disorders as these individuals may have challenging and complex peri- and postoperative hospital courses. Evidence-based literature supports optimizing nonpharmacologic interventions and providing multimodal management of pain, including the behavioral approaches of mindfulness, breathing relaxation, guided imagery, aromatherapy, and biofeedback. For patients with persistent pain after discharge from the hospital, treatments like cognitive behavioral therapy may improve coping skills and provide cognitive restructuring. In addition, yoga, tai chi, physical/occupation/recreational therapy, hypnosis, and modalities such as acupuncture, battlefield acupuncture, transcutaneous electrical stimulation may be useful and should be considered.

Enhanced recovery after surgery
The ERAS is a multimodal, patient-centered, perioperative protocol that was developed to achieve early recovery after surgical procedures. This program was first described in the 1990s by Dr. Henrik Kehlet, a colorectal surgeon at Copenhagen University in Denmark. His work has been shown to decrease length of stay, decrease complications, and improve economic costs. Although the ERAS program was initially described in colorectal surgery, the program has been introduced and accepted in a variety of surgical specialties. The various algorithms for specific surgeries include preoperative, intraoperative, and postoperative protocols that are incorporated into care plans that decrease surgical stress, maintain physiologic function, and expedite return to physical baseline. The algorithm included avoidance of prolonged perioperative fasting, perioperative nutrition (preoperative fluid and carbohydrate loading up to 2 h preoperatively), avoidance of intraoperative drain placement, avoidance of salt/water

overload, early postoperative mobilization, early catheter removal, and the promotion of oral nutrition. The ERAS program begins with behavior modifications such as smoking and alcohol cessation and presurgical counseling with patients and families about reasonable postsurgical expectations.[52] An example of an orthopedic analgesic protocol is shown below.

MICHIGAN MEDICINE ORTHOPEDIC ANALGESIC PROTOCOL

Pre-op	Celecoxib 400 mg, acetaminophen 1000 mg, gabapentin 600 mg, clonidine 0.1 mg patch (avoid SPB <100 and HR < 50). Intraoperative neuraxial anesthesia, dexamethasone 4 mg IV, periarticular hip injection, ketorolac 30 mg IV at skin closure.
Post-op	Dexamethasone 10 mg IV q8hour x 2 doses, ketorolac 15 mg IV q6hr x 3 doses, magnesium gluconate 400 mg daily prn muscle spasms, omeprazole 40 mg daily, ondansetron 4 mg q8hr prn, oxycodone 5–10 mg q4hr prn pain, advance POD#1 celecoxib 200 mg, gabapentin 100 mg TID, acetaminophen 500 mg q4.[43]

SIDE EFFECTS MANAGEMENT

Nausea/vomiting	Tolerance typically develops after several doses and offer antiemetics.
Pruritis	Counsel to avoid scratching, avoid irritating soaps, offer trial of antihistamine.
Constipation	Consider premedicating with a bowel regimen, consider polyethylene glycol.

FUTURE CONSIDERATIONS

There are many ideas to consider for the future of inpatient pain medicine. Precision medicine may help to customize pain regimens specifically for each individual. For example, pharmacogenomic biomarkers can be utilized to match an individual to the optimal medication, dosage, and timing.[53–55] Genetic testing is now widely available, and screening may become more cost-effective and accessible. The results of genetic tests may assist providers to recognize genetic enzyme deficiencies or chromosomal abnormalities (i.e., P450 defects) and optimize patient-specific pain regimens. The combination of pharmacogenomic and genetic information may assist providers in tailoring medications but needs to be more fully developed prior to commercial use.[56–59] Regulatory agencies, such as the Joint Commission on Accreditation of Healthcare Organizations (JCAHO), have regularly provided guidance on performance improvement and management in the

hospital setting for pain, which highlight education, safety, and collaboration.[60]

CONCLUSION

Pain care of the hospitalized patient continues to be a top priority for clinicians, administrators, and oversight committees, including the JCAHO. These oversight groups suggest hospitals provide a multipronged and multilevel approach that prioritizes individualized pain care. The literature suggests poorly managed pain increases patient distress, anxiety, length of stay, and potentially adds to the chronification of pain. To this end, routine pain assessment in the acute medical or surgical setting should be population specific and involve continuous quality improvement. A focus on patient and staff education, monitoring, safety, and rational polypharmacy may reduce future complications. In addition, the concerns related to excess opioid prescription have become increasingly apparent, some of which started with inpatient opioid prescribing. As such, management in the hospital setting should focus on providing multimodal and multidisciplinary approaches that employ both pharmacologic and nonpharmacologic pain therapies.

REFERENCES

1. Krebs EE, Lorenz KA, Bair MJ, et al. Development and initial validation of the PEG, a three-item scale assessing pain intensity and interference. *J Gen Intern Med.* 2009;24(6): 733–738. https://doi.org/10.1007/s11606-009-0981-1.
2. Donaldson G, Chapman CR. *Pain Is More Than Just a Number.* University of Utah Health Care/Department of Anesthesiology; 2013.
3. Buckenmaier CC, Galloway KT, Polomano RC, McDuffie M, Kwon N, Gallagher RM. Preliminary validation of the defense and Veterans pain rating scale (DVPRS) in a military population. *Pain Med.* January 2013;14(1):110–123. https://doi.org/10.1111/j.1526-4637.2012.01516.x.
4. Botting R. Mechanism of action of acetaminophen: is there a cyclooxygenase 3? *Clin Infect Dis.* October 2000; 31(Suppl 5):S202–S210.
5. Chen JY, Wu GJ, Mok MS, et al. Effect of adding ketorolac to intravenous morphine patient-controlled analgesia on bowel function in colorectal surgery patients—a prospective, randomized, double-blind study. *Acta Anaesthesiol Scand.* 2005;49:546–551.
6. Schlachta CM, Burpee SE, Fernandez C, et al. Optimizing recovery after laparoscopic colon surgery (ORAL-CS): effect of intravenous ketorolac on length of hospital stay. *Surg Endosc.* 2007;21:2212–2219.
7. Derry S, Conaghan P, Da Silva JA, Wiffen PJ, Moore RA. Topical NSAIDs for chronic musculoskeletal pain in adults. *Cochrane Database Syst Rev.* 2016;4(4):CD007400. https://doi.org/10.1002/14651858.CD007400.pub3.

8. Bosek V, Miguel R. Comparison of morphine and ketorolac for intravenous patient-controlled analgesia in postoperative cancer patients. *Clin J Pain.* 1994;10:314−318.

9. Brown CR, Mazzulla JP, Mok MS, et al. Comparison of repeat doses of intramuscular ketorolac tromethamine and morphine sulfate for analgesia after major surgery. *Pharmacotherapy.* 1990;10:45S−50S.

10. Cataldo PA, Senagore AJ, Kilbride MJ. Ketorolac and patient controlled analgesia in the treatment of postoperative pain. *Surg Gynecol Obstet.* 1993;176:435−438.

11. Spindler JS, Mehlisch D, Brown CR. Intramuscular ketorolac and morphine in the treatment of moderate to severe pain after major surgery. *Pharmacotherapy.* 1990; 10:51S−58S.

12. Hill MV, McMahon ML, Stucke RS, Barth RJ. Wide variation and excessive dosage of opioid prescriptions for common general surgical procedures. *Ann Surg.* 2017;265(4): 709−714. https://doi.org/10.1097/SLA.0000000000001993.

13. Fujii MH, Hodges AC, Russell RL, et al. MacLeanpostdischarge opioid prescribing and use after common surgical procedure. *J Am Coll Surg.* June 2018;226(6): 1004−1012.

14. Overton HN, Hanna MN, Bruhn WE, et al. Opioidprescribing guidelines for common surgical procedures: an expert panel consensus. *J Am Coll Surge.* 2018;227(4).

15. Brummett CM, Waljee JF, Goesling J, et al. New persistent opioid use after minor and major surgical procedures in US adults. *JAMA Surg.* 2017;152(6):e170504. https://doi.org/10.1001/jamasurg.2017.0504.

16. Ballotpedia. *Opioid Prescription Limits and Policies by State*; February 11, 2019. https://ballotpedia.org/Opioid_prescription_limits_and_policies_by_state#cite_note-ncslopioid-2.

17. Beers MH. Explicit criteria for determining potentially inappropriate medication use by the elderly. *Arch Intern Med.* 1997:1571531−1571536.

18. American Geriatrics Society Beers Criteria Update Expert Panel. American Geriatrics Society 2019 updated AGS Beers Criteria(R) for potentially inappropriate medication use in older adults. *J Am Geriatr Soc.* 2019;67(4): 674−694.

19. Ballantyne J. *The Massachusetts General Hospital Handbook of Pain Management. Section V Chapter 21 Acute Pain.* Philadelphia: Lippincott Williams & Wilkins; 2006.

20. Moslemi F, Rasooli S, Baybordi A, Golzari SE. A comparison of patient controlled epidural analgesia with intravenous patient controlled analgesia for postoperative pain management after major gynecologic oncologic surgeries: a randomized controlled clinical trial. *Anesthesiol Pain Med.* 2015;5(5):e29540. https://doi.org/10.5812/aapm.29540.

21. https://www.oregonpainguidance.org/opioidmedcalculator/.

22. Dowell D, Haegerich TM, Chou R. CDC guideline for prescribing opioids for chronic pain — United States, 2016. *MMWR Recomm Rep.* 2016;65(RR-1):1−49. https://doi.org/10.15585/mmwr.rr6501e1external icon.

23. Veterans Affairs. *VA/DoD Clinical Practice Guideline for Opioid Therapy for Chronic Pain.* 2017.

24. Manchikanti L, et al. Responsible, safe, and effective prescription of opioids for chronic non-cancer pain: American Society of Interventional Pain Physicians (ASIPP) guidelines. *Pain Physician.* 2017;20(2S):S3−S92.

25. Benzon H. *Practical Management of Pain.* Philadelphia, PA: Elsevier/Saunders; 2014.

26. https://www.practicalpainmanagement.com/resource-centers/opioid-monitoring-2nd-ed/buprenorphine-surgery-what-protocol.

27. https://www.samhsa.gov/medication-assisted-treatment/treatment#medications-used-in-mat. Center for Substance Abuse Treatment. *Key Application Program (KAP) Keys for Physicians: Based on TIP 40, Clinical Guidelines for the Use of Buprenorphine in the Treatment of Opioid Addiction.* Rockville, MD: Substance Abuse and Mental Health Services Administration; 2005. Available from: https://store.samhsa.gov/shin/content/KAPT40/KAPT40.pdf. (Accessed July 25, 2017).

28. Wolff RF, Aune D, Truyers C, et al. Systematic review of efficacy and safety of buprenorphine versus fentanyl or morphine in patients with chronic moderate to severe pain. *Curr Med Res Opin.* 2012;28:833−845.

29. Müller-Lissner S, Bassotti G, Coffin B, et al. Opioid-induced constipation and bowel dysfunction: a clinical guideline. *Pain Med.* 2017;18(10):1837−1863. https://doi.org/10.1093/pm/pnw255.

30. Kumar L, Barker C, Emmanuel A. Opioid-induced constipation: pathophysiology, clinical consequences, and management. *Gastroenterol Res Pract.* 2014;2014:141737.

31. Lynch ME. Antidepressants as analgesics: a review of randomized controlled trials. *J Psychiatry Neurosci.* 2001; 26(1):30−36.

32. Max M. Antidepressants as analgesics. In: *Progress in Pain Research and Management.* Seattle: IASP Press; 1994.

33. https://www.micromedexsolutions.com/micromedex2. https://www.micromedexsolutions.com/micromedex2/librarian/CS/A6AABE/ND_PR/evidencexpert/ND_P/evidencexpert/DUPLICATIONSHIELDSYNC/D3A8E6/ND_PG/evidencexpert/ND_B/evidencexpert/ND_AppProduct/evidencexpert/ND_T/evidencexpert/PFActionId/pf.HomePage?navitem=topHome&isToolPage=true.

34. Smith HS, Smith EJ, Smith BR. Duloxetine in the management of chronic musculoskeletal pain. *Therapeut Clin Risk Manag.* 2012;8:267−277. https://doi.org/10.2147/TCRM.S17428.

35. Reus VI, Rawitscher L. Possible interactions of tramadol and antidepressants. *Am J Psychiatry.* 2000;157:839.

36. Issa MA, Marshall Z, Wasan AD. *Essentials of Pain Medicine*, Chapter 48, 427−436.e2.

37. Beal BR, Wallace MS. An overview of pharmacologic management of chronic pain. *Med Clin N Am.* 2016;100(1): 65−79. https://doi.org/10.1016/j.mcna.2015.08.006.

38. Tzellos TG, Papazisis G, Amaniti E, Kouvelas D. Efficacy of pregabalin and gabapentin for neuropathic pain in spinal-cord injury: an evidence-based evaluation of the literature. *Eur J Clin Pharmacol.* 2008;64: 851−858.

39. Huang-Lionnet JH, Brummett C, Raja SN. *Essentials of Pain Medicine*, Chapter 30, 251−260.e2.

40. https://www.hhs.gov/ash/advisory-committees/pain/repo rts/2018-12-draft-report-on-updates-gaps-inconsistencies-recommendations/index.html#2.1.1-acute-pain.

41. History of anaesthesia: the ketamine story – past, present and future. *Eur J Anaesthesiol.* 2017;34(9):571–575. Copyright: (C) 2017 European Society of Anaesthesiology.

42. Schwenk ES, Viscusi ER, Buvanendran A, et al. Consensus guidelines on the use of intravenous ketamine infusions for acute pain management from the American Society of Regional Anesthesia and Pain Medicine, The American Academy of Pain Medicine, and The American Society of Anesthesiologists. *Reg Anesth Pain Med.* 2018;43(5):456–466. https://doi.org/10.1097/AAP.0000000000000806.

43. Michelet D, Brasher C, Horlin AL, et al. Dahmani Ketamine for chronic non-cancer pain: a meta-analysis and trial sequential analysis of randomized controlled trials. *S. Eur J Pain.* 2017. https://doi.org/10.1002/ejp.1153 [Epub ahead of print] Review.

44. Jonkman K, Dahan A, van de Donk T, Aarts L, Niesters M, van Velzen M. Ketamine for pain. *F1000Res.* 2017;6. https://doi.org/10.12688/f1000research.11372.1. F1000 Faculty Rev-1711.

45. Vadivelu N, Schermer E, Kodumudi V, Belani K, Urman RD, Kaye AD. J Role of ketamine for analgesia in adults and children. *Anaesthesiol Clin Pharmacol.* 2016;32(3):298–306. https://doi.org/10.4103/0970-9185.168149._Review.

46. Peltoniemi MA, Hagelberg NM, Olkkola KT, Saari TI. Ketamine: a review of clinical pharmacokinetics and pharmacodynamics in anesthesia and pain therapy. *Clin Pharmacokinet.* 2016 Sep;55(9):1059–1077. https://doi.org/10.1007/s40262-016-0383-6.

47. Fine PG. Low dose ketamine in the management of opioid nonresponsive terminal cancer pain. *J Pain Symptom Manag.* 1999;17(4):296–300.

48. Schwartzman R, Alexander G, Grothusen J, Paylor T, Reichenberger E, Perreault M. Outpatient intravenous ketamine for the treatment of complex regional pain syndrome: a double blind placebo-controlled study. *Pain.* 2009;2009. https://doi.org/10.1016/j.pain.2009.08.015.

49. Campbell-Flemming JM, Williams A. The use of ketamine as adjuvant therapy to control severe pain. *Clin J Oncol Nurs.* 2008;12(1):102–107.

50. Rakic AM, Golembiewski J. Low-dose ketamine infusion for postoperative pain management. *Journal of Perianesthesia Nurse.* 2009;24(4):25–27.

51. Chan AK, Cheung CW, Chong YK. Alpha-2 agonists in acute pain management. *Expert Opin Pharmacother.* 2010;11:2849–2868.

52. Fearon KC, Ljungqvist O, Von Meyenfeldt M, et al. Enhanced recovery after surgery: a consensus review of clinical care for patients undergoing colonic resection. *Clin Nutr.* 2005;24:466–477.

53. *Precision Medicine*: U.S. Food and Drug Administration. https://www.fda.gov/medicaldevices/productsandmedical procedures/invitrodiagnostics/precisionmedicine-medical devices/default.htm.

54. *Frequently Asked Questions About Pharmacogenomics.* National Human Genome Research Institute. http://www.genome.gov/27530645.

55. *Pharmacogenomics*: National Institute of General Medical-Sciences. https://www.nigms.nih.gov/education/Pages/factsheet-pharmacogenomics.aspx.

56. Holmquist GL. Opioid metabolism and effects of cytochrome P450. *Pain Med.* 2009;10:S1–S29.

57. Tennant FS. Opioid blood levels in high dose, chronic pain patients. *Prac Pain Manag.* 2006;6(2):28–30.

58. Tennant FS. Genetic screening for defects in opioid metabolism: historical characteristics and blood levels. *Prac Pain Manag.* 2015.

59. Agarwal D, Udoji MA, Trescot A. Genetic testing for opioid pain management: a primer. *Pain Ther.* 2017;6(1):93–105. https://doi.org/10.1007/s40122-017-0069-2.

60. The Joint Commission. *R3 Report Issue 11: Pain Assessment and Management Standards for Hospitals*; August 29, 2017. https://www.jointcommission.org/-/media/tjc/documen ts/standards/r3-reports/r3_report_issue_11_2_11_19_re v.pdf.

CHAPTER 13

Pain Care Essentials: Interventional Pain

ALLEN S. CHEN, MD, MPH • ADAM HINTZ, MD

INTRODUCTION

Treatment of pain, acute, subacute, or chronic, often involves a continuum of treatment options. Initially, conservative options such as physical therapy, medications, and alternative/complimentary treatments should be considered. If these modalities provide inadequate pain control, interventional procedures, which inherently carry more risk, can be considered. In this chapter, we review relevant anatomy, theory, indications, and provide an overview of how common pain procedures are performed. This chapter is not meant to be a comprehensive guide or instructional manual. The landscape of interventional pain practice continues to evolve and change; as such we highly recommend that providers pursue an accredited fellowship in interventional pain, and stay current on the latest techniques, limitations, and literature. Given this, we present a broad outline and theoretical basis of commonly utilized pain procedures.

LUMBAR MEDIAL BRANCH BLOCKS

Lumbar facet (zygapophyseal) joints (z-joints) are an important potential source of low back pain. The most frequent etiology of lumbar facet pain derives from degenerative disease.[1] Surgical fusion of two vertebrae can also lead to accelerated degeneration of adjacent levels of facet joints.[2,3] Another frequent cause is trauma secondary to whiplash injuries, although more common in the cervical region.[4,5]

Degenerative facet arthropathy is the most common cause of facet-mediated pain and occurrence increases with age. Up to 40% of elderly patients with chronic low back pain have facet-mediated pain. As such, diagnostic confidence of a medial branch block is increased when performed on an older patient with chronic low back pain in comparison with a younger patient, who may have other sources of low back pain[6]. Axial,

nonradicular low back pain may be consistent with pain from the facet joints. Facet pain referral patterns have been well studied, and although they can vary, typically follow predictable patterns. Pain radiating below the knee is a negative predictor of facet-mediated pain[7,8]. Stiffness, pain worsened with prolonged standing and relieved by recumbency is consistent with lumbar facet pain[9]. Imaging, including X-ray, CT, and MRI, is helpful in excluding other diagnoses; however no radiographic finding is sensitive or specific for facet-mediated pain. The correlation of facet joint arthropathy and a positive response to diagnostic medial branch blocks is not clear.[10,11] Given the ambiguous nature of diagnosing facet-mediated pain via patient history, physical exam, and radiographic findings, medial branch blocks have become the gold standard for diagnosis.

Relevant Anatomy

Facet joints are paired synovial joints located posterolateral to the vertebral body and comprised of the superior articular process at and the inferior articular process below that level. The two facet joints and intervertebral disc at each level make up the "three-joint complex" which stabilizes and supports the spine. In the lumbar spine, the facet joints are generally oriented in the sagittal plane. The sensory innervation to each lumbar facet joint is supplied by the medial branch of the posterior rami. The medial branch of the posterior rami also innervates the multifidus muscle, interspinous muscle and ligament, and the periosteum of the neural arch. Each facet joint receives dual innervation from the medial branch at, and the medial branch above, the level of the facet joint. For example, the L4–L5 facet joint receives its innervation from the L3 and L4 medial branch nerves. Each of the L1–L4 medial branches travels across the transverse process at the junction of the transverse process and the superior articular process.

Pain Care Essentials and Innovations. https://doi.org/10.1016/B978-0-323-72216-2.00013-2

As the nerve passes medially, the medial branch is covered by the mamillo-accessory ligament which can become calcified.[12] Due to its course and the mamillo-accessory ligament, the target for the lumbar medial branches is the junction of the transverse and superior articular process (Fig. 13.1). A variant of innervation of the facet joints in the lumbar spine is the innervation of the L5—S1 facet joint, which is innervated by the medial branch of L4 above and the L5 dorsal ramus. The L5 dorsal ramus travels along a course where it is accessible at the junction of the superior articular process of S1 and the sacral ala.

Theoretical Basis of Procedure

Due to the high prevalence of false-positive responses to a single medial branch block, two confirmatory blocks done on separate occasions should be performed.[13,14] Although there is some debate, all guidelines and position papers to date by major interventional pain and spine societies recommend a double block paradigm. The block should produce significant relief following each injection. Criteria for success per Spine Intervention Society Guidelines are 80% relief of pain. To avoid false-positive responses to blocks, low volumes of anesthetic are used, typically between 0.3 and 0.5 mL of volume.[15] The concern with higher volumes is that

anesthetic may spread to block adjacent nerves including the lateral and intermediate branches which innervate the paraspinal muscles, ligaments, sacroiliac joints, and skin. False-negative responses due to vascular uptake, and the low sensitivity of aspiration prior to injection, argue for the use of contrast prior to injection of the anesthetic.[16] The dual innervation of each level of facet joint requires the block of both medial branches innervating each joint (e.g., L3 and L4 medial branches for the L4—L5 facet joint) to achieve a successful block.

Procedure: L1—L4 Medial Branch Blocks

The patient is placed in the prone position and an anteroposterior (AP) view of the desired vertebral level is obtained in the center of the X-ray beam. The beam should be tilted cephalad or caudad to line up the superior endplate at the target level. Next, the C-arm is obliqued in the ipsilateral direction to optimize the junction of the superior articular and transverse processes. There should be clear visualization of the transition area between the transverse process and the superior articular process. The target for final needle placement should be the junction of the superior articular and transverse process (Fig. 13.2). 22- or 25-gauge 3 ½-inch or 5-inch spinal needles are inserted into the skin with close attention to the desired trajectory to

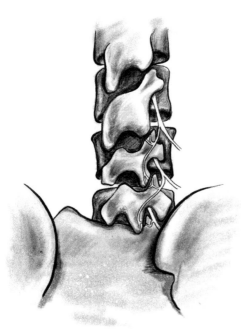

FIG. 13.1 Oblique view of medical branches along the junction of the superior articular process and transverse process. Illustration by Susie S. Kwon, MD.

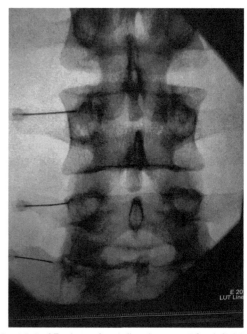

FIG. 13.2 AP view of needle placement for left L3, L4 medial branch blocks and L5 dorsal rami block (Image: A. Chen, MD, MPH).

the optimal endpoint at the inflexion of the superior articular process and transverse process. 25-gauge needles may be used without skin anesthesia.[17] If the target is well-identified and the needle insertion site is well-chosen, this can be efficiently achieved by inserting the spinal needle coaxially with the intensifier, i.e., the spinal needle should be parallel with the beam of the intensifier. Careful attention should be paid to prevent the needle from migrating cephalad to the transverse process, so as to not enter the intervertebral foramen. After aspiration, a small aliquot of contrast is injected under live fluoroscopy to confirm location and ensure there is no vascular uptake (Fig. 13.3). If vascular flow is detected, the needle should be redirected and confirmed that contrast remains over the medial branch. Once confirmed, 0.3–0.5cc of anesthetic is injected at each level and the needles removed.

Procedure: L5 Dorsal Rami Block

For the L5 dorsal ramus, the target is the groove between the sacral ala and the superior articular process of the L5–S1 joint. The dorsal rami run caudad from this groove, ultimately splitting into the lateral and medial branches. Thus, this block is of the dorsal rami prior to the division. On fluoroscopic view, the target is generally best viewed with ipsilateral obliquity in order to move the superior articular process medially in relation to the sacrum, thus exposing the target. Particular attention should be paid to the iliac crest when optimizing this view as it may obscure direct access to the target. Once the target is visualized and identified, a 22- or 25-gauge spinal needle is inserted and advanced to the target using coaxial alignment. A small aliquot of contrast is injected to confirm location and ensure no vascular uptake. If vascular flow is noted, redirect the needle and reinject to confirm that contrast remains over the dorsal rami. Once confirmed, 0.3–0.5cc of anesthetic is injected and needles are removed.

Cervical Medial Branch Blocks

Cervical facet (zygapophyseal) joints (z-joints) are potential causes of neck pain, shoulder pain, upper back pain, and headaches. Degenerative disease and whiplash injuries account for the majority of facet-mediated pain in the cervical spine.[4]

Neck pain referred from the facet joints follows predictable patterns that correspond to levels of facet joints. Each joint is innervated by the medial branches of the cervical dorsal rami. For those suffering with chronic neck pain, the most common cause is of facet joint origin and the prevalence of facet-mediated chronic neck pain has been reported as high as 55%.[18] The most common cervical joints identified as the source of pain have been C2–C3, C5–C6, and C6–C7, respectively.[19] Studies conducted by Bogduk, Dwyer, and Aprill originally mapped referral patterns of pain from the different facet joint levels. This distribution of pain has been confirmed in other studies and serves as the basis for targeting joint levels.[20–22] These pain referral patterns are useful when the pain is thought to be derived from the facet joint; however, these referral patterns do not necessarily exclude other potential causes of neck pain. Headaches associated with upper cervical joint disease are indicative of the C2–C3 facet joint.[23,24] Although there is some debate, all guidelines and position papers to date by major interventional pain and spine societies recommend using a double block paradigm.

Relevant Anatomy

The innervation of the facet joints C3–C4 to C7–T1 receive dual innervation from the medial branches of the posterior rami at the same level and the level below (e.g., the C6–C7 facet joint is innervated by the C6 and C7 medial branch).[25] The path of the medial branches innervating C3–4 to C7–T1 is targeted as they cross the waist of the articular pillars. In general, a diagonal line should be drawn from corner to corner of the

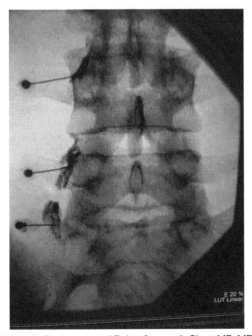

FIG. 13.3 Post-contrast AP view (Image: A. Chen, MD, MPH).

articular pillars. The intersection of these lines indicates the target for the medial branch block. The medial branch of the C2 dorsal rami, also known as the greater occipital nerve, receives a communicating branch from the third occipital nerve (TON), and together with a separate articular branch of the third occipital nerve innervates the C2–C3 facet joint. This level and the C7 medial branch differ in their approach. The third occipital nerve is accessible to block at the junction of the C2 and C3 articular pillars, and generally will be adequately blocked with two targets: just above and just below the C2–3 joint line, taking care not the enter the joint itself. The C7 medial branch is much more variable in its path and often does not cross the lateral mass in the same fashion as the other cervical medial branches. Instead the medial branch of the C7 dorsal rami courses over the superior-lateral transverse process and can vary in its course.

Theoretical Basis of Procedure

Medial branch blocks are diagnostic in nature; they do not provide long-term pain relief and are a means to an end, which is radiofrequency ablation (RFA). If the medial branches, which supply innervation to a painful joint, are anesthetized and provide pain relief, one would expect that destruction of those nerves with thermal RFA to provide longer-term relief. One of the most important aspects of medial branch blocks is communication with patients and ensuring that patients understand the purpose and expectations of the procedure. These blocks should only be done if patients are open to an ablative procedure, which might provide longer-term relief; if not, pursuing diagnostic medial branch blocks is a futile effort.

Procedure

The patient may be positioned in either prone or lateral decubitus, depending on operator preference. A true lateral is necessary for procedure safety and proper placement of needles. For the medial branches of the C3 through C6 vertebral levels, the target is the center of the lateral cervical mass, which can be visualized as the intersection of two lines each going diagonally from the superior corner of the articular pillar to the opposite inferior corner. The target for the third occipital nerve is at the junction of the articular pillars of C2 and C3. The C7 medial branch dorsal rami target is the superior articular process. Given the smaller target for C7, it is imperative to keep the needle over the target of the superior articular process as to not go too ventrally and enter the C7–T1 intervertebral foramen or too dorsally and enter the C6–C7 facet joint. AP views confirm that the needle tip has not moved medial to the lateral mass. The needle target should be placed in the center of the image to avoid imaging parallax. Once identified, a 25-gauge 2 ½ or 3 ½ inch spinal needle, depending on patient body habitus, is introduced into the skin and advanced in coaxial view to the target. A small amount of contrast (0.3 mL) is then injected to ensure lack of vascular uptake. After confirmation, 0.3–0.5 mL of local anesthetic is injected with careful stabilization of the needle against os and the needle is removed.

RADIOFREQUENCY ABLATION

Relevant Anatomy

The target of RFA is also the medial branch, and as such anatomy is the same as outlined in the medial branch section above.

Theoretical Basis of Radiofrequency Ablation

RFA of the medial branches of the primary dorsal ramus has long been accepted as a safe and effective way to treat axial low back pain due to painful facet joints. The theory behind the procedure was initially described by Shealy in 1974 after reviewing the results presented by Rees in 1972 who used a tenotomy blade to sever the innervation of the facet joints and successfully treat pain in 998 of his 1000 patients.[26,27] After Shealy encountered numerous hematomas with this approach, he used a technique of RFA to lesion the nerve with the aid of fluoroscopic guidance. The initial results of this procedure produced "good" or "excellent" results in 100 of 140 patients with no complications. RFA, or radiofrequency rhizotomy, of a nerve is performed using an insulated needle with an exposed metal tip through which a current is applied. This creates heat and thermal damage to the intended target tissues.[28] In the case of facet-mediated low back pain, the target nerves are medial branches of the dorsal rami that supply the painful facet joints. By lesioning the neural pathway of painful sensory transmission from the painful joints, longer-term pain relief is achieved. This procedure is not curative, but rather provides a palliative treatment for pain; after several months, the nerves reinnervate the facet joint and pain can return. Pain relief following RFA of the medial branch nerve for facet-mediated pain has been reported to extend up to 12 months.[29] This relief is longer than one would expect from typical nerve regrowth after lesioning, which is at a rate of 1 mm per day. It is believed that the heat lesioning by RFA causes a coagulation seal at the lesioning site which requires increased time for repair by endocellular processes, ultimately prolonging symptom improvement.[30] The amount of heat generated to lesion the tissue is a combination of power supplied to the needle and time of lesioning.[28] Two main electrodes are currently marketed to produce the lesion: conventional and water-cooled RFA. Given the more common usage of conventional RFA, the mechanism and procedural techniques discussed further will refer to this design. Subtypes of continuous and pulsed RFA also exist and depend on the pain etiology and targeted nerve. An important technical characteristic of conventional probes is that the burn created by the electrode is in an elliptical pattern with the majority of the lesioning occurring at a maximal distance at the midportion of the shaft of the exposed electrode with very little occurring at the tip.[31] Shape of the RF lesion must be considered during lesioning of the nerve, and in conventional RF the needle should be placed parallel to the nerve rather than perpendicular to it.[32]

Efficacy of RF for Lumbar

With careful patient selection and two successful medical branch blocks, lumbar medial branch RFA can provide substantial long-lasting pain reduction. Dreyfuss (2000) found that 60% of patients reported 90% pain relief and close to 90% of patients achieved at least 60% pain relief at 12 months.[29] A prospective double-blind randomized controlled trial performed by van Kleef et al. (1999) reported improvement in "highest pain" and "mean pain" scores in the RFA treatment group when compared with sham procedure at 8 weeks.[33] Following successful RFA treatment, if pain returns, RFA can be repeated with similar outcomes for pain relief and duration of relief as the initial procedure.[34,35]

Lumbar Radiofrequency Procedure

If using traditional radiofrequency probes, this procedure is ideally done using a parallel approach. As discussed above, the burn area for a traditional probe is in an ovoid shape, without limited lesioning beyond the tip of the probe. As such, in order to maximize nerve ablation, the probe should be placed parallel to the course of the medial branch.

L1–L4 Medial Branch RFA

The patient is placed in prone position, and after sterile prep and drape, an AP view of the level of interest is obtained. Once the target level is centered, the C-arm is obliqued ipsilaterally to visualize the inflection between the superior articular process and the transverse process. Next, progressive caudal tilt of the C-arm is performed

until a groove is visualized between the superior articular process and the transverse process. This groove is the target for the radiofrequency probe. This caudal view and subsequent coaxial placement allows for the electrode to approach from an inferolateral angle and ultimately lie in parallel to the medial branch. After a proper view of the target is visualized, the skin is anesthetized. Generally, an 18- or 20-gauge RFA electrode is inserted and advanced in coaxial fashion to the target location aiming for the groove where the caudal aspect of the superior articular process and the superior medial edge of the transverse process meet. Larger diameter needles increase burn area, and gauge should be considered carefully in conjunction with increased needle trauma with larger diameter needles. The needle is advanced so it lies in the groove between the superior articular process and the transverse process, lying parallel to the medial branch nerve. Once ideal placement is obtained, the fluoroscope is rotated to obtain an AP view, in which the active tip should be visualized along the junction of the superior articular process and the transverse process. A lateral view is then obtained to ensure appropriate depth, and to confirm that the active tip is outside of the intervertebral foramen. Lesioning then occurs for 90 s at 80°C.

L5 Dorsal Rami RFA

For the L5 dorsal ramus, the target is the groove between the sacral ala and the superior articular process of the L5–S1 joint. The fluoroscopy arm is rotated ipsilaterally and tilted caudally as the groove at the sacral ala becomes clear. This groove is the target for the radiofrequency probe. This caudal view and subsequent coaxial placement allow for the electrode to approach from an inferolateral angle and ultimately lie in parallel to the dorsal rami. After a proper view of the target is visualized, the skin and subcutaneous tissue along the intended track of the RFA needle is anesthetized. An 18- or 20-gauge RFA electrode is inserted and advanced in coaxial fashion to the target location. The needle is advanced so it lies on the sacral ala, parallel to the L5 dorsal ramus. Once ideal placement is obtained, the fluoroscope is rotated to obtain an AP view and the tilt is removed, and the active tip should be visualized running parallel to the dorsal rami at the sacral ala. A lateral view is then obtained to ensure appropriate depth, and to confirm that the active tip is outside of the intervertebral foramen.

Cervical Radiofrequency Procedure

Correct placement of the electrodes is paramount in order to achieve successful lesioning of the medial branches in the cervical spine and to avoid complications. Depending on which level is being targeted, it is essential to understand and recognize the typical course of each target level as described previously.

The patient is placed in the prone position, and after sterile prep and drape, an initial AP view is obtained to identify target levels. A caudal tilt on fluoroscopy ensures that as the electrodes are placed in coaxial view, they will lie parallel to the direction of the medial branch along the articular pillar. Skin is anesthetized, and an 18- or 20-gauge radiofrequency probe needle is inserted and advanced using intermittent fluoroscopic guidance to maintain needle position parallel to the fluoroscopy beam. The electrode is then advanced in coaxial fashion to the lateral aspect of the articular pillar until os is reached. Once bone is felt and location confirmed with imaging, the RFA needle is redirected laterally to slip past the lateral margin of the articular pillar. The RFA needle is then advanced along the articular pillar while maintaining contact with the lateral aspect of the pillar. A lateral view is then obtained to confirm appropriate depth of the RFA active tip over the target. Further adjustments can be made while using the above technique to ensure that the active tip of the radiofrequency probe is in adequate position. After this is achieved, an AP view is obtained to ensure that the RFA needle is still in contact with the lateral aspect of the pillar.

Stimulation and Lesioning

With precise parallel placement of the radiofrequency probe, the value of sensory and motor stimulation is debated. Motor stimulation can confirm that the needle is not placed in close proximity to nerve roots. During this time, the multifidi should also contract, confirming proper placement. Sensory stimulation can confirm that the probe is stimulating at or near the area of axial pain, and that none is noted into the arm. The probes are then removed, and anesthetic injected before lesioning. Lesioning is then conducted for 90 s at 80°C. If the patient reports any symptoms down the extremity, the lesioning should be immediately discontinued. Although some practitioners choose to inject steroid to avoid possible neuritis, this practice is based primarily on theory, without much evidence to support it.

EPIDURAL STEROID INJECTIONS
Relevant Anatomy

The cervical spine is composed of seven cervical vertebrae and eight paired cervical nerve roots which supply the upper extremity. C1, which has an anterior and posterior arch but no vertebral body, is commonly referred to as the atlas and C2 as the axis. C2 has a unique feature from other vertebral levels as a bony projection called the dens (or odontoid process) which articulates with C1 allowing for rotation of the head. The remaining cervical vertebrae are overall similar to other vertebrae throughout the spinal column in that they have an anterior vertebral body, posterior spinous process, and paired pedicles, laminae, transverses processes, and articular pillars. The articular pillars are comprised of the pars interarticularis and the superior and inferior articular processes. Between two levels of vertebrae, the superior articular process of the inferior level and the inferior articular process of the superior level form the facet joint on either side. Intervertebral discs separate each of the vertebral bodies. Nerve roots exit the spinal canal through the intervertebral foramen which is comprised in the cervical spine of the pedicles, superior articular process, uncinate process, and vertebral body. In the cervical spine, the intervertebral foramen opens in an oblique, anterolateral direction with the nerve root located posteriorly and inferiorly. The numbering of the cervical nerve roots differs in the cervical spine in comparison to the thoracic and lumbar levels. The cervical nerve roots are named by the vertebral level below the exiting nerve root (i.e., C6 nerve root exits between the C5–C6 intervertebral foramen). The nomenclature differs at the C7–T1 intervertebral foramen where the exiting nerve root is designated C8. Throughout the rest of the spine, the exiting nerve roots derive their name from the vertebral level above (i.e., L4 nerve root exits the L4–L5 intervertebral foramen).

The lumbar spine is composed of five lumbar vertebrae and five paired lumbar nerve roots which supply the lower extremity. The lumbar vertebrae have similar anatomy and have an anterior vertebral body, posterior spinous process, and paired pedicles, laminae, transverses processes, and articular pillars. In the lumbar spine, the nerve root exits the canal posterolaterally via the intervertebral foramen, passing underneath the pedicle.[36,37] The lumbar nerve roots are named by the vertebral level above the exiting nerve root (i.e., L4 nerve root exits between the L4–L5 intervertebral foramen).

The spinal cord is covered by three meninges: the innermost pia, arachnoid, and dura mater. The epidural space is a potential space between the ligamentum flavum posteriorly and the dura anteriorly. Posterior to the ligamentum flavum is the interspinous ligament which attaches to the spinous process at the level above and below each level, and the supraspinous ligament which runs along the posterior aspects of the spinous process. These ligaments may be encountered prior to engagement with the ligamentum flavum when performing an epidural injection. The depth of the cervical epidural space, between the ligamentum flavum and the dura, is much smaller than in the lumbar spine. The epidural space at C7–T1 is less than 2–3 mm,[38] whereas the depth of the lumbar epidural space, between the ligamentum flavum and the dura, has been reported to be 4–6 mm.[39,40]

Theoretical Basis of Epidural Injections

Epidural injections are used in the treatment of pain from cervical and lumbar nerve root irritation. Cervical and lumbar radicular pain may occur along the dermatome of the extremity supplied by the nerve root affected.[41] Sensory symptoms can include pain, paresthesias, or numbness.[42] Motor weakness may also be present affecting the muscles innervated by the nerve root involved. Nerve root irritation can occur from a number of different causes: disc herniation, spondylosis, instability, trauma, or tumors.[42] Based on the affected nerve root, symptoms and exam follow a predictable pattern.

Evidence for Cervical Interlaminar Epidural Injections

A prospective study by Castagenera et al. (1994) reported that over 70% of patients with chronic radicular cervical pain obtained at least 75% or greater pain relief at 3, 6, and 12 months following cervical epidural steroid injection.[43] Stav et al. (1993) conducted a randomized prospective study where patients with cervical radicular pain were randomized into receiving local anesthetic with methylprednisolone into the cervical epidural space or cervical muscles. In patients that had the injectate placed into the epidural space, 68% reported greater than 50% pain relief at 1 year from injection compared with less than 12% of patients who had the steroid injected into the cervical muscles.[44] Cicala et al. (1989) found similar results as Stave et al. (1993) at 1-year follow-up.[45] Although promising with their results, the previously stated studies have various shortcomings. None of the studies employed fluoroscopic guidance and all relied solely on the loss of resistance technique to achieve epidural access. Additionally, patient selection in these studies based on symptoms, physical exam, or radiographic imaging was either absent or had a mix of pathophysiology. One prospective study looked at those differences in radicular arm pain at 1, 3, and 6 months between groups randomized to conservative management (gabapentin and/or nortriptyline and physical therapy), cervical interlaminar epidural steroid injection, or combination of both treatments.[46] The only statistically significant positive outcome found by the investigators was at 3 months for those who were in the combination treatment arm.

A single-blind, prospective, randomized, comparative trial by McCormick et al. (2017) evaluated whether using a catheter to deliver steroid to the site of pathology in the cervical spine versus depositing the medication at the site of the standard interlaminar approach (C7–T1) had improved efficacy. Seventy-six patients were randomized, and at 1 month follow-up, the difference between the two groups was not statistically significant.[47] Choi et al. (2016) retrospectively analyzed medical records of 128 patients who underwent fluoroscopically guided cervical epidural steroid injections. Overall, almost 70% of patients had greater than 50% reduction in pain on visual analog scale at second visit (average approximately 1 month later). This was a statistically significant improvement in symptoms across all groups analyzed. The authors also found a statistically significant better response in patients with acute radicular pain secondary to a herniated disc versus patients with chronic neck pain and spinal stenosis.[48]

In a randomized, double-blind, active control trial for patients who had interlaminar epidural injections for cervical disc herniations using lidocaine 0.5% with or without betamethasone, Manchikanti et al. (2013) reported that 72% of patients in the lidocaine group and 68% of patients in the lidocaine and betamethasone group had 50% improvements in pain and function at 2 years.[49]

Evidence for Lumbar Epidural Steroid Injections

Manchikanti et al. (2012) performed a randomized double-blind controlled trial evaluating the effectiveness of interlaminar epidural steroid injections for patients with radicular pain secondary to disc herniations with anesthetic and steroid versus anesthetic alone. Significant improvement was defined as at least 50% improvement with pain relief and functional status. At 1-year follow-up, 67% of patients receiving anesthetic only versus 85% of those who received anesthetic plus steroid reported improvement, with a statistically significant difference. There were also statistically significant improvements found at 3- and 6-month follow-up in the steroid treatment group.[50] Manchikanti et al. (2014) continued to follow these patients and published their findings. At 2 years, they found significant improvement in 70% of patient who received the steroid and anesthetic versus 60% who received the anesthetic alone.[51] In a 2011 study by Kim and Brown, patients with lumbar radicular pain were randomized to receive anesthetic mixed with equipotent doses of either dexamethasone or methylprednisolone. The VAS scores were documented at an average follow-up day of 51.1 for the methylprednisolone group and 41.1 for the dexamethasone group, which was not statistically significant. Decreases in VAS from preprocedure to follow-up were 19.7% and 27.2% for dexamethasone and methylprednisolone, respectively, but the differences were not statistically significant.[52]

Cervical Epidural Injection Procedure

The patient is placed in prone position, and after sterile prep and drape, an AP view of the level of interest is obtained. Once the target level is centered, typically the C7–T1 interlaminar space, the endplates of the vertebrae above and below are squared off. The initial target should be the superior aspect of the lamina at the level below the interlaminar space of intended entry, just lateral to the spinous process. Skin is anesthetized and the needle is then advanced to the superior aspect of the inferior lamina until os is reached. Targeting os of the lamina allows safe advancement of the needle. Once os is reached, the needle is then redirected superiorly and advanced until the ligamentum flavum is engaged. Next, loss of resistance technique is used until the epidural space is entered.

A contralateral oblique image should then be obtained to check depth. Lateral views can be difficult given the patient's shoulders may obstruct fluoroscopic visualization, so a contralateral oblique is recommended. The fluoroscope is typically obliqued 45–55° contralateral to needle tip to clearly view the laminar line. Once the needle tip approaches the ventral aspect of the lamina, one can start to expect loss of resistance.

Lumbar Interlaminar Epidural Steroid Injection Procedure

The patient is placed in prone positioning with a pillow placed under the abdomen to reduce lumbar lordosis and help open the interlaminar space for easier visualization and entry. After sterile prep and drape, an AP view of the level of interest is obtained. Once the target level is centered, the superior endplate of the vertebrae below the target space and the inferior endplate of the vertebrae above are squared off. In this view, the

interlaminar space should be maximally accessible. Given the variation in patient anatomy, the fluoroscope may need to be tilted either cephalad or caudad to increase accessibility of the interlaminar space. The initial target should be the superior aspect of the lamina at the level below the interlaminar space of intended entry, just lateral to the spinous process. The final needle target may be paramedian or directed midline. After proper identification, the skin is anesthetized. Then a Tuohy needle is advanced to the superior aspect of the inferior lamina until os is reached. Targeting the lamina helps determine depth and provides a firm endpoint. Once os is reached, the needle is then redirected superiorly and advanced until the ligamentum flavum is engaged. Next, loss of resistance technique is used until the epidural space is entered.

Depending on preference, either a lateral or contralateral oblique image can be obtained to check depth. If a lateral is used, as with the cervical spine, knowledge of the lumbar lamina is necessary to understand how the imaging relates to the true needle depth. For an accurate view of needle depth, the needle must be lateral to midline and extra care should be taken to obtain a contralateral, rather than an ipsilateral, view otherwise the image will not show appropriate depth. Once the needle tip approaches the ventral aspect of the laminar line, one can start to expect loss of resistance.

Loss of Resistance Technique for Interlaminar Epidural Steroid Injections

A loss of resistance technique is used to determine when the needle tip has entered the epidural space. This technique uses a loss of resistance syringe which can be plastic or glass, using air, saline, or both. The loss of resistance technique is performed by advancing a Tuohy needle through the skin, subcutaneous tissue, and posterior muscles. When the ligamentum flavum is reached, the stylet is removed from the needle and the loss of resistance syringe is attached. The ligament provides resistance and prevents the plunger from advancing in the syringe. The needle is then advanced slowly while pressure is applied to the plunger. When the needle tip enters the epidural space, a loss of resistance will be felt. If loss of resistance begins prior to the needle being at the level of the ligament, a false loss is the likely source. A false loss can also occur if the needle tip is advanced too far and goes through the dura into the subdural space. Care should be taken not to advance the needle past the epidural space to avoid potential complications of neural injury, and post dural puncture headache.

After loss of resistance is achieved, the syringe is removed from the needle, with observation for cerebrospinal fluid or blood flow from the needle. If CSF or blood flow is encountered, the procedure should be abandoned at that location and the procedure should be rescheduled or another location should be attempted. If no CSF or blood is encountered, extension tubing is attached to the Tuohy needle and 0.5–1 mL of contrast is injected under live fluoroscopy to confirm the needle tip is not placed intravascularly and epidural spread is seen. After appropriate epidural contrast spread is confirmed, nonparticulate steroid is injected, and the needle is removed.

LUMBAR TRANSFORAMINAL EPIDURAL STEROID INJECTIONS

Relevant Anatomy

The lumbar intervertebral foramen is formed between the pedicles of the vertebrae superiorly and inferiorly. The lamina and facet joint form the posterior border and the vertebral bodies and intervertebral disc anteriorly. In the lumbar spine, the intervertebral foramen is directed laterally with the nerve root exiting under the superior pedicle. The nerve roots enter the intervertebral foramen from the spinal cord along the medial and inferior aspect of the superior pedicle and travel obliquely, inferiorly, and laterally. Reinforcing medullary arteries traverse the intervertebral foramen along with the nerve root. The largest and most clinically relevant of these is the artery of Adamkiewicz (arteria radicularis magna). This artery typically arises from the T5 to L5 levels and is on the left side in 69%–85% of the population.[53]

Theoretical Basis of Transforaminal Epidural Injections

Lumbar transforaminal epidural steroid injections are used for the treatment of lumbar radicular pain. Patient selection for transforaminal steroid injections is similar to that for interlaminar epidural steroid injections; however, this procedure should generally be done with unilateral symptoms. The advantage of the transforaminal approach compared with interlaminar or caudal techniques is that the transforaminal route target is more specific to the intended nerve root. In addition, it has the advantage that the injectate reaches the ventrolateral epidural space.[54] The disadvantage of the transforaminal approach, when compared with interlaminar, is that it conveys more risk, particularly of arterial injection and subsequent paraplegia.[55–59] This is frequently thought to occur due to intraarterial injection into the artery of Adamkiewicz. Additionally, particulate steroid preparations are thought to convey higher risk of spinal cord infarction than nonparticulate steroids.[58]

Evidence

Vad et al. (2002) conducted a prospective, randomized study with participants receiving either a transforaminal epidural steroid injection or a saline trigger-point injection. Successful outcomes were determined by subjective report of "good" or "very good" improvement and a 50% reduction in their pain. At an average follow-up of 1.4 years, the transforaminal epidural group had a statistically significant success rate of 84% compared with 48% of the saline trigger-point group.[60] Ackerman and Ahmad (2007) compared different approaches to the epidural space in three separate groups: caudal, interlaminar, or transforaminal. Ninety participants were randomly assigned to each group and were evaluated at 24 weeks by reporting "complete relief," "partial relief," or "no relief." At 24 weeks, 25 of the 30 patients who underwent transforaminal epidural steroid injection reported either "complete relief" or "partial relief" which was statistically significant when compared with the other two approaches.[61] A prospective, randomized study comparing interlaminar and transforaminal epidural steroid injections for chronic unilateral radicular pain by Rados et al. (2010) found that 63% of patients in the transforaminal group achieved at least 50% pain relief at 24 weeks compared with 53% in the interlaminar group. They did not find these differences to be statistically significant.[62] Jeong et al. (2007) evaluated the effectiveness of injections at the level of disc herniation (preganglionic) affected the nerve root or at the level where the nerve root exited the foramen (ganglionic) at 3 and 6 months follow-up. At 3 months follow-up, 88% of patients reported subjective pain relief with injection at the level of the disc herniation and 71% reported improvement with injection at the level of the nerve root exiting. At 6 months, no statistical significance was found between the two groups with 60% reporting "good" or "excellent" outcomes in the preganglionic group versus 67% in the ganglionic group.[63] A similar study by Lee et al. (2006) found that 90% of patients who received a preganglionic epidural steroid injection and 69% of patients receiving a ganglionic injection after 2 weeks obtained a greater than 50% reduction of pain by visual assessment scale.[64] In a randomized, double-blind controlled trial by Karppinen (2001) comparing transforaminal injection of either steroid or saline found only a favorable difference between the two groups at

2 weeks follow-up. At 4 weeks, there was no significant difference between the two groups. At 3- and 6-month follow-up, there was a statistically significant effect in favor of the saline group. At 1 year, no statistical significance between the two groups was found.[65] This study has been often criticized for not using a true placebo as the control group had an injection of saline.[66] Ghahreman et al. (2010) designed a prospective, randomized study of 150 patients comparing the efficacy of transforaminal steroid injection or intramuscular erector spinae muscle injection using local anesthetic, local anesthetic with steroid or normal saline. At 1 month, the number of responders (at least 50% reduction of radicular pain) in the group who received transforaminal epidural steroid injections (54%) was significantly greater than the other groups. Patients who responded to transforaminal normal saline (19%), transforaminal local anesthetic (7%), intramuscular steroids (18%), or intramuscular saline (13%) did not have a significant difference between groups.[67]

Procedure for Transforaminal Epidural Steroid Injections

The patient is placed in prone position and after sterile prep and drape, AP view of the target level is obtained. The superior endplate of the vertebra of the intended foramen is aligned. In order to optimally enter the foramen, the C-arm should be obliqued ipsilaterally. The final needle tip position below the inferior and midline portion of the pedicle, or the six o'clock position. The "safe triangle" is formed by the borders of the exiting nerve root, the inferior border of the pedicle, and an imaginary sagittal line from the lateral aspect of the pedicle. Of note, the safety triangle is generally considered safe as it reduces the chance of an inadvertent nerve injury. It does not, however, prevent potential injury to blood vessels in the vicinity of the nerve root.

A 22-gauge 3 ½- or 5-inch needle is then inserted and advanced to the inferior border at the six o'clock position of the pedicle using multiplanar fluoroscopy. The needle is then redirected inferiorly and advanced into the foramen (Fig. 13.4). An AP view is then used to confirm needle position (Fig. 13.5). Next, a lateral view is obtained to verify the depth of the needle in the foramen. Correct placement should visualize the needle tip just inside the foramen (Fig. 13.6). The C-arm is then positioned in an AP view, and under continuous fluoroscopy, contrast is injected through extension tubing to confirm epidural spread without vascular or intrathecal uptake (Fig. 13.7). Steroid and often local anesthetic are then injected and the needle is withdrawn.

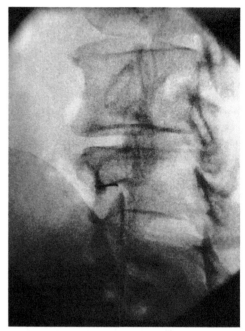

FIG. 13.4 Oblique view, needle placement for subpedicular transforaminal epidural injection (Image: A. Chen, MD, MPH)

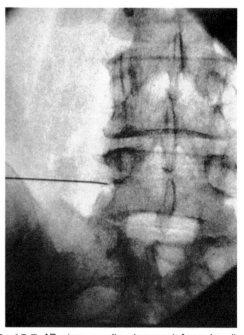

FIG. 13.5 AP view, needle placement for subpedicular transforaminal epidural injection (Image: A. Chen, MD, MPH)

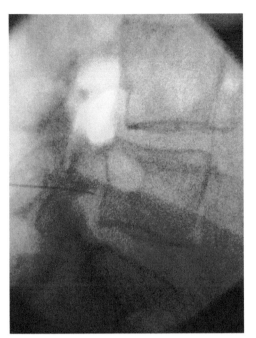

FIG. 13.6 Lateral view, needle placement for subpedicular transforaminal epidural injection (Image: A. Chen, MD, MPH).

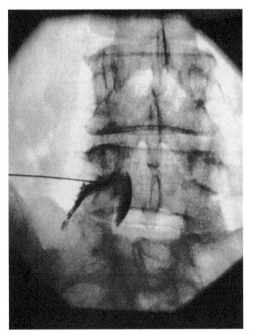

FIG. 13.7 Post-contrast AP view, subpedicular transforaminal epidural injection (Image: A. Chen, MD, MPH).

SACROILIAC JOINT INJECTION

Relevant Anatomy

The sacroiliac (SI) joint is a diarthrodial joint in which the inferior aspect of the joint is composed of synovial membrane and the cranial aspect is more fibrous in nature.[68-70] The auricular surfaces of the sacroiliac joint have considerable variation with regard to their size, shape, and contour between individuals.[71,72] It is typically formed from the first three sacral vertebrae and the iliac bone with the sacral contribution often concave and the iliac portion convex.[40,69] The auricular surface creates an L shape with the longer aspect in a dorsocaudal direction and the shorter portion positioned dorsocranially or can be present as more in the shape of a "C."[69,71] The SI joint lies in an oblique angle lateral to medial in a ventral to dorsal direction.[72] When visualized radiographically on an anteroposterior view, the more ventral part of the SI joint appears more lateral in relation to the medially dorsal aspect of the joint. The ligament complex of the SI joint are the strongest ligaments in the human body and are composed of the anterior sacroiliac ligament, interosseous sacroiliac ligament, posterior sacroiliac ligament, sacrotuberous ligament, and the sacrospinous ligament.[72] The volume of the SI joint is around typically 1−2 ml.[73] In the majority of individuals, innervation of the SI joint is supplied by the dorsal ramus of L5, S1, S2, and S3.[72,74−76]

Theoretical Basis for Sacroiliac Joint Injections

Pain arising from the sacroiliac joint generally follows a predictable pain pattern. Most commonly, pain arising from the SI joint is reported in the buttock, lower lumbar region, and the posterolateral thigh.[77−80] Other less common areas of referred pain from the SI joint include the groin and the lower leg.[80−82]

Reliable aggravating and alleviating factors, or other aspects of the patient's history, associated with sacroiliac joint pain, have not been found.[83−86] Radiographic investigation of the sacroiliac joint has not been found to be a reliable predictor of patients with SI joint pain[87−89]. However, imaging can be helpful in ruling out other causes of low back pain.

Evidence

In a retrospective study by Slipman et al. (2001), 29 patients who underwent SI joint steroid injections had a decrease in their Oswestry disability index by 10.9 points and a decrease in their visual analogue pain scores by 57% at 2 years.[90] Hawkins et al. (2009) reviewed charts of 155 patients and found that of patients who had relief at 2 weeks, the average duration of relief for patients extended to greater than 9 months.[91] A prospective case series by Liliang et al. (2009) found that out of 39 patients with confirmed SI joint pain by two independent blocks, two-thirds achieved at least 50% pain relief for more than 6 weeks with a mean duration of almost 37 weeks after injection of anesthetic and triamcinolone.[92]

Sacroiliac Joint Injection Procedure

The patient is positioned prone, and after sterile prep and drape, an AP fluoroscopic view of the pelvis is taken. The target of needle placement is the inferior one-third of the posterior joint. The SI joint most commonly has a medial oblique configuration going from anterior to posterior, which may cause two joint lines to be visualized in the AP view—the anterior and posterior margins of the joint. To obtain needle entry, the fluoroscopic view should demonstrate clear joint margins with lucency of the joint space. This joint lines should begin to approximate as the C-arm is rotated in a contralateral oblique fashion to the joint of interest. After proper view of the target is visualized, the skin and subcutaneous tissue along the intended track of the needle is anesthetized. A 22-gauge spinal needle is then advanced in coaxial technique to the lateral edge of the sacrum, medial to the joint. Once bone is reached, the needle is withdrawn slightly and redirected laterally into the joint. Tactile confirmation can be made as the needle advances through the posterior ligaments. After negative aspiration, a small amount of contrast is injected and checked with an image confirming intraarticular placement of the needle tip (Figs. 13.8, 13.9). After correct placement has been achieved, injectate containing anesthetic and steroid is performed, and the needle is removed.

SPINAL CORD STIMULATION: A BRIEF REVIEW

Spinal cord stimulation (SCS) has been widely accepted to treat a number of chronic neuropathic pain conditions.[93] The first reported use of SCS was by Shealy et al. (1967) to treat lower chest and upper abdominal pain secondary to metastatic cancer.[94] This proof of concept has led to the application being used for conditions such as failed back surgery syndrome, complex regional pain syndrome, postherpetic pain, peripheral neuropathy, phantom limb pain, angina, and ischemic limb pain[93,95,96]. Initially, SCS was thought to work based on the Gate Control Theory by Melzack and Wall; however, the actual mechanism, or mechanisms, behind SCS still remains unknown.[93,97] Using

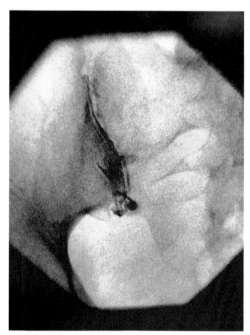

FIG. 13.8 Post-contrast Sacroiliac joint injection (Image: A. Chen, MD, MPH).

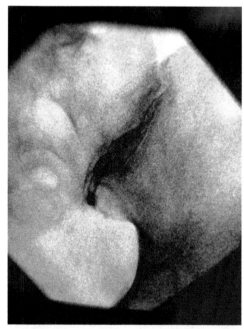

FIG. 13.9 Post-contrast Sacroiliac joint injection (Image: A. Chen, MD, MPH).

stimulation of large myelinated A-β fibers in the dorsal horn to inhibit transmission of A-δ and C was the proposed mechanism of relief.[93] Further studies have suggested other mechanisms of action as well such as decreasing the hyperexcitability of certain types of neurons in the dorsal horn (wide-dynamic range neurons) and the release of various transmitters.[93,98]

The components of SCS include an electrode lead, an implantable pulse generator (IPG), and a programmer. Today, leads come in a number of arrays that provide better coverage of pain at lower amplitudes allowing longer battery lives.[93,99] IPGs, with a battery, can be either nonrechargeable or rechargeable. The advantage of rechargeable units is their longer lifespans (dependent on usage and settings), however, require regular charging of the unit which some patients may deem as an inconvenience. Nonrechargeable batteries can last up to 3–5 years.[100] Once the battery becomes nonfunctional, the battery can be replaced without having to manipulate the leads.

After the appropriate screening process, which includes psychological evaluation, patients undergo a trial to ensure efficacy prior to permanent implantation. During the trial, the leads are placed percutaneously and the IPG is externalized. Percutaneous leads are placed via a Tuohy needle using an interlaminar epidural approach. Target lead placement for lower extremity and low back symptoms are commonly between T8 and T11.[101] The trial lasts 7–10 days and the patient records any improvement in their pain intensity and functional gains. After the trial has concluded, the leads are removed. If the trial is successful, the patient can undergo permanent placement of the leads and IPG. The IPG is placed subcutaneously in a location most comfortable for the patient, most commonly the lumbar flank or buttocks. The permanent leads can be placed either percutaneously or surgically via laminectomy.

Three different adjustments can be made to the stimulation delivered by the leads: frequency, amplitude, and pulse width. By manipulating these variables and the different contacts of the lead array, the programmer can target various anatomic areas of the body and maximize pain control. Originally, stimulation created paresthesia and were mapped to the patient's symptoms. With the advent of higher frequency settings for SCS, paresthesia-free options are now available. Lower frequencies used that produce paresthesias are typically between 40 and 60Hz with paresthesia-free settings being 1–10,000 kHz.[102] Numerous reviews of the literature have reported the long-term efficacy and safety of SCS to improve chronic neuropathic pain[103–106].

INTRATHECAL DRUG-DELIVERY SYSTEMS: A BRIEF REVIEW

Delivery of pain medications to the intrathecal space is used to selectively target receptors in the spinal cord.[107] Intrathecal therapy is typically used to treat severe cancer or chronic noncancer pain that is refractory to conservative treatments. Careful patient selection is required given the risks, maintenance, and high cost. The evaluation for patient candidacy should at minimum include determination of the pain etiology, prior therapies, comorbidities, compliance, technical considerations, as well as psychological and social factors. Psychological screening and addressing patient expectations need to be discussed prior to proceeding with this invasive treatment. A bolus trial injection prior to implantation is commonly performed and recommended.[108,109] Three methods exist to provide pain medication to the intrathecal space: externalized systems, partially externalized systems, and implanted infusion pumps.[110] Various patient criteria determine which approach is most appropriate, and variables such as life expectancy[110] should be considered. A number of medications can be used depending on the indication and desired effect including opioids, antispasmodics, calcium channel blockers, and anesthetics. Intrathecal systems consist of a programmable reservoir that can infuse medication over a fixed or variable rate, and a catheter to deliver the medication to the intended location. Complications can include infection, bleeding, catheter migration, and neurological injury. Opioid medications have been associated with granuloma formation around the tip of the catheter over time, which may require surgical intervention and/or replacement of the system or catheter.[111] Other risks are associated with infused medications, such as respiratory depression with opioids, particularly if the medication travels more rostrally. During refills, if medication is inadvertently injected into the subcutaneous tissue (i.e., pocket fill) instead of through the reservoir port, complications can lead to serious adverse events including death.

A 2002 study by Smith et al. randomized 202 patients with cancer to receive either intrathecal delivery of morphine or hydromorphone in addition to conventional therapy or conventional therapy alone. Clinical success was determined by at least 20% decrease in VAS pain scores from baseline to 4 weeks or at least a 20% decrease in reduction in toxicity. Both groups showed improvements in their VAS pain scores (51.5% and 39.1%, respectively) which was not statistically significant between the two arms. A statistically significant decrease in toxicity was found in the intrathecal drug-delivery group when compared with the conventional therapy only group (50.3% vs. 17.1%).[112] Paice et al. conducted a retrospective study of more than 400 patients with intrathecal drug therapy and found a greater than 60% improvement in mean pain reduction. In that same study, 87% of patients reported that they were very or moderately satisfied with their therapy, while 12% reported being very, moderately, or slightly dissatisfied.[113]

As of 2012, it has been reported that close to 100,000 intrathecal drug-delivery systems have been implanted worldwide.[111] As with any interventional procedure to treat painful conditions, careful examination of risks, benefits, and alternatives must be thoroughly considered.

CONCLUSION

Our ability to treat pain with interventional procedures continues to evolve as further research into techniques and approaches develop. Appropriate patient selection is paramount. This chapter discussed the theory, evidence, and techniques of the more common procedures used by pain interventionalists. As with all fields in medicine, practitioners are encouraged to continually update their knowledge as new information arises to provide the highest quality of care to their patients in a safe and effective manner.

REFERENCES

1. Gellhorn AC, Katz JN, Suri P. Osteoarthritis of the spine: the facet joints. *Nat Rev Rheumatol.* 2012;9(4):216–224. https://doi.org/10.1038/nrrheum.2012.199.
2. Lee JC, Choi S-W. Adjacent segment pathology after lumbar spinal fusion. *Asian Spine J.* 2015;9(5):807. https://doi.org/10.4184/asj.2015.9.5.807.
3. Little JS, Ianuzzi A, Chiu JB, Baitner A, Khalsa PS. Human lumbar facet joint capsule strains: II. Alteration of strains subsequent to anterior interbody fixation. *Spine J.* 2004;4(2):153–162. https://doi.org/10.1016/j.spinee.2003.07.002.
4. Derby R. Point of view: chronic cervical zygapophysial joint pain after whiplash: aplacebo-controlled prevalence study. *Spine.* 1996;21(15):1744. https://doi.org/10.1097/00007632-199608010-00006.
5. Pennie B, Agambar L. Patterns of injury and recovery in whiplash. *Injury.* 1991;22(1):57–59. https://doi.org/10.1016/0020-1383(91)90166-c.
6. Schwarzer AC, Wang SC, Bogduk N, Mcnaught PJ, Laurent R. Prevalence and clinical features of lumbar zygapophysial joint pain: a study in an Australian population with chronic low back pain. *Ann Rheum Dis.* 1995;54(2):100–106. https://doi.org/10.1136/ard.54.2.100.
7. Manchikanti L, Singh V, Pampati V, et al. Evaluation of the relative contributions of various structures in chronic low back pain. *Pain Physician.* 2001;4(4):308–316.
8. Perolat R, Kastler A, Nicot B, et al. Facet joint syndrome: from diagnosis to interventional management. *Insights Imag.* 2018;9(5):773–789. https://doi.org/10.1007/s13244-018-0638-x.
9. Eisenstein S, Parry C. The lumbar facet arthrosis syndrome. Clinical presentation and articular surface changes. *J Bone Jt Surg Br.* 1987;69-B(1):3–7. https://doi.org/10.1302/0301-620x.69b1.2950102.
10. Stojanovic MP, Sethee J, Mohiuddin M, et al. MRI analysis of the lumbar spine: can it predict response to diagnostic and therapeutic facet procedures? *Clin J Pain.* 2010;26(2):110–115. https://doi.org/10.1097/ajp.0b013e318 1b8cd4d.
11. Schütz U, Cakir B, Dreinhöfer K, Richter M, Koepp H. Diagnostic value of lumbar facet joint injection: aprospective triple cross-over study. *PloS One.* 2011;6(11). https://doi.org/10.1371/journal.pone.0027991.
12. Bogduk N. The lumbar mamillo-accessory ligament. *Spine.* 1981;6(2):162–167. https://doi.org/10.1097/00007632-198103000-00010.
13. Schwarzer AC, Aprill CN, Derby R, Fortin J, Kline G, Bogduk N. The false-positive rate of uncontrolled diagnostic blocks of the lumbar zygapophysial joints. *Neurosurg Q.* 1995;5(4):287–288. https://doi.org/10.1097/00013414-199512000-00009.
14. Manchikanti L, Boswell MV, Singh V, Pampati V, Damron KS, Beyer CD. Prevalence of facet joint pain in chronic spinal pain of cervical, thoracic, and lumbar regions. *BMC Muscoskel Disord.* 2004;5(1). https://doi.org/10.1186/1471-2474-5-15.
15. Dreyfuss P, Schwarzer AC, Lau P, Bogduk N. Specificity of lumbar medial branch and L5 dorsal ramus blocks. *Spine.* 1997;22(8):895–902. https://doi.org/10.1097/00007632-199704150-00013.
16. Lee CJ, Kim YC, Shin JH, et al. Intravascular injection in lumbar medial branch block: a prospective evaluation of 1433 injections. *Anesth Analg.* 2008;106(4):1274–1278. https://doi.org/10.1213/ane.0b013e318162c358.
17. Chen AS, Miccio VF, Smith CC, Christolias GC, Blanchard AR. Procedural pain during lumbar medial branch blocks with and without skin wheal anesthesia aprospective comparative observational study. *Pain Med.* 2019;20(4):779–783. https://doi-org.archer.luhs org/10.1093/pm/pny322.
18. Bogduk N. *Practice Guidelines for Spinal Diagnostic and Treatment Procedures.* 2nd ed. San Francisco, CA: International Spine Intervention Society; 2013.
19. Lee MJ, Riew KD. The prevalence cervical facet arthrosis an osseous study in a cadveric population. *Spine J.* 2009;9(9):711–714. https://doi.org/10.1016/j.spinee 2009.04.016.
20. Aprill C, Mb AD, Mb NB. Cervical zygapophyseal joint pain patterns II. *Spine.* 1990;15(6):458–461. https://doi.org/10.1097/00007632-199006000-00005.

21. Cooper G, Bailey B, Bogduk N. Cervical zygapophysial joint pain maps. *Pain Med.* 2007;8:344−353.
22. Mb AD, Aprill C, Bogduk N. Cervical zygapophyseal joint pain patterns I. *Spine.* 1990;15(6):453−457. https://doi.org/10.1097/00007632-199006000-00004.
23. Wang E, Wang D. Treatment of cervicogenic headache with cervical epidural steroid injection. *Curr Pain Headache Rep.* 2014;18(9). https://doi.org/10.1007/s11916-014-0442-3.
24. Bovim G, Berg R, Dale LG. Cervicogenic headache: anesthetic blockades of cervical nerves (C2-C5) and facet joint (C2/C3). *Pain.* 1992;49(3):315−320. https://doi.org/10.1016/0304-3959(92)90237-6.
25. Bogduk N. The clinical anatomy of the cervical dorsal rami. *Spine.* 1982;7(4):319−330. https://doi.org/10.1097/00007632-198207000-00001.
26. Shealy CN. The role of the spinal facets in back and sciatic pain. *Headache J Head Face Pain.* 1974;14(2):101−104. https://doi.org/10.1111/j.1526-4610.1974.hed1402101.x.
27. Mcculloch J. Percutaneous radiofrequency lumbar rhizolysis (rhizotomy). *Stereotact Funct Neurosurg.* 1976;39(2):87−96. https://doi.org/10.1159/000102481.
28. Ball RD. Technical aspects of conventional and water-cooled monopolar lumbar radiofrequency rhizotomy. *Tech Reg Anesth Pain Manag.* 2015;19(3−4):96−108. https://doi.org/10.1053/j.trap.2016.10.001.
29. Dreyfuss P, Halbrook B, Pauza K, Joshi A, Mclarty J, Bogduk N. Efficacy and validity of radiofrequency neurotomy for chronic lumbar zygapophysial joint pain. *Spine.* 2000;25(10):1270−1277. https://doi.org/10.1097/00007632-200005150-00012.
30. Bogduk N. Evidence-informed management of chronic low back pain with facet injections and radiofrequency neurotomy. *Spine J.* 2008;8(1):56−64. https://doi.org/10.1016/j.spinee.2007.10.010.
31. Lord SM, Bogduk N. Radiofrequency procedures in chronic pain. *Best Pract Res Clin Anaesthesiol.* 2002;16(4):597−617. https://doi.org/10.1053/bean.2002.0250.
32. Rosenthal R, Ipson B. Clinical applications of radiofrequency lesioning for back and neck pain. *Pract Pain Manag.* 2005;12(5).
33. Kleef MV, Barendse GAM, Kessels A, Voets HM, Weber WEJ, Lange SD. Randomized trial of radiofrequency lumbar facet denervation for chronic low back pain. *Spine.* 1999;24(18):1937. https://doi.org/10.1097/00007632-199909150-00013.
34. Son JH, Kim SD, Kim SH, Lim DJ, Park JY. The efficacy of repeated radiofrequency medial branch neurotomy for lumbar facet syndrome. *J Korean Neurosurg Soc.* 2010;48(3):240. https://doi.org/10.3340/jkns.2010.48.3.240.
35. Schofferman J, Kine G. Effectiveness of repeated radiofrequency neurotomy for lumbar facet pain. *Spine.* 2004;29(21):2471−2473. https://doi.org/10.1097/01.brs.0000143170.47345.44.
36. Standring S. Gray's anatomy. 41st edition. London: Elsevier; 2016. In: Bogduk N, ed. *Practice Guidelines for Spinal Diagnostic and Treatment Procedures.* 2nd ed. San Francisco, CA: International Spine Intervention Society; 2013.
37. Husemeyer R, White D. Topography of the lumbar epidural space. *Anaesthesia.* 1980;35(1):7−11. https://doi.org/10.1111/j.1365-2044.1980.tb03712.x.
38. Fujinaka MK, Lawson EF, Schulteis G, Wallace MS. Cervical epidural depth: correlation between needle angle, cervical anatomy, and body surface area. *Pain Med.* 2012;13(5):665−669. https://doi.org/10.1111/j.1526-4637.2012.01361.x.
39. Fyneface-Ogan S. *Anatomy and Clinical Importance of the Epidural Space.* Epidural Analgesia − Current Views and Approaches. 2012. https://doi.org/10.5772/39091.
40. Nickalls R, Kokri M. The width of the posterior epidural space in obstetric patients. *Anaesthesia.* 1986;41(4):432−433. https://doi.org/10.1111/j.1365-2044.1986.tb13240.x.
41. Carette S, Fehlings MG. Cervical radiculopathy. *N Engl J Med.* 2005;353(4):392−399. https://doi.org/10.1056/nejmcp043887.
42. Caridi JM, Pumberger M, Hughes AP. Cervical radiculopathy: a review. *HSS J.* 2011;7(3):265−272. https://doi.org/10.1007/s11420-011-9218-z.
43. Castagnera L, Maurette P, Pointillart V, Vital JM, Erny P, Sénégas J. Long-term results of cervical epidural steroid injection with and without morphine in chronic cervical radicular pain. *Pain.* 1994;58(2):239−243. https://doi.org/10.1016/0304-3959(94)90204-6.
44. Stav A, Ovadia L, Sternberg A, Kaadan M, Weksler N. Cervical epidural steroid injection for cervicobrachialgia. *Acta Anaesthesiol Scand.* 1993;37(6):562−566. https://doi.org/10.1111/j.1399-6576.1993.tb03765.x.
45. Cicala RS, Thoni K, Angel JJ. Long-term results of cervical epidural steroid injections. *Clin J Pain.* 1989;5(2):143−146. https://doi.org/10.1097/00002508-198906000-00003.
46. Cohen SP, Hayek S, Semenov Y, et al. Epidural steroid injections, conservative treatment, or combination treatment for cervical radicular pain. *Anesthesiology.* 2014;121(5):1045−1055. https://doi.org/10.1097/aln.0000000000000409.
47. Mccormick ZL, Nelson A, Bhave M, et al. A prospective randomized comparative trial of targeted steroid injection via epidural catheter versus standard C7-T1 interlaminar approach for the treatment of unilateral cervical radicular pain. *Reg Anesth Pain Med.* 2017;42(1):82−89. https://doi.org/10.1097/aap.0000000000000521.
48. Choi JW, Lim HW, Lee JY, et al. Effect of cervical interlaminar epidural steroid injection: analysis according to the neck pain patterns and MRI findings. *Korean J Pain.* 2016;29(2):96. https://doi.org/10.3344/kjp.2016.29.2.96.
49. Manchikanti L, Cash KA, Pampati V, et al. A randomized, double-blind, active control trial of fluoroscopic cervical interlaminar epidural injections in chronic pain of cervical disc herniation: results of a 2-year follow-up. *Pain Physician.* 2013;16:465−478.

50. Manchikanti L, Singh V, Cash KA, Pampati V, Falco FJE. The role of fluoroscopic interlaminar epidural injections in managing chronic pain of lumbar disc herniation or radiculitis: a randomized, double-blind trial. *Pain Pract.* 2012; 13(7):547−558. https://doi.org/10.1111/papr.12023.

51. Manchikanti L, Singh V, Cash kA, Pampati V, Falco FJE. A randomized, double-blind, active-control trial of the effectiveness of lumbar interlaminar epidural injections in disc herniation. *Pain Physician.* 2014;17:61−74.

52. Kim D, Brown J. Efficacy and safety of lumbar epidural dexamethasone versus methylprednisolone in the treatment of lumbar radiculopathy. *Clin J Pain.* 2011;27(6): 518−522. https://doi.org/10.1097/ajp.0b013e31820c53e0.

53. Lu J, Ebraheim NA, Biyani A, Brown JA, Yeasting RA. Vulnerability of great medullary artery. *Spine.* 1996; 21(16):1852−1855. https://doi.org/10.1097/00007632-199608150-00003.

54. Benoist M, Boulu P, Hayem G. Epidural steroid injections in the management of low-back pain with radiculopathy: an update of their efficacy and safety. *Eur Spine J.* 2011;21(2): 204−213. https://doi.org/10.1007/s00586-011-2007-z.

55. Glaser S, Falco F. Paraplegia following a thoracolumbar transforaminal epidural steroid injection. *Pain Physician.* 2005;8:309−314.

56. Houten JK, Errico TJ. Paraplegia after lumbosacral nerve root block. *Spine J.* 2002;2(1):70−75. https://doi.org/10.1016/s1529-9430(01)00159-0.

57. Lyders E, Morris P. A case of spinal cord infarction following lumbar transforaminal epidural steroid injection: MR imaging and angiographic findings. *Am J Neuroradiol.* 2009;30(9):1691−1693. https://doi.org/10.3174/ajnr.a15676.

58. Kennedy DJ, Dreyfuss P, Aprill CN, Bogduk N. Paraplegia following image-guided transforaminal lumbar spine epidural steroid injection: two case reports. *Pain Med.* 2009;10(8):1389−1394. https://doi.org/10.1111/j.1526-4637.2009.00728.x.

59. Somayaji HS, Saifuddin A, Casey AT, Briggs TW. Spinal cord infarction following therapeutic computed tomography-guided left L2 nerve root injection. *Spine.* 2005;30(4). https://doi.org/10.1097/01.brs.0000153400.67526.07.

60. Vad VB, Bhat AL, Lutz GE, Cammisa F. Transforaminal epidural steroid injections in lumbosacral radiculopathy. *Spine.* 2002;27(1):11−15. https://doi.org/10.1097/00007632-200201010-00005.

61. Ackerman WE, Ahmad M. The efficacy of lumbar epidural steroid injections in patients with lumbar disc herniations. *Anesth Analg.* 2007;104(5):1217−1222. https://doi.org/10.1213/01.ane.0000260307.16555.7f.

62. Rados I, Sakic K, Fingler M, Kapural L. Efficacy of interlaminar vs transforaminal epidural steroid injection for the treatment of chronic unilateral radicular pain: prospective, randomized study. *Pain Med.* 2011;12(9): 1316−1321. https://doi.org/10.1111/j.1526-4637.2011.01213.x.

63. Jeong HS, Lee JW, Kim SH, Myung JS, Kim JH, Kang HS. Effectiveness of transforaminal epidural steroid injection by using a preganglionic approach: a prospective randomized controlled study. *Radiology.* 2007;245(2): 584−590. https://doi.org/10.1148/radiol.2452062007.

64. Lee JW, Kim SH, Choi J-Y, et al. Transforaminal epidural steroid injection for lumbosacral radiculopathy: preganglionic versus conventional approach. *Korean J Radiol.* 2006;7(2):139. https://doi.org/10.3348/kjr.2006.7.2.139.

65. Karppinen J, Malmivaara A, Kurunlahti M, et al. Periradicular infiltration for sciatica. *Spine.* 2001;26(9): 1059−1067. https://doi.org/10.1097/00007632-200105010-00015.

66. Manchikanti L, Buenaventura R, Manchikanti K, et al. Effectiveness of therapeutic lumbar transforaminal epidural steroid injections in managing lumbar spinal pain. *Pain Physician.* 2012;15:E199−E245.

67. Ghahreman A, Ferch R, Bogduk N. The efficacy of transforaminal injection of steroids for the treatment of lumbar radicular pain. *Pain Med.* 2010;11(8):1149−1168. https://doi.org/10.1111/j.1526-4637.2010.00908.x.

68. Cohen SP. Sacroiliac joint pain: a comprehensive review of anatomy, diagnosis, and treatment. *Anesth Analg.* 2005; 101(5):1440−1453. https://doi.org/10.1213/01.ane.0000180831.60169.ea.

69. Vleeming A, Schuenke MD, Masi AT, Carreiro JE, Danneels L, Willard FH. The sacroiliac joint: an overview of its anatomy, function and potential clinical implications. *J Anat.* 2012;221(6):537−567. https://doi.org/10.1111/j.1469-7580.2012.01564.x.

70. Cole JD, Blum DA, Ansel LJ. Outcome after fixation of unstable posterior pelvic ring injuries. *Clin Orthop Relat Res.* 1996;329:160−179. https://doi.org/10.1097/00003086-199608000-00020.

71. Schunke GB. The anatomy and development of the sacroiliac joint in man. *Anat Rec.* 1938;72(3):313−331. https://doi.org/10.1002/ar.1090720306.

72. Solonen KA. The sacroiliac joint in the light of anatomical, roentgenological and clinical studies. *Acta Orthop Scand.* 1957;28(suppl 27):3−127. https://doi.org/10.3109/ort.1957.28.suppl-27.01.

73. Fortin J, Tolchin R. Sacroiliac arthrograms and postarthrography computerized tomography. *Pain Physician.* 2003;6:287−290.

74. Fortin J, Kissling R, O'Connor B, Vilensky J. Sacroiliac joint innervation and pain. *Am J Orthoped.* 1999:687−690.

75. Forst L, Wheeler M, Fortin J, Vilensky J. The sacroiliac joint: anatomy, physiology and clinical significance. *Pain Physician.* 2006;9:61−68.

76. Cox R, Fortin J. The anatomy of the lateral branches of the sacral dorsal rami: implications for radiofrequency ablation. *Pain Physician.* 2014;17:459−464.

77. Fortin J, Dwyer A, West S, Pier J. Sacroiliac joint: pain referral maps upon applying a new injection/arthrography technique. Part I: asymptomatic volunteers. *Spine.* 1994;19(13):1475−1482.

78. Fortin J, April C, Ponthieux B, Pier j. Sacroiliac joint: pain referral maps upon applying a new injection/arthrography technique. Part II: clinical evaluation. *Spine*. 1994; 19(13):1483–1489.
79. Murakami E, Aizawa T, Noguchi K, Kanno H, Okuno H, Uozumi H. Diagram specific to sacroiliac joint pain site indicated by one-finger test. *J Orthop Sci*. 2008;13(6): 492–497. https://doi.org/10.1007/s00776-008-1280-0.
80. Slipman CW, Jackson HB, Lipetz JS, Chan KT, Lenrow D, Vresilovic EJ. Sacroiliac joint pain referral zones. *Arch Phys Med Rehabil*. 2000;81(3):334–338. https://doi.org/ 10.1053/apmr.2000.0810334.
81. Depalma MJ, Ketchum JM, Trussell BS, Saullo TR, Slipman CW. Does the location of low back pain predict its source? *PM R*. 2011;3(1):33–39. https://doi.org/ 10.1016/j.pmrj.2010.09.006.
82. Laslett M. Evidence-based diagnosis and treatment of the painful sacroiliac joint. *J Man Manip Ther*. 2008;16(3): 142–152. https://doi.org/10.1179/jmt.2008.16.3.142.
83. Dreyfuss P, Michaelsen M, Pauza K, Mclarty J, Bogduk N. The value of medical history and physical examination in diagnosing sacroiliac joint pain. *Spine*. 1996;21(22): 2594–2602. https://doi.org/10.1097/00007632-19961 1150-00009.
84. Schwarzer AC, Aprill CN, Bogduk N. The sacroiliac joint in chronic low back pain. *Spine*. 1995;20(1):31–37. https://doi.org/10.1097/00007632-199501000-00007.
85. Laslett M, Aprill CN, Mcdonald B, Young SB. Diagnosis of sacroiliac joint pain: validity of individual provocation tests and composites of tests. *Man Ther*. 2005;10(3): 207–218. https://doi.org/10.1016/j.math.2005.01.003.
86. Maigne J-Y, Aivaliklis A, Pfefer F. Results of sacroiliac joint double block and value of sacroiliac pain provocation tests in 54 patients with low back pain. *Spine*. 1996;21(16):1889–1892. https://doi.org/10.1097/000 07632-199608150-00012.
87. Bäcklund J, Dahl EC, Skorpil M. Is CT indicated in diagnosing sacroiliac joint degeneration? *Clin Radiol*. 2017; 72(8). https://doi.org/10.1016/j.crad.2017.03.006.
88. Elgafy H, Semaan HB, Ebraheim NA, Coombs RJ. Computed tomography findings in patients with sacroiliac pain. *Clin Orthop Relat Res*. 2001;382:112–118. https://doi.org/10.1097/00003086-200101000-00017.
89. Dreyfuss P, Dreyer SJ, Cole A, Mayo K. Sacroiliac joint pain. *J Am Acad Orthop Surg*. 2004;12(4):255–265. https://doi.org/10.5435/00124635-200407000-00006.
90. Slipman CW, Lipetz JS, Plastaras CT, et al. Fluoroscopically guided therapeutic sacroiliac joint injections for sacroiliac joint syndrome. *Am J Phys Med Rehabil*. 2001; 80(6):425–432. https://doi.org/10.1097/00002060-200 106000-00007.
91. Hawkins J, Schofferman J. Serial therapeutic sacroiliac joint injections: apractice audit. *Pain Med*. 2009;10(5):850–853. https://doi.org/10.1111/j.1526-4637.2009.00651.x.
92. Liliang P-C, Lu K, Weng H-C, Liang C-L, Tsai Y-D, Chen H-J. The therapeutic efficacy of sacroiliac joint blocks with triamcinolone acetonide in the treatment of sacroiliac joint dysfunctionwithout spondyloarthropathy. *Spine*.

2009;34(9):896–900. https://doi.org/10.1097/brs.0b01 3e31819e2c78.
93. Jeon YH. Spinal cord stimulation in pain management: areview. *Korean J Pain*. 2012;25(3):143. https://doi.org/ 10.3344/kjp.2012.25.3.143.
94. Shealy CN, Mortimer JT, Reswick JB. Electrical inhibition of pain by stimulation of the dorsal columns. *Anesth Analg*. 1967;46(4). https://doi.org/10.1213/00000539-196707000-00025.
95. Waszak PM, Modrić M, Paturej A, et al. Spinal cord stimulation in failed back surgery syndrome: review of clinical use, quality of life and cost-effectiveness. *Asian Spine J*. 2016; 10(6):1195. https://doi.org/10.4184/asj.2016.10.6.1195.
96. Meglio M. Spinal cord stimulation in chronic pain management. *Neurosurg Clin*. 2004;15(3):297–306. https://doi.org/10.1016/j.nec.2004.02.012.
97. Melzack R, Wall PD. Pain mechanisms: a new theory. *Science*. 1965;150(3699):971–978. https://doi.org/10.11 26/science.150.3699.971.
98. Linderoth B, Stiller C-O, Gunasekera L, et al. Release of neurotransmitters in the CNS by spinal cord stimulation: survey of present state of knowledge and recent experimental studies. *Stereotact Funct Neurosurg*. 1993;61(4): 157–170. https://doi.org/10.1159/000100634.
99. North RB, Kidd DH, Olin JC, Sieracki JM. Spinal cord stimulation electrode design: prospective, randomized, controlled trial comparing percutaneous and laminectomy electrodes—Part I: technical outcomes. *Neurosurgery*. 2002;51(2):381–390. https://doi.org/10.1227/ 00006123-200208000-00015.
100. Hornberger J, Kumar K, Verhulst E, Clark MA, Hernandez J. Rechargeable spinal cord stimulation versus nonrechargeable system for patients with failed back surgery syndrome: acost-consequences analysis. *Clin J Pain*. 2008;24(3): 244–252. https://doi.org/10.1097/ajp.0b013e318160 216a.
101. Tiede J, Brown L, Gekht G, Vallejo R, Yearwood T, Morgan D. Novel spinal cord stimulation parameters in patients with predominant back pain. *Neuromodulation*. 2013;16(4):370–375. https://doi.org/10.1111/ner.12032.
102. Morales A, Yong RJ, Kaye AD, Urman RD. Spinal cord stimulation: comparing traditional low-frequency tonic waveforms to novel high frequency and burst stimulation for the treatment of chronic low back pain. *Curr Pain Headache Rep*. 2019;23(4). https://doi.org/10.1007/ s11916-019-0763-3.
103. Taylor RS, Buyten J-PV, Buchser E. Spinal cord stimulation for chronic back and leg pain and failed back surgery syndrome: a systematic review and analysis of prognostic factors. *Spine*. 2005;30(1):152–160. https://doi.org/ 10.1097/01.brs.0000149199.68381.fe.
104. Frey M, Manchikanti L, Benyamin R, Schultz D, Smith H, Cohen S. Spinal cord stimulation for patients with failed back surgery syndrome: a systematic review. *Pain Physician*. 2009;12:379–397.
105. Grider J, Manchikanti L, Carayannopoulos A, et al. Effectiveness of spinal cord stimulation in chronic spinal pain: a systematic review. *Pain Physician*. 2016;19:E33–E54.

106. Kapural L, Peterson E, Provenzano DA, Staats P. Clinical evidence for spinal cord stimulation for failed back surgery syndrome (FBSS). *Spine*. 2017;42. https://doi.org/10.1097/brs.0000000000002213.

107. Yaksh T, Rudy T. Analgesia mediated by a direct spinal action of narcotics. *Science*. 1976;192(4246):1357—1358. https://doi.org/10.1126/science.1273597.

108. Deer T, Smith H, Cousins M, et al. Consensus guidelines for the selection and implantation of patients with non-cancer pain for intrathecal drug delivery. *Pain Physician*. 2010;13:E175—E213.

109. Stempien L, Tsai T. Intrathecal baclofen pump use for spasticity. *Am J Phys Med Rehabil*. 2000;79(6):536—541. https://doi.org/10.1097/00002060-200011000-00010.

110. Benzon HT. *Practical Management of Pain*. Philadelphia, PA: Elsevier/Saunders; 2014.

111. Deer TR, Prager J, Levy R, et al. Polyanalgesic consensus conference-2012: consensus on diagnosis, detection, and treatment of catheter-tip granulomas (inflammatory masses). *Neuromodulation*. 2012;15(5):483—496. https://doi.org/10.1111/j.1525-1403.2012.00449.x.

112. Smith TJ, Staats PS, Deer T, et al. Randomized clinical trial of an implantable drug delivery system compared with comprehensive medical management for refractory cancer pain: impact on pain, drug-related toxicity, and survival. *J Clin Oncol*. 2002;20(19):4040—4049. https://doi.org/10.1200/jco.2002.02.118.

113. Paice JA, Penn RD, Shott S. Intraspinal morphine for chronic pain: a retrospective, multicenter study. *J Pain Symptom Manag*. 1996;11(2):71—80. https://doi.org/10.1016/0885-3924(95)00099-2.

CHAPTER 14

Rehabilitation in Pain Medicine

JOSEPH SOLBERG, DO • HUNTER VINCENT, DO • WILLIAM WHITE, DO

The goals of rehabilitation in patients suffering from acute or chronic pain can be quite variable. However, the foundation of successful rehabilitation always focuses on functional and analgesic optimization. Patients can have pain for a multitude of reasons and a proper diagnosis is essential in directing the appropriate rehabilitation protocol. Physical Medicine and Rehabilitation specialists utilize a comprehensive approach in diagnosing and managing patients with acute and chronic function-limiting or painful conditions.[1]

A vast majority of patients suffering from pain will present for evaluation of low back, neck, or joint pain. Rehabilitation-based therapies include physical and occupational therapy, therapeutic exercise, modalities, manual therapies, and bracing. Ideal treatment of any one condition is likely to be multimodal and include both rehabilitation-therapies as well as other treatments such as oral medications, topical medications, or possibly interventional procedures which can help facilitate participation in rehabilitation treatments. It is also important to address both the psychological and behavioral aspects of pain in addition to the physical impairments. As such, instituting a multidisciplinary, multimodal treatment plan will provide the most sustainable improvements in both pain and function.[2]

PART 1: THERAPIES

The most fundamental component of pain rehabilitation is therapy. When considering a specific therapy prescription, it is essential to first establish an accurate diagnosis and to determine the goals of treatment. Although therapies can come in many shapes and forms, emphasis should always be placed on improving function and independence. Where acute and chronic pain exists, decline in function is typically seen. Therapies serve as a way to emphasize increased activity levels and/or encourage movement where it is often avoided. As such, improved function can be accompanied by both decreased pain levels and enhanced ability to cope with any persisting pain. Finally, it is important

to set realistic goals. In cases where complete pain resolution may not be feasible, improving overall function should always be emphasized.

Physical Therapy is a discipline of rehabilitation medicine that aims to help individuals develop, maintain, and restore maximum body movement and physical function. The ultimate goal of physical therapy is to improve health and quality of life by enhancing mobility and balance, reducing pain, and preventing disability. Physical therapists use many techniques to improve strength, range of motion, and coordination, specifically catered to an individual's medical condition. They also train patients to improve body mechanics that may be contributing to exacerbation of pain symptoms. Physical therapists may use modalities and manual techniques to facilitate rehabilitation which are discussed later in the chapter.

Occupational Therapy (OT) is another discipline of rehabilitation medicine that aims to enhance functional independence through therapeutic performance of activities of daily living. OT aims to enable people, including those with chronic pain, to overcome their ailments through maximizing individual functionality. Occupational therapists typically focus on fine and gross motor movements, particularly flexibility and coordination of the upper extremities. Occupational Therapists are especially adept at teaching energy conservation techniques and emphasizing ergonomics and posture to maximize function and minimize pain.

Psychology also plays a large role in rehabilitation. Specifically, pain psychology can play a pivotal role in an individual's ability to overcome chronic pain. Pain is comprised of both sensory and emotional components that affect one's perception of pain. Therefore, the interpretation of pain can be modified by regulating one's thoughts and/or emotions. This principle is of utmost importance to pain rehabilitation and is a crucial component of the multidisciplinary approach to treating chronic pain. It should be noted that many patients suffering from chronic pain may be apprehensive about a psychological referral and are more likely to

Pain Care Essentials and Innovations. https://doi.org/10.1016/B978-0-323-72216-2.00014-4

be willing to proceed with evaluation after receiving an appropriate explanation and rationale of treatments such as cognitive behavioral therapy (CBT) and mindfulness-based stress reduction.

Movement-Based Therapies

Introducing activity where it may otherwise be lacking is an important step in the process of overcoming both acute and chronic pain alike. Physiologically, movement and exercise do not directly reduce pain. However, it is clear that staying active plays an important role in reducing the musculoskeletal sequelae, including pain, which often accompanies inactivity. Relative rest should be emphasized in the acute inflammatory phase of an injury and physical activity should be rapidly reintroduced unless there is an obvious risk of structural damage. As the patient becomes more active, tolerance for functional activities increases and overall wellness typically improves.

McKenzie approach

The McKenzie Approach[3,4] is a popular standardized method to evaluate, treat and prevent low back pain that is typically used in patients with acute low back pain accompanied by radicular leg pain. A key component of the McKenzie Approach is to identify the directional preference of movement. This approach divides the diagnosis of back pain into three "syndromes": (1) derangement, (2) dysfunction, and (3) postural.

1. Derangement—the most common syndrome classification—the goal in this treatment is to perform exercises that cause *centralization* of radicular pain. Specifically, an individual with low back pain that radiates in the buttocks or leg can be taught to move the pain more proximally into the low back. This can be induced with the use of extension-based exercises and is a common choice of physical therapists when approaching back pain. This principal can be applied to other areas of the body as well.[5] The figure below (Fig. 14.1)[5] is a visual representation of the McKenzie centralization phenomenon—the gradual movement of radicular symptoms (aka sciatica) to isolated low back pain.
2. Dysfunction—determined by mechanical impairments and deformities of affected tissue within the body (e.g.,: scar tissue). Treatment is performed with the goal of remodeling the affected tissue via engagement/mobilizing through exercise.
3. Postural—goal of treatment is to avoid improper end-range positions (e.g.,: slouching) by education and proper posture training.

Complimentary movement therapies. Several movement-based therapies have been found to be potentially helpful in the treatment of low back pain. More common activities, such as Pilates, yoga, and tai chi, already have strong participation among the general population. Lesser known techniques, such as

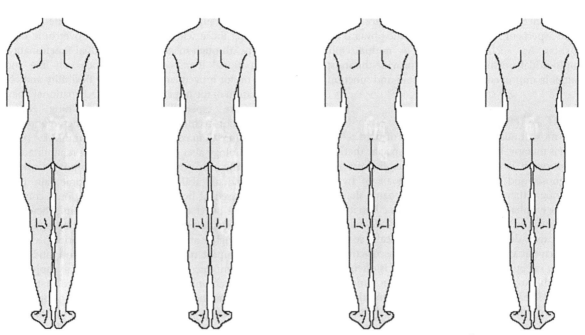

FIG. 14.1 McKenzie centralization phenomenon (Musculoskeletal Key, 2017)[5].

Feldenkrais and Alexander, also offer significant utility in certain subsets of patients. While most of the research surrounding Pilates, yoga, and tai chi is characterized by inconsistent findings and significant variability among studies, the risk for potential harm is quite low with these forms of exercise and they should be considered as a recommendation for patients with chronic pain, especially low back pain[6].

Pilates

A form of core-strengthening exercises that emphasize proper form, muscle activation, and alignment. Although Pilates exercises were originally designed for performance artists, the beneficial effects have led to wider popularity in recent years. Several randomized studies have indicated the beneficial effects of Pilates on the treatment of back pain including lower disability scores and pain ratings after the intervention that are maintained at 1-year follow-up.[7] However, it is unclear whether Pilates offers greater benefit than other forms of exercise.[8]

Yoga

An exercise and lifestyle philosophy that promotes relaxation, breathing techniques, flexibility, and strengthening. Throughout the years, yoga has gained mainstream popularity and is a frequently chosen form of exercise for men and women alike. Yoga is commonly advocated as a treatment for musculoskeletal conditions including arthritis and back pain[9]. Although there is some research indicating that yoga may be more beneficial than strength training,[6] the evidence for yoga compared with other forms of exercise in the treatment of chronic back pain is mixed in regard to both improvements in pain[10] and quality of life.[11] However, a recent Cochrane systematic review in 2017 concluded that there is low to moderate evidence that yoga may provide low to moderate improvements in back-related function and may be slightly more effective for pain relief at 3−6 months when compared with no exercise at all.[12] In addition, the same review noted that while yoga is associated with more adverse events when compared with no exercise, none of the events were considered serious and it was found to have the same risk of adverse events as other exercise modes for back pain. It remains unclear if adding yoga to existing exercise programs is more beneficial than exercise alone (Table 14.1).

Tai Chi

Tai chi is a form of exercise dating back to ancient China, which emphasizes slow purposeful total body movements synchronized with breathing. It has been

TABLE 14.1
Yoga and Pilates Comparison.

Yoga	Pilates
Mental and spiritual well-being	Fitness and physical well-being
Breathing techniques	Strengthening
Flexibility	Core exercises
Meditation	Toning
Utilizes body weight techniques and simple props	Utilizes equipment such as medicine balls and free weights

proposed to help with balance and fall prevention, flexibility, as well as cardiovascular fitness, particularly in elderly populations.[13] Tai chi has also been favored over no exercise, backward walking, and jogging for chronic low back pain[14]. In addition, some research has shown tai chi to be more effective than traditional physical rehabilitation for chronic pain[15].

Feldenkrais method

This technique was developed from the study of biomechanics and the interrelationship between muscle contraction and motion. Specifically, there are two complementary components of awareness through movement which consists of verbal cues to movement, and functional integration which involves touch to facilitate movement. The goal is learned mindfulness of unnecessary muscle contractions during routine motor patterns. This helps form new neuromuscular patterns of movement and leads to development of efficient and pain-free motion. Feldenkrais therapy can be performed by patients at any functional level and can even be performed in gravity-eliminated positions such as lying down.[16]

Alexander technique

This technique is a psychophysical educational approach to improving balance, coordination, and ease of movement. Emphasis is placed on adjusting movement patterns built into everyday activities that may be unknowingly resulting in pain or discomfort. The technique involves examination of posture, breathing, and movement fluidity. There are three underlying principles: (1) an organism functions as a whole; (2) a person's ability to function optimally is dependent on the relationship of the head, neck, and spine; and (3) body function is affected by habitual patterns of use.[17]

Manual Techniques

Manual medicine refers to a variety of hands-on therapies ranging from gentle, passive joint stretching to forceful mobilization to enhance range of motion. These techniques are most commonly utilized to treat musculoskeletal disorders, particularly neck and low back pain. Many physicians and other providers use hands-on skills in their approach to treat acute and chronic pain. Understanding the indications, principles, applications, and potential complications of manipulation, traction, and massage is an essential component to prescribing the appropriate treatment. While there is some debate about the reproducible benefits of such treatments, there is no shortage of significant, subjective benefit to individual patients.

Doctors of Osteopathic Medicine (D.O.), Chiropractors (D.C.), and Physical Therapists are practitioners that most often utilize manual techniques. D.O.s are trained in the administration of osteopathic manipulative medicine (OMM), which is founded on the concept that the body possesses self-healing mechanisms and that structure and function are interrelated. The goal is to promote optimal structural alignment to allow for self-healing to take place. Chiropractic philosophy describes a fundamental relationship between overall health and the spine. Specifically, mechanical impairments of the spine are thought to impair health, and the corrections of spinal misalignment can bring about improvements in health.[18]

Manipulation refers to the use of hands on a patient to encourage maximal, painless movement of the musculoskeletal system and to improve motion in restricted areas. The primary goal is to improve the function and well-being of the patient through reduction of pain and improved biomechanical range of motion. Techniques are evaluated for success based on comparison of structural evaluation before and after treatment.

The treatments vary in their anatomical area of focus or in the type of force utilized. Specific names of each technique or discrepancies in style may vary heavily based on region, provider, or discipline. However, classification of the techniques is most easily summarized as (1) soft tissue technique, (2) articulatory technique, or (3) mobilization with thrust.

Types of Manipulation

Soft Tissue Technique. The goal of soft tissue treatment is to mobilize muscles and fascia. The forces utilized are typically directed in a way that muscle fibers are stretched laterally or longitudinally. Forces are applied slowly and released slowly to avoid potentiating spasm or exacerbating painful symptoms. An experienced practitioner is capable of assessing the response of the tissue to treatment through palpation. While soft tissue treatment can be used as the primary treatment (such as with massage), it can also be used to facilitate movement of edema or lymphatic fluid, reduce/modify pain, or prepare an area for specific mobilization. This is similar to massage; however, the focus with soft tissue treatment is on moving tissue rather than relaxing muscles.[19]

Articulatory Treatment. This technique involves the repeated movement of a joint within its anatomical planes of movement to increase range of motion. This type of treatment is frequently used in patients with decreased joint range of motion such as for adhesive capsulitis or frozen shoulder. Specific techniques such as Spencer's technique and Mulligan's technique are frequently used in patients with adhesive capsulitis, with existing research showing Mulligan's technique to potentially be more effective than Spencer's and traditional rehab at 6 weeks intervention.[20] The force is described as "low velocity, high amplitude" and can treat deep musculature by targeting the origin and insertion sites of individual muscles.

Mobilization With Thrust. This technique is also referred to as HVLA ("high velocity, low amplitude"). Typically, these techniques are the quickest form of addressing restriction of joint motion. Specifically, a barrier is engaged and moved beyond a set point via a low amplitude (short distance) thrust. This is sometimes accompanied by an audible "pop." The pop, although frequently sought after, has no effect on the treatment outcome.

The tissues should be prepared for thrusting technique. Soft tissue treatment is often a precursor to thrust technique. If the tissues are not properly prepared, it is more difficult to engage the barrier and more force is required. Most importantly, the patient must be relaxed. Often, the thrust is given during exhalation, as it is believed that the tissues are more relaxed and receptive to motion at that time. With improper administration, the force will be dissipated by muscles and fascia rather than the mechanical barrier. Understandably, this redistribution of energy can result in iatrogenic injury. Perhaps the most serious complication of cervical manipulation is stroke associated with vertebrobasilar artery dissection. While a majority of vertebrobasilar dissections occur in the absence of cervical manipulation (either spontaneously or after trivial trauma with common daily movements), the estimated risk for an adverse outcome after cervical spine manipulation ranges from 1 in 400,000 manipulations to 1 in 3.85 million manipulations.[21] Additional complications are listed below (Box 14.1).

BOX 14.1
Reported Complications of Spinal Manipulation

THORACIC/LUMBAR
- Cauda equina syndrome
- Lumbar pedicle fracture
- Lumbar/thoracic compression fracture
- Rib fracture
- Lumbar/thoracic disk herniation

CERVICAL
- Vertebrobasilar insufficiency/stroke
- Lateral medullary infarction
- Internal carotid artery dissection
- Cerebral infarct
- Cervical myelopathy
- Cervical radiculopathy
- Long thoracic nerve palsy
- Diaphragmatic palsy
- Central retinal artery occlusion
- Cervical fracture/dislocation
- Epidural hematoma
- Intervertebral disk herniation
- Tracheal rupture

BOX 14.2
Contraindications for High-Velocity Manipulation Techniques

- Unstable fractures
- Severe osteoporosis
- Multiple myeloma
- Osteomyelitis
- Primary bone tumors
- Paget disease
- Any progressive neurologic deficit
- Spinal cord tumors
- Cauda equina compression
- Central cervical intervertebral disk herniation
- Hypermobile joints
- Rheumatoid arthritis
- Inflammatory phase of ankylosing spondylitis
- Psoriatic arthritis
- Reiter syndrome
- Anticoagulant therapy
- Congenital bleeding disorder
- Acquired bleeding disorder
- Inadequate physical and spinal examination
- Poor manipulative skills

BOX 14.3
Contraindications to Spinal Manipulation

ABSOLUTE CONTRAINDICATIONS
- Active inflammatory arthropathy
- Acute spondyloarthropathy
- Demineralization
- Ligamentous laxity with subluxation/dislocation
- Tumor/metastasis
- Spinal infection/osteomyelitis
- Acute fracture/dislocation
- Severe osteoporosis
- Acute myelopathy
- Cauda equina syndrome

RELATIVE CONTRAINDICATIONS
- Severe spondylosis
- Known malignancy
- Benign bone tumor
- Spinal trauma
- Spinal hypermobility
- Acute disk herniation
- Ankylosing spondylitis/spondyloarthropathy
- History of spinal surgery
- Acute soft tissue injury
- Blood dyscrasia
- Anticoagulation
- History/symptoms of vertebrobasilar insufficiency
- Bone demineralization/osteopenia

Various contraindications to HLVA exist. The most common and important to remember include atlantoaxial (C1−C2) ligamentous instability. Patients with rheumatoid arthritis and those with Trisomy 21 are particularly vulnerable. Additional contraindications are listed in Boxes 14.2 and 14.3.

Additional Treatments/OMM Techniques

Muscle Energy is a technique that utilizes the patient's active participation to voluntarily move a muscle and restore range of motion beyond a diagnosed barrier. This technique has been used extensively by therapists and is often referred to as contract-relax technique or Proprioceptive Neuromuscular Facilitation.[22] The patient is positioned into the barrier (restricted range of motion component) and is asked to contract away from the barrier against an isometric, holding force. The muscle contraction is held for 3−5 s. Then there is a period of postisometric relaxation, during which the new barrier (with increased ROM) is passively reengaged. This is repeated until no further incremental improvements are achieved.

Myofascial Release is a technique founded on the premise that the body is encased in fascia, a type of connective tissue that interconnects all bones, muscles, nerves, and internal structures. Because of this interconnectivity, injury in one area can result in pain and dysfunction at a distant point. Direct myofascial technique involves loading the myofascial tissues, holding the tissues in position, and waiting for release. The release is perceived by the practitioner treating the patient. This results in increased range of motion and reduced pain symptoms.[19]

Massage is a general technique of soft tissue manipulation with the goal of producing beneficial effects on the nervous and muscular systems as well as optimizing circulatory flow of both blood and lymph.[23] There are multiple techniques which are typically categorized based on geographic region of origin.

Western techniques—"Swedish massage"

* Effleurage—gliding of hands/fingers over the skin in a rhythmic, circular pattern with varying degrees of pressure (Fig.14.2).
* Petrissage—kneading motion involving compression of skin between the thumb and fingers, typically by alternating hands in a rhythmic, rolling motion (Fig. 14.3).
* Tapotement—percussion massage—includes hacking, clapping, beating, pounding, and vibration (Figs. 14.4 and 14.5).
* Friction—small surface area pressure performed in a circular, longitudinal, or transverse motion with the goal of breaking down adhesions/scar tissue, loosening ligaments, and disabling trigger points (Fig. 14.6).

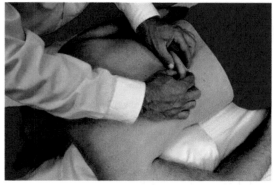

FIG. 14.3 Pétrissage massage: "rolling." In this form of pétrissage, the skin or muscle is gathered up between the fingers and thumb and rolled continuously, gathering new skin and muscle.

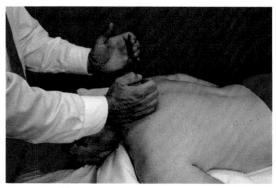

FIG. 14.4 Tapotement massage: "hacking." Hacking involves striking the body at right angles with the ulnar aspect of the hands.

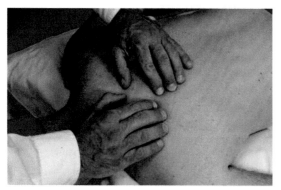

FIG. 14.2 Effleurage massage. This type of massage being performed on the patient's posterior shoulder is a rhythmic, circular motion with the fingertips. Pressure can be varied to massage deeper structures.

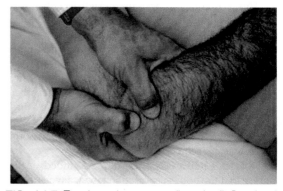

FIG. 14.5 Tapotement massage: "cupping." Cupping is frequently performed over the rib cage to loosen secretions in the lungs.

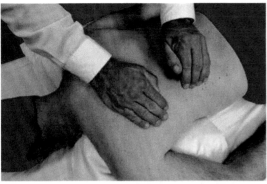

FIG. 14.6 Friction massage. Friction massage being performed on the lateral epicondyle to promote tendon healing.

Eastern techniques

- ### Acupressure

Acupressure is similar to acupuncture in terms of its analysis of the human body, but it uses pressure rather than needles to achieve its effects. There are benefits including the elimination of potential complications of bleeding and infection and expands the range of patients who might benefit from this treatment to include individuals receiving anticoagulants, those with needle phobia, and those who are severely immunosuppressed. Acupressure can also be taught to the patient who can then apply this technique as self-treatment on a more frequent basis. This can be very helpful in the early stages of treatment when the duration of the relief from acupressure may be short-lived.[2]

- ### Reflexology

Reflexology is a healing art based on the theory that there are reflexes in the feet and hands that correspond to every part of the body. The theory behind the treatment is that the entire body has been comprehensively mapped on the hands and feet, similar to topographic mapping of the brain. Pressure can be applied to specific parts of the hands and feet to influence the parts of the body being treated. At this time, evidence of its benefit in the treatment of any particular condition is limited.[24]

Rolfing

A therapy technique similar to massage based on "structural integration." The goal of treatment is to achieve proper vertical alignment and efficient movement. A typical regimen involves superficial massage with progression to deeper friction massage in an attempt to stretch fascia and allow muscles to relax and lengthen. Preliminary clinical studies with small samples of patients with chronic musculoskeletal pain and chronic fatigue syndrome suggest positive effects on gait, pain reduction, improved ROM, functional status, and subjective well-being.[25]

Traction

Traction is a technique used to stretch soft tissues with the goal of separating joint surfaces by the use of pulling force.[26] The forces can be delivered by various methods, including manual, mechanical, motorized, hydraulic, or with the assistance of gravity. Duration of force can range from continuous (long duration), sustained, or intermittent (cycled, short duration). In order for the treatment to be effective, the surface resistance of the targeted area must be overcome. The physiologic effects of traction have been extensively evaluated and reported. Traction can stretch muscles and ligaments, tighten the posterior longitudinal ligament to exert a centripetal force on the annulus fibrosis, enlarge the intervertebral space and intervertebral foramina, and separate apophyseal joints. Specific types of traction are demonstrated below for both cervical (Fig. 14.7) and lumbar spine (Fig. 14.8) (Table 14.2).

There is no consensus on the definitive indications for traction, but the condition having the most evidence for its use is cervical radiculopathy. The use of traction with lumbar radiculopathy, neck pain, and low back pain is more controversial.[27] The popularity of lumbar traction in treating low back pain, with or without radicular features, has declined in favor of more active treatment programs. In the absence of contraindications, traction can be used to treat any condition in which the physiologic effects of traction would theoretically be beneficial.

Absolute contraindications to traction include malignancy, infection such as osteomyelitis or diskitis, osteoporosis, inflammatory arthritis, unstable fracture, cord compression, and uncontrolled hypertension or cardiovascular disease in the setting of carotid or vertebral artery disease. Traction should be discontinued if there is exacerbation of symptoms, discomfort from the traction device (especially over the abdomen), or with production of systemic symptoms such as dizziness. Additional contraindications are listed below (Box 14.4).

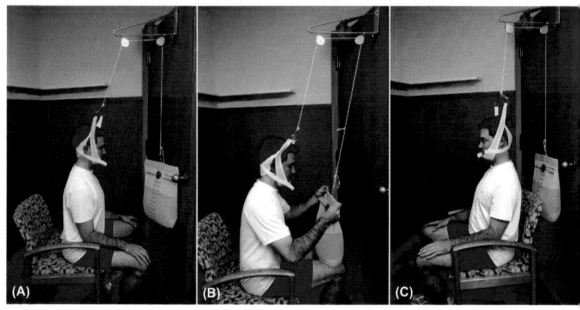

FIG. 14.7 Home cervical traction. (A), Cervical traction performed using an over-the-door pulley system. This type of traction is performed with the patient facing the door to allow for the cervical spine to be slightly flexed. Movement of the door should be avoided during treatment. (B), Intermittent traction can be performed by resting the weight (water bag) on the patient's lap, producing a slack in the tension rope. The cervical posture is maintained throughout the course of traction. (C), The patient is improperly positioned, with the back to the door. This can lead to extension and possible worsening of the cervical condition.

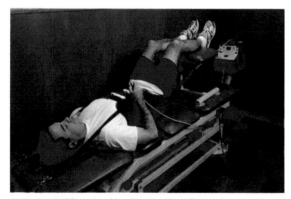

FIG. 14.8 Motorized lumbar traction. The patient is placed in a supine position with the hips and knees flexed. The distraction force is mechanically created by pulling on a pelvic belt. The upper body is stabilized by another strap around the chest. Additional distraction force can be accomplished on a traction table that allows the upper and lower segments to separate.

TABLE 14.2
Cervical and Lumbar Traction Comparison.

	Cervical	**Lumbar**
Equipment	Head or Chin Sling	Thoracic or chest belt Inversion table, split traction table, or autotraction table
Positioning	20–30 degrees of cervical flexion Supine or seated	Neutral Supine
Force	Intermittent forces 25 lbs or more is required to overcome normal cervical lordosis	Sustained forced Requires significantly greater forces to create distraction

BOX 14.4
Contraindications to Traction

GENERAL TRACTION
Osteomyelitis or diskitis
Osteoporosis
Spinal cord compression
Malignancy
Unstable fracture
Uncontrolled hypertension
Severe cardiovascular disease

CERVICAL TRACTION
Central disk herniation
Hypermobility
Rheumatoid arthritis
Carotid or vertebral artery disease
Temporomandibular joint dysfunction (with chin strap)

LUMBAR TRACTION
Pregnancy
Hemorrhoids and intraabdominal conditions that may be
    affected by increased intraabdominal pressure
Cauda equina syndrome

Writing a Therapy Prescription

A crucial skill to develop as a provider is the ability to accurately write a therapy prescription. A thorough and proper prescription should provide the therapist with pertinent information to safely and effectively treat the patient. The components for a comprehensive therapy prescription are as follows:

1. Identify to discipline of therapy. This will usually be either physical therapy or occupational therapy. See the beginning of the "Therapies" section to better choose the correct discipline.
2. Provide the diagnosis and laterality. It is also helpful to include pertinent history such as "status post lumbar discectomy."
3. Specify the frequency and duration of treatment. For chronic low back pain, this may be 1–2 times per week for 6 weeks.
4. Specify the treatment being recommended. Treatments include therapeutic modalities, manual therapies, therapeutic exercises, and other specialized treatments. Additionally, instructing the therapist to provide guidance in the creation of a home exercise program (HEP) is essential.
   a. Therapeutic exercises: Range of motion, stretching, strengthening, balance/proprioception, etc.
   b. Manual therapies: Massage, soft tissue mobilization, traction, myofascial release, etc.
   c. Therapeutic modalities: Transcutaneous electrical nerve stimulation (TENS), ultrasound (US), diathermy, cryotherapy, etc.
   d. Specialized treatments: Assistance with bracing, orthotics, kinesio-taping, aquatic therapy, etc.
5. Importantly, any safety precautions or contraindications to certain exercises or modalities should be listed. This can include cardiovascular and pulmonary considerations or limitations in their weight-bearing status. Additionally, contraindications for certain modalities for specific situations should be included (see Modalities section). A patient's appropriateness for physical therapy should be determined based on a thorough evaluation of their medical history and physical examination.

Sample physical therapy prescription

Physical therapy. *Diagnosis*: 42-year-old male with low back pain secondary to discogenic and myofascial pain.
Duration: 1–2 visits per week for 6 weeks.
Therapeutic exercises: ROM, core strengthening, postural alignment, hamstring stretching, and instruct on HEP.
Manual therapies: soft tissue mobilization.
Therapeutic modalities: none.
Specialized treatments: none.
Precautions: avoid lumbar flexion-based exercises.

In this sample prescription, we are limiting the time spent with passive modalities and focusing on therapeutic exercises. Because the patient's pain is thought to be coming from the intervertebral discs, we instruct the therapist to avoid exercises that put increased stress on the offending structures. This template serves as comprehensive approach to writing therapy orders for any condition.[28]

PART 2: MODALITIES

A proper multidisciplinary rehabilitation program in pain medicine incorporates the use of modalities to assist with pain relief, in an effort to provide relief and help facilitate adherence to a therapeutic exercise regimen. A modality can be classified as any physical agent or technique used to produce a therapeutic response.[29] Modalities are commonly used by therapists, athletic trainers, and chiropractors to assist with participation in a coordinated rehabilitation program. In general, modalities are low risk and can provide varying levels of benefit for a variety of painful conditions, depending on both chronicity and severity. The most commonly used modalities include ice, heat, diathermy/US, and TENS. While the below information is by no means comprehensive, it is a brief overview of the most common modalities used for pain relief in rehab. It is also important to understand the appropriate indications and contraindications for specific modalities, to ensure proper use and minimize harm to the patient.

Heat and Cold

The age old question of whether to use ice or heat is often confusing for patients, and proper understanding of these modalities will help to educate patients on their appropriate use. Both heat and ice have the potential to provide analgesia in a variety of pain disorders, although primarily for musculoskeletal joint and soft tissue-related injuries. Changes in tissue temperature have been shown to create various physiologic effects, including altered hemodynamics, neuromuscular activity, and connective tissue elasticity (Box 14.5 and 14.6). These features are believed to play a vital role in their therapeutic characteristics.[30]

Cold exposure has specifically been shown to produce a decrease in gamma motor neuron activity, which has been correlated with a reduction in muscle spasms.[31] The use of cryotherapy is often best in the acute phase of soft tissue injuries because of its greater depth of penetration, causes vasoconstriction, and produces better antiinflammatory effects. However, it can also be used in the rehabilitative phase due to its pain relieving qualities, which can facilitate earlier, more consistent, and higher intensity exercise.[32]

BOX 14.6
Physiologic Effects of Cold

HEMODYNAMIC
- Immediate cutaneous vasoconstriction
- Delayed reactive vasodilatation
- Decreased acute inflammation

NEUROMUSCULAR
- Slowing of conduction velocity
- Conduction block and axonal degeneration with prolonged exposure
- Decreased group 1 a fiber tiring rates (muscle spindle)
- Decreased group 2 fiber firing rates (muscle spindle)
- Decreased group 1b fiber firing rates (Golgi tendon organ)
- Decreased muscle stretch reflex amplitudes
- Increased maximal isometric strength
- Decreased muscle fatigue
- Temporarily reduced spasticity

JOINT AND CONNECTIVE TISSUE
- Increased joint stiffness
- Decreased tendon extensibility
- Decreased collagenase activity

MISCELLANEOUS
- Decreased pain
- General relaxation

BOX 14.5
Physiologic Effects of Heat

HEMODYNAMIC
- Increased blood flow
- Decreased chronic inflammation
- Increased acute inflammation
- Increased edema
- Increased bleeding

NEUROMUSCULAR
- Increased group 1a fiber firing rates (muscle spindle)
- Decreased group 2 fiber firing rates (muscle spindle)
- Increased group 1b fiber firing rates (Golgi tendon organ)
- Increased nerve conduction velocity

JOINT AND CONNECTIVE TISSUE
- Increased tendon extensibility
- Increased collagenase activity
- Decreased joint stiffness

MISCELLANEOUS
- Decreased pain
- General relaxation

On the contrary, heat is best used as a comfort measure for patients with subacute and chronic pain conditions. Heat has been shown to increase collagen extensibility, increase blood flow, indirectly decrease muscle spindle excitability, and increase pain tolerance.[33] These qualities of heat application make it best suited for chronic joint and inflammatory conditions, particularly those resulting in stiffness and reduced range of motion.

Therapeutic cryotherapy

The use of cryotherapy has been indicated in a variety of conditions ranging from acute musculoskeletal injuries to myofascial pain, and even minor burns (Box 14.7). Contrary to therapeutic heat, all forms of cryotherapy are considered superficial. However, there are many forms of therapeutic cryotherapy which can be applied to either a local region or to the entire body (Box 14.8).

There is significant variability in the mode, duration, and frequency of cryotherapy application. The mode of cryotherapy application can be in the form of ice pack,

BOX 14.7
General Uses of Cryotherapy in Physical Medicine

- Musculoskeletal conditions (sprains, strains, tendonitis, tenosynovitis, bursitis, capsulitis, etc.)
- Myofascial pain
- After certain orthopedic surgeries
- Component of spasticity management
- Emergency treatment of minor burns

TABLE 14.3
Types of Cryotherapy—Localized versus Whole Body.

TYPES OF CRYOTHERAPY	
Localized	**Whole Body**
Superficial ice pack	Ice bath
Ice massage	Whirlpool
Topical vapocoolant	Cryotherapy chamber

BOX 14.8
General Precautions for the Use of Cold

- Cold intolerance
- Cryotherapy-induced neurapraxia or axonotmesis
- Arterial insufficiency
- Impaired sensation
- Cognitive or communication deficits that preclude reporting of pain
- Cryopathies
- Cryoglobulinemia
- Paroxysmal cold hemoglobinuria
- Cold hypersensitivity
- Raynaud disease or phenomenon

TABLE 14.4
Types of Heat—Superficial versus Deep.

TYPES OF HEAT	
Superficial	**Deep**
Heating pad	Shortwave diathermy
Hydrocollator packs	Ultrasound
Paraffin baths	Microwave diathermy
Heat lamp	
Hydrotherapy	
Fluidotherapy	

crushed ice bags, vapocoolant spray, ice massage, cold whirlpool, or cold compression device. The duration and frequency of treatment can vary, typically ranging from 10 to 20 min three times per day, up to 30—45 min every 2 hours. Currently, there is no consensus on proper mode, duration, or frequency of cryotherapy and clinical practice varies by provider or patient preference. Research has demonstrated a very wide range of clinical effectiveness.[34] A tissue temperature reduction of 10—15°C appears to be necessary to achieve local analgesia and lower metabolism, in order to maximize the benefits of cryotherapy.[35] (Table 14.3).

Therapeutic heat

Heating modalities come in a variety of forms, classified as either deep or superficial, to target different tissue layers.[29] Superficial heat modalities include heating pad, hydrocollator packs, heat lamps, paraffin wax, and whirlpools. The most common deep heat modalities are US and shortwave diathermy (SWD) (Table 14.4). The use of superficial heat is generally very safe and well tolerated by most patients; however,

the general precautions of heat are listed below (Box 14.9).

Superficial Heat

Superficial heating modalities typically penetrate less than 2 cm from the skin surface, primarily affecting the skin and subcutaneous fat layers.[29] Tissue temperatures have been shown to increase 5—6°C after 6 minutes

BOX 14.9
General Precautions for the Use of Heat

- Acute trauma, inflammation
- Impaired circulation
- Bleeding diatheses
- Edema
- Large scars
- Impaired sensation
- Malignancy
- Cognitive or communication deficits that preclude reporting of pain

of heat application, with sustained effects for approximately 30 min.[30] Using superficial heat for approximately 15–30 min has been shown to increase muscle temperature by 1°C at a depth up to 3 cm.[36] Superficial applications of heat have been shown to be potentially beneficial for a range of musculoskeletal pathologies including joint pain, low back pain, muscle pain, myofascial pain, and many others.[37,38] It is also important for patients to utilize a skin barrier, such as a towel or pillow case, to minimize risk of skin burn (Fig.14.9).

Diathermy

The term *diathermy*, meaning "through heat," encompasses several heating modalities targeting deeper structures while minimizing temperature changes of the more superficial layers. The most commonly used forms of diathermy include US and SWD, while microwave diathermy (MD) is a less commonly used. With better penetration to deeper tissue layers, diathermy elicits the benefits of heat to deeper layers of muscle, tendon, and large peripheral joints. The most effective target temperature has been shown to range from 104 to 113°F. This temperature range maximizes tissue vasodilation and metabolic changes while minimizing tissue damage and pain [39]. We will primarily cover US and SWD in this section, as these tend to be the most clinically applicable.

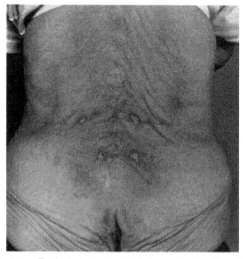

FIG.14.9 Typical heating pad burn. Note the focal hypopigmentation from burns at areas of increased pressure. Also note the more diffuse hyperpigmentation changes (erythema ab igne).

Ultrasound

Therapeutic US is one of the most popular methods for providing diathermy. US is a form of sound wave that occurs at a frequency above the limit of audible human hearing. Most therapeutic US operates between 0.8 and 3 MHz, with the most common range between 0.8 and 1.1 MHz. While US waves can also be used for diagnostic imaging, therapeutic US sends high frequency acoustic waves through tissue to provide a variety of both thermal and nonthermal benefits to deeper levels of tissue including changes in temperature, pressure, and cellular function. As US waves travel through tissue, the energy of the sound waves dissipates via a process known as *attenuation* which results from absorption of waves into tissue, beam divergence, or beam deflection. The absorption of US waves into target tissue creates molecular vibration within the target tissue, ultimately converting the sound energy into heat.[40]

The depth of penetration varies depending on the amount of beam attenuation in tissue and specific factors such as wave frequency, beam orientation, and tissue type. Typically, higher frequency beams will not penetrate as deep as lower frequency, because higher frequency acoustic waves are attenuated more rapidly. In addition, a coupling medium is used on the surface of the skin to minimize reflection of US waves at the skin surface and enhance wave transmission. Although there are many comparable options, the best medium is one with similar acoustic impedance as target tissue, resulting in minimal beam attenuation and maximal transmission of US waves from transducer to tissue. Furthermore, tissue type has a significant impact on penetration with approximately 50% of a US beam penetrating several centimeters into muscle, only a few tenths of a millimeter into bone, and 7–8 cm in fat.[41] Although results can vary, it is common for deeper tissue layers such as large peripheral joints and the bone-muscle interface to reach temperatures of 114.8°F.[42,43]

US can be performed in either continuous or pulsed modes. Pulsed US delivers acoustic waves in brief intervals, which can have a customized pulse intensity, duration, and patterned frequency. However, pulsed US does not produce the same thermal effects as continuous US and is presumed to maximize nonthermal effects of US on target tissue. Additionally, the most common technique for administration of US is known as "stroking technique," which involves a practitioner slowly moving the US transducer in a circular or linear pattern over a small area of tissue (approximately 4 square inches). This technique is theorized to provide more energy distribution to target tissue and minimize risk of focal burning, as compared with a stationary technique.[2]

There are a plethora of techniques for therapeutic US with very minimal data to support one use over the other. While therapeutic US in the setting of ongoing therapy has a low risk of detriment to the patient, some research for its clinical benefits has failed to show conclusive evidence.[44]

Other variants of US exist. One technique, known as indirect US, can be performed to a specific area without the probe directly touching the skin. Additionally, phonophoresis is a technique which utilizes US waves to drive biologically active medication to deeper tissue layers. The most commonly used phonophoresis agent is corticosteroid—its antiinflammatory effects are thought to have synergistic benefits with US. Iontophoresis is a technique similar to phonophoresis but uses an electrical field to drive ionic solutions (such as corticosteroids or anesthetics) subcutaneously into soft tissues. Specific benefits from such techniques have not been consistently validated and existing research thus far is mixed.[45–47]

Shortwave diathermy

SWD is a modality that creates heat via emitted electromagnetic radio waves. The heat is produced by oscillation of high frequency electric and magnetic fields, most commonly at 27.2 MHz. Traditionally, there are two types of SWD units which create heat in different ways. Inductive SWD units contain coils which creates a magnetic field. This field projects forward into the body and generates a circular, electric field within the target tissue. Typically, the coils are confined to flexible cables or within a rigid drum.[39] In comparison, capacitive SWD units use condenser plates to transfer oscillations of electric field between the plates. The target tissue is placed between the condenser plates and acts as a capacitor to store electrical charge, resulting in local heating of the tissue.

Generally, SWD can produce therapeutic heat as deep as 3–5 cm; however, this can vary widely depending on applicator type, setup, and amount of subcutaneous fat.[37,48] Muscle temperature has been shown to rise 9.5 °C with less than 1 cm of subcutaneous fat, versus only 5.6 °C with greater than 2 cm of subcutaneous fat.[38] In addition, research has shown heat to be better distributed with only air between tissue and applicator, compared to a barrier with a cotton terrycloth.[38]

The indications for use of SWD are similar with those of US and it is typically used to help with extensibility of soft tissue and improve myofascial.[49] SWD treatments typically last between 20 and 30 min, with the intensity being adjusted based on patient tolerance and subjective pain intensity.

BOX 14.10
Ultrasound Precautions

- General heat precautions
- Near brain, eyes, reproductive organs
- Gravid or menstruating uterus
- Near pacemaker
- Near spine, laminectomy sites
- Malignancy
- Skeletal immaturity
- Arthroplasties
- Methyl methacrylate or high-density polyethylene

Comprehensive precautions for US and SWD are listed in Box 14.10 and 14.11. One important consideration in the use of SWD versus US is that SWD *cannot* be used near metallic implants, whereas US does not have this limitation. SWD should also not be used in patients with implantable pacemakers or deep brain stimulators, as the electromagnetic waves can cause device malfunction and potential patient harm.[50]

Microwave diathermy

A variant of diathermy also exists known as MD, which uses electromagnetic radio waves with frequencies between 915 and 2456 Mhz to generate heat. The frequency of MD tends to be lower than SWD which allows for better penetration into tissue, but this allows for more dispersion of the electromagnetic beam. Understandably, this creates a far less localized effect. Although MD was once quite popular, it has fallen out of favor in clinical practice, partially due to the need for protective eyewear to minimize cataract formation.[29]

Transcutaneous Electrical Nerve Stimulation

TENS is one of the most commonly used modalities for pain relief. TENS as a method of electroanalgesia was

---

BOX 14.11
Shortwave Precautions

- General heat precautions
- Metal (jewelry, pacemakers, intrauterine devices, surgical implants, deep brain stimulators, etc.)
- Contact lenses
- Gravid or menstruating uterus
- Skeletal immaturity

initially proposed in 1965 by Melzack and Wall, theorized to be effective via the "gate control theory" of pain[51]. The gate control theory states that stimulation of large somatosensory afferent peripheral nerve fibers can inhibit the transmission of nociceptive signals carried via the small, unmyelinated C fibers. Subsequent studies have added further complexity to this theory, and the exact mechanistic explanation of TENS remains partially unknown to this day.

A TENS unit consists of a battery powered electronic pulse generator that creates a low voltage electrical current. This current is transmitted through transcutaneous patches placed over the desired area of treatment and is highly customizable to the patient's symptomatic response. Conventional TENS units are typically classified as high stimulation frequency (>100 Hz), low intensity (10−30 mA), and short pulse duration (50−100 ms).[48] Other forms of TENS applications exist in the form of acupuncture-TENS (the electrical stimulation is transmitted through an acupuncture needle), as well as Pulsed or Burst TENS (where the frequency oscillates between high and low stimulation).

Most clinical trials have examined the effectiveness of TENS in chronic pain conditions. Evidence is minimal for use in acute pain states. Metaanalyses have shown positive trends toward improvements in pain and overall function with TENS application compared with placebo;[52] however, the efficacy of TENS in any pain disorder continues to be largely controversial and the evidence is overall mixed. In a 2019 overview of Cochrane reviews by Gibson et al., the study was unable to conclude that TENS is beneficial for pain control, disability, health-related quality of life, or use of pain relieving medicines in patients with chronic pain[53].

Furthermore, the effectiveness of different TENS application, such as acupuncture or burst, remains controversial—there is no significant research available to date suggesting improved outcomes with either method. Despite the lack of significant evidence, due to its noninvasive and low risk nature, TENS is a frequently used modality for chronic musculoskeletal pain. See below for a list of indications and contraindications with transcutaneous electrical stimulation [Table 14.5].

Low Level Laser Therapy

The word "laser" is actually an acronym for Light Amplification by Stimulated Emission of Radiation. While both high (HLLT) and low (LLLT) powered lasers have a multitude of clinical applications, only low energy (<90 mW) lasers are used for pain relief in various musculoskeletal pathologies. While the mechanism of action for low energy lasers is not well understood, their effects on pain relief are believed to work via changes in tissue metabolism and physiology at the cellular level. Research has been unsuccessful in demonstrating that lasers create significant tissue temperature changes.[54] While LLLT has been used experimentally for various musculoskeletal conditions, there is no consensus on optimal use or indication, creating a wide range of viable applications. While some recent literature suggests LLLT may be an effective modality for pain relief in musculoskeletal disorders,[55] the research is overall mixed in regard to its clinical efficacy.[56]

Multidisciplinary Chronic Pain Programs

In refractory cases of chronic pain, where patients have failed trials of several interventions, the utilization of a

---

TABLE 14.5
TENS—Indications versus Contraindications.[48].

Indications	Contraindications

1. Neurogenic pain:
  a. Phantom pain
  b. Sympathetically mediated pain
  c. Postherpetic neuralgia
  d. Trigeminal neuralgia
  e. Radiculopathy or radiculitis
2. Musculoskeletal pain
  a. Peripheral joint-mediated pain
  b. Osteoarthritis
  c. Rheumatoid arthritis
	1. Do not place on or near the eyes, in the mouth, or transcerebrally
	2. Do not place over the carotid sinuses (vasovagal reflex), anterior neck (laryngospasm)
	3. Do not use on areas of significantly reduced or absent sensation
	4. Do not use over the trigeminal nerve if history of herpes zoster induced trigeminal neuralgia
	5. Avoid in epilepsy or pregnancy
	6. Avoid in patients with an implanted cardiac pacemaker or defibrillator

multidisciplinary pain program may be considered. Patients experiencing chronic pain commonly have other psychosocial stressors or behavioral changes such as disturbances in sleep, changes in mood, kinesiophobia, and other pain-avoidance beliefs and behaviors which add to the complexity of managing chronic pain. While treating potential pain-generating sources with interventional procedures is an important component of comprehensive care, multidisciplinary pain program are capable of addressing many of the underlying psychological, behavioral, and environmental components that may be preventing a patient from making functional progress.[1]

Multidisciplinary pain programs typically consist of a wide spectrum of practitioners and the structure can fluctuate depending on the specific program. Care teams can include pain physicians, physical therapists, occupational and vocational therapists, pain psychologists, biofeedback specialists, massage therapists, acupuncturists, and chiropractors to name a few. The use of CBT,[57] Eye Movement Desensitization and Reprocessing (EMDR),[58] and virtual reality[59,60] has also been shown to be potentially helpful in chronic pain programs with some populations. Moreover, a pain medicine specialist should also consider the use of adjuvant medications such as antidepressants, sleep aids, and other pain medications to help with baseline pain control during the intensive pain program. The suggested frequency and duration is patient-dependent and often correlates with the severity of symptoms. In the most severe cases, patients can receive 7–8 h of treatment per day for 4 weeks,[1] with some research suggesting that more intensive pain rehab programs (>100 h of treatment) are more effective than less intensive programs.[61]

The National Pain Strategy strongly supports the use of interdisciplinary pain management involving primary care, pain specialists, and tertiary care.[62] An interdisciplinary approach with proper communication between practitioners and patients can provide a robust support system to improve psychological, emotional, and physical well-being, which ultimately fosters improved independence and maximizes overall patient function.

PART 3: BRACING

The concept of bracing for pain relief is often confusing for many practitioners and can be complicated depending on severity and acuity. In the setting of more serious clinical situations such as acute nonoperative vertebral fractures, severe scoliosis/kyphosis, trauma, or postsurgical

patients, options available for bracing are quite numerous. As it pertains to this section, we will briefly discuss some of the most common options for bracing in patients with back or neck pain, without spinal instability, to assist with pain control and help facilitate a patient's rehabilitative process.

Lumbar supports are often used both as a preventative measure and for conservative treatment in acute and chronic low back pain. In regard to its preventative qualities, the use of lumbar support has been shown to have little to no effect when compared with patients who received no intervention, in terms of number of days with low back pain or reduction of sick days. In addition, the research supporting the use of lumbar support for treatment of low back pain is mixed. Some research has shown no difference in regard to short-term pain relief and variable results in terms of benefit over no intervention for return to work, functional improvement, or subacute and chronic pain relief.[63] Although the literature supporting use of lumbar support is quite poor and highly variable, utilization of lumbar bracing is common because of its relatively low cost and low risk to the patient.

The most common type of braces used for patients with acute and chronic low back pain are a soft lumbosacral orthosis (LSO), lumbar binder, or lumbar corset. While there are slight differences in the designs of these braces and a plethora of options available, the rationale for their use is similar. Wrapping an LSO or corset around the abdominal and lumbar region has been theorized to increase intraabdominal pressure, which subsequently increases stability of the lumbar region. This mimics the effects of engaging core postural muscles and can beneficially alter posture and spine biomechanics, resulting in pain relief.[64] It has long been suspected that prolonged use of a lumbar binder or LSO could result in weakening and reduced activation of lumbar or core musculature; however, some recent research has disputed this theory.[65,66] Lumbar corsets may also provide benefit by providing sensory feedback that encourages use of proper biomechanics during activities and avoiding painful positions. Common mistakes patients make are wearing the lumbar support to high in the abdominal region or overlapping the rib cage. An important consideration is that lumbar braces can be difficult to use in patients with significant abdominal obesity, because of a tendency for the brace to migrate.

Acute osteoporotic vertebral compression fractures can cause significant pain. Most fractures are nonoperative, especially when they do not cause any significant neural compression resulting in weakness, numbness,

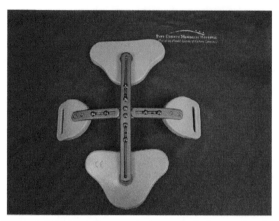

FIG. 14.10 Cruciform anterior spinal hyperextension thoracolumbosacral orthosis.

or other neurologic sequelae of spinal cord or nerve root compression. Extension bracing can be considered for pain control in acute vertebral compression fractures. Cruciform anterior spinal hyperextension aka CASH braces (Fig. 14.10) and Jewett braces (Fig. 14.11) are two types of extension braces that can be used for thoracolumbar osteoporotic vertebral compression fractures to keep the spine in extension. Unstable fractures should be evaluated by an orthopedist for surgical considerations before performing any long-term bracing.

Cervical bracing also has mixed clinical efficacy. In general, cervical collars have not proven to be effective in nontraumatic acute or chronic neck pain. For whiplash injuries, patients that have early mobilization fared better in the long term than those patients immobilized

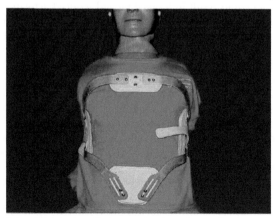

FIG. 14.11 Jewett hyperextension thoracolumbosacral orthosis.

with a cervical collar. As such, early mobilization is recommended. Hard collar immobilization in acute radicular pain lacks clinical evidence. There is insufficient data for the use of neck collars in chronic neck pain. Use of soft cervical collars in chronic neck pain may encourage a lack of mobility and lead to loss of cervical ROM.[67]

CONCLUSION

Rehabilitation plays a critical role in the treatment of painful conditions as part of a multimodal, multidisciplinary pain program. Therapeutic exercise and physical and occupational therapies can improve strength, ROM, and aerobic capacity with the goal of improving function and reducing pain. There is a vast array of other rehabilitative therapies which include manual techniques, modalities, and bracing, all of which can play a role in a pain rehabilitation program. Some patients suffering from chronic pain may benefit from a formal intensive multidisciplinary rehabilitation pain program focusing on the social, psychological, and physical aspects of chronic pain. Rehabilitation remains paramount in treating both acute and chronic painful conditions.

REFERENCES

1. Benzon HT. *Essentials of Pain Medicine.* Elseiver; 2018.
2. Braddom R, Peterson A, Marcus D, Saulino M, Hung C, Kornbluth I. *Handbook of Physical Medicine and Rehabilitation.* Philadelphia: Saunders; 2004:427–497.
3. McKenzie R, May S. *The Lumbar Spine: Mechanical Diagnosis and Therapy.* vol. 2. Waikanae, New Zealand: Spinal Publications; 2003.
4. van Tulder M, Malmivaara A, Esmail R, et al. Exercise therapy for low back pain: a systematic review within the framework of the Cochrane collaboration back review group. *Spine.* 2000;25(21):2784–2796.
5. "Lumbar Syndrome." *Musculoskeletal Key;* 2017. https://musculoskeletalkey.com/lumbar-syndrome/.
6. *The Diagnosis and Treatment of Low Back Pain Work Group. VA/DoD Clinical Practice Guideline for Diagnosis and Treatment of Low Back Pain.* 2017. Version 2.
7. Rydeard R, Leger A, Smith D. Pilates-based therapeutic exercise: effect on subjects with nonspecific chronic low back pain and functional disability: a randomized controlled trial. *J Orthop Sports Phys Ther.* 2006;36:472–484.
8. Yamato TP, Maher CG, Saragiotto BT, et al. Pilates for low back pain: complete republication of a cochrane review. *Spine.* 2016;41(12):1013–1021.
9. Sherman KJ, Cherkin DC, Erro J, et al. Comparing yoga, exercise, and a self-care book for chronic low back pain: a randomized, controlled trial. *Ann Intern Med.* 2005;143: 849–856.

10. Chou R, Deyo R, Friedly J, et al. *AHRQ Comparative Effectiveness Reviews. Noninvasive Treatments for Low Back Pain.* Rockville (MD): Agency for Healthcare Research and Quality (US); 2016.

11. Aboagye E, Karlsson ML, Hagberg J, Jensen I. Cost-effectiveness of early interventions for nonspecific low back pain: a randomized controlled study investigating medical yoga, exercise therapy and self-care advice. *J Rehabil Med.* 2015;47(2):167–173.

12. Wieland LS, Skoetz N, Pilkington K, Vempati R, D'Adamo CR, Berman BM. Yoga treatment for chronic non-specific low back pain. *Cochrane Database Syst Rev.* 2017;(1). CD010671.

13. Wang C, Collet JP, Lau J. The effect of tai chi on health outcomes in patients with chronic conditions: a systematic review. *Arch Intern Med.* 2004;164:493–501.

14. Wu G. Evaluation of the effectiveness of Tai Chi for improving balance and preventing falls in the older population: a review. *J Am Geriatr Soc.* 2002;50:746–754.

15. Kong LJ, Lauche R, Klose P, et al. Tai chi for chronic pain conditions: a systematic review and metaanalysis of randomized controlled trials. *Sci Rep.* 2016;6:25325.

16. Lundblad I, Elert J, Gerdle B. Randomized controlled trial of physiotherapy and Feldenkrais interventions in female workers with neck-shoulder complaints. *J Occup Rehabil.* 1999;9:179–194.

17. Jain S, Janssen K, DeCelle S. Alexander technique and Feldenkrais method: a critical overview. *Phys Med Rehabil Clin N Am.* 2004;15(4):811–825.

18. Cherkin DC, Deyo RA, Battie M, et al. A comparison of physical therapy, chiropractic manipulation, and provision of an educational booklet for the treatment of patients with low back pain. *N Engl J Med.* 1998;339(15):1021–1029.

19. Savarese RG, Capobianco JD, Adesina AT, Reed G. *OMT Review: A Comprehensive Review in Osteopathic Medicine.* Legis Press; 2018.

20. Haveela B, Dowle P, Chandrasekar P. Effectiveness of Mulligan's technique and Spencer's technique in adjunct to conventional therapy in frozen shoulder: a randomised controlled trial. *Int J Adv Res Dev.* 2018;3(1):253–260.

21. Koss R. Quality assurance monitoring of osteopathic manipulative treatment. *J Am Osteopath Assoc.* 1990;90(5):427–433.

22. Hindle KB, Whitcomb TJ, Briggs WO, Hong J. Proprioceptive neuromuscular facilitation (PNF): its mechanisms and effects on range of motion and muscular function. *J Hum Kinet.* 2012;31:105–113. https://doi.org/10.2478/v10078-012-0011-y.

23. Cotter AC, Schulman RA. An overview of massage and touch therapies. In: *Manual Medicine: State of the Art Reviews.* Vol. 14. Philadelphia: Hanley & Belfus; 2000.

24. Wang MY, Tsai PS, Lee PH, Chang WY, Yang CM. The efficacy of reflexology: systematic review. *J Adv Nurs.* 2008;62(5):512–520.

25. Jacobson E. Structural integration, an alternative method of manual therapy and sensorimotor education. *J Alternative Compl Med.* 2011;17(10):891–899.

26. Hinterbuchner C. In: Basmajian JV, ed. *Manipulation, Traction and Massage.* Baltimore: Williams & Wilkins; 1985.

27. Harte AA, Baxter GD, Gracey JH. The efficacy of traction for back pain: a systematic review of randomized controlled trials. *Arch Phys Med Rehabil.* 2003;84(10):1542–1553.

28. Wyss, James, Patel A, Malhotra G. *Therapeutic Programs for Musculoskeletal Disorders. "Guide to Therapy Prescription Writing.* Demos Medical Publishing; 2013:28–35.

29. Grabois M, Benny B, Kwai-tung C. *Physical Medicine Techniques in Pain Management.* Practical Management of Pain; 2014:p629–642.

30. Therapeutic heat and cold. In: Michlovitz SL, von Nieda K, Behrens BJ, Michlovitz SL, eds. *Physical Agents: Theory and Practice.* 2nd ed. Philadelphia: FA Davis; 2006:37–54.

31. Lehmann JF, Delateur BJ. Therapeutic heat. In: Lehmann JF, ed. *Therapeutic Heat and Cold.* 4th ed. Baltimore, MD: Williams & Wilkins; 1990.

32. Bleakley C, McDonough S, MacAuley D. The use of ice in the treatment of acute soft-tissue injury. *Am J Sports Med.* 2004;32:251–261.

33. Mense S. Effects of temperature on the discharge of muscle spindles and tendon organs. *Pflügers Archiv.* 1978;375:159–166.

34. MacAuley DC. Ice therapy: how good is the evidence? *Int J Sports Med.* 2001;22:379–384.

35. Galiuto L. The use of cryotherapy in acute sports injuries. *Ann Sports Med Res.* 2016;3(2):1060.

36. Weinberger A, Fadilah R, Lev A, et al. Intra-articular temperature measurements after superficial heating. *Scand J Rehabil Med.* 1989;21:55–57.

37. Lehmann JF, McDougall JA, Guy AW, et al. Heating patterns produced by shortwave diathermy applicators in tissue substitute models. *Arch Phys Med Rehabil.* 1983;64:575–577.

38. Lehmann JF, DeLateur BJ, Stonebridge JB. Selective muscle heating by shortwave diathermy with a helical coil. *Arch Phys Med Rehabil.* 1969;50:117–123.

39. Guy AW, Lehmann JF, Stonebridge JB. Therapeutic applications of electromagnetic power. *Proc IEEE.* 1974;62:55–75.

40. Ziskin MC. Fundamental physics of ultrasound and its propagation in tissue. *Radiographics.* 1993;13:705–709.

41. Goldman DE, Heuter TF. Tabular data of the velocity and absorption of high-frequency sound in mammalian tissues. *J Acoust Soc Am.* 1956;28:35–37.

42. Lehmann JF, DeLateur BJ, Warren CG, et al. Heating of joint structures by ultrasound. *Arch Phys Med Rehabil.* 1968;49:28–30.

43. Lehmann JF, DeLateur BJ, Warren CG, et al. Heating produced by ultrasound in bone and soft tissue. *Arch Phys Med Rehabil.* 1967;48:397–401.

44. Miller DL, Smith NB, Bailey MR, et al. Overview of therapeutic ultrasound applications and safety considerations. *J Ultrasound Med.* 2012;31(4):623–634.

45. Bare AC, McAnawa MB, Pritchard AE, et al. Phonophoretic delivery of 10% hydrocortisone through the epidermis of humans as determined by serum cortisol concentrations. *Phys Ther.* 1996;76(7):738–745. discussion 746–739.

46. Rosim G, Barieri C, Lancas F, et al. Diclofenac phonophoresis in human volunteers. *Ultrasound Med Biol.* 2005;31: 337–343.

47. Penderghest C, Kimura I, Gulick D. Double-blind clinical efficacy study of pulsed phonophoresis on perceived pain associated with symptomatic tendinitis. *J Sport Rehabil.* 1998;7:9–19.

48. Frontera W, Delisa J. *Delisa's Physical Medicine and Rehabilitation: Principles and Practices.* 5th ed. Vol. 1. Wolters Kluwer Health; 2012:1–2432.

49. Mitchell S, Trowbridge C, Fincher A, et al. Effect of diathermy on muscle temperature, electromyography, and mechanomyography. *Muscle Nerve.* 2008;38: 992–1004.

50. Nutt J, Anderson V, Peacock J, et al. DBS and diathermy interaction induces severe CNS damage. *Neurology.* 2001; 56:1384–1386.

51. Melzack R, Wall PD. Pain mechanisms: a new theory. *Science.* 1965;150:971–979.

52. Brosseau L, Milne S, Robinson V, et al. Efficacy of the transcutaneous electrical nerve stimulation for the treatment of chronic low back pain: a meta-analysis. *Spine.* 2002;27(6): 596–603.

53. Gibson W, Wand BM, Meads C, Catley MJ, O'Connell NE. Transcutaneous electrical nerve stimulation (TENS) for chronic pain – an overview of Cochrane Reviews. *Cochrane Database Syst Rev.* 2019;(2).

54. Yousefi-Nooraie R, Schonstein E, Heidari K, et al. Low level laser therapy for nonspecific low-back pain. *Cochrane Database Syst Rev.* 2007;(2).

55. Clijsen R, Brunner A, Barbero M, Clarys P, Taeymans J. Effects of low-level laser therapy on pain in patients with musculoskeletal disorders: a systematic review and meta-analysis. *Eur J Phys Rehabil Med.* 2017;53(4): 603–610.

56. Gam A, Thorsen H, Lonnberg F. The effect of low-level laser therapy on musculoskeletal pain: a meta-analysis. *Pain.* 1993;52:63–66.

57. Vlaeyen J, Morley S. Cognitive-behavioral treatments for chronic pain: what works for whom? *Clin J Pain.* 2005; 21(1):1–8.

58. Tesarz J, Leisner S, Gerhardt A, et al. Effects of eye movement desensitization and reprocessing (EMDR) treatment in chronic pain patients: a systematic review. *Pain Med.* 2014;15(2):247–263.

59. Wiederhold BK, Gao K, Sulea C, Wiederhold MD. Virtual reality as a distraction technique in chronic pain patients. *Cyberpsychol, Behav Soc Netw.* 2014;17(6):346–352.

60. Brenda W, Kenneth G, Camelia S, Mark W. Virtual reality as a distraction technique in chronic pain patients. *Cyberpsychol, Behav Soc Netw.* 2014;17(6).

61. Guzmán J, Esmail R, Karjalainen K, et al. Multidisciplinary rehabilitation for chronic low back pain: systematic review. *BMJ.* 2001;322(7301):1511–1516.

62. Department of Health and Human Services. *National Pain Strategy: A Comprehensive Population Health Strategy for Pain.* Available at: https://iprcc.nih.gov/docs/HHSNational_Pain_Strategy.pdf. Accessed 15 June 2017.

63. Van Duijvenbode I, Jellema P, Van Poppel M, Van Tulder MW. Lumbar supports for prevention and treatment of low back pain. *Cochrane Collab.* 2008;(2).

64. Miyamoto K, Linuma N, Maeda M, et al. Effects of abdominal belts on intra-abdominal pressure, intramuscular pressure in the erector spinae muscles and myoelectrical activities of trunk muscles. *Clin Biomech.* 1999;14(2):79–87.

65. Fayolle-minon I, Calmels P. Effect of wearing a lumbar orthosis on trunk muscles: study of the muscle strength after 21 days of use on healthy subjects. *Joint Bone Spine.* 2008;75(1):58–63.

66. van Poppel M, de Looze M, Koes B, et al. Mechanisms of action of lumbar supports: asystematic review. *Spine.* 2000;25(16):2103–2113.

67. Muzin S, Isaac Z, Walker J, Abd OE, Baima J. When should a cervical collar be used to treat neck pain? *Curr Rev Musculoskelet Med.* 2008;1(2):114–119. https://doi.org/10.1007/s12178-007-9017-9.

Comorbid Chronic Pain and Posttraumatic Stress Disorder: Current Knowledge, Treatments, and Future Directions

DAVID E. REED, II, PHD • BRIANA COBOS, MA • PAUL NABITY, PHD • JESSE DOOLIN, MS • DONALD D. MCGEARY, PHD

UNDERSTANDING COMORBID POSTTRAUMATIC STRESS DISORDER AND CHRONIC PAIN: CURRENT TREATMENTS AND FUTURE DIRECTIONS

It is crucial for providers, researchers, and consumers to understand chronic pain through a comprehensive model that accounts for both the complexity of the pain experience and the complicated changes in the pain experience and phenotype with in the context of trauma. Early theories of pain, which are covered later in this chapter, failed to adequately account for pain complexity and are insufficient to guide diagnosis, understanding, and treatment of trauma-related pain (i.e., pain and comorbid posttraumatic stress disorder [PTSD]). The first part of this chapter will describe the evolution of understanding pain from unidimensional Cartesian models to more complex models that culminated in the predominant contemporary biopsychosocial model. The biopsychosocial model accurately acknowledges that the experience of pain cannot be explained solely through the physical experience and that the physical experience is affected by factors seemingly unrelated to one's physical pain. Hence, any proposed explanatory models of chronic pain comorbidity must also acknowledge this fact. Finally, the chapter will explore existing treatments for comorbid pain and PTSD (both pharmacological and non-pharmacological) and will offer suggestions on future directions for research and clinical care that may guide ongoing efforts to effectively treat these complex patient populations.

PREVALENCE OF CHRONIC PAIN AND POSTTRAUMATIC STRESS DISORDER

Up to 40% of adults in the United States experience chronic pain, defined as persistent pain lasting for at least 6 months,[1] with costs estimated at $560 billion.[2] Chronic pain may occur within several contexts, including musculoskeletal injury, cancer, and traumatic events.[3-5] Indeed, pain is highly comorbid with PTSD, a disorder characterized by avoidance, hypervigilance, negative cognitions and affect, and intrusive symptoms (e.g., flashbacks).[6] Moreover, those with chronic pain are more likely to endorse PTSD symptoms than their counterparts without chronic pain.[7,8] Military populations are particularly susceptible to this comorbidity and are more likely to be diagnosed with PTSD and/or chronic pain compared with the civilian population.[7,9] With advancements in battlefield technology, and medicine more generally, current military personnel have a better chance at surviving than those in the Vietnam era; nevertheless, physical and mental health conditions persist beyond their time of service.[10] Similarly, civilians who have experienced a traumatic event are also more likely to survive due to advancements in medicine. Therefore it is pertinent to examine the current state of the science as it relates to how these two common health conditions (i.e., chronic pain and PTSD) are understood and treated, the historical context from which this thinking evolved, and the innovations that may lie ahead.

Pain Care Essentials and Innovations. https://doi.org/10.1016/B978-0-323-72216-2.00015-6

HISTORICAL AND MODERN PERSPECTIVES OF PAIN TREATMENT

In order to understand current pharmacologic treatments for pain, it is important to place these treatments within the context, evolution, and acquired knowledge of earlier biomedical models dating back to Descartes.[11–13] Descartes viewed pain as one of the principal perceptual and physical bodily experiences that test the existence of the body.[11] He believed that pain was a disturbance passed through nerve fibers throughout the body until it reached the brain and was evidence that the mind and body are dualistic mechanisms responding in tandem to specific stimuli such as temperature and pain.[11] Not only did this promote thought from philosophers, it also subsequently led scientists to attempt to locate pain nerve fibers within the body that transferred pain sensations.[11] Descartes' theory, also now known as the *specificity theory*, was essential in promoting research related to specific functions of nerve pathways to the brain in response to pain. The two-step process consists of the (1) body integrating a pain signal into one bodily sensation and (2) traveling to the brain where it is mechanically perceived. This influenced the practice of medicinal usage, whereby practitioners pursued physical pain treatments, such as herb usage for analgesic effects or physicians severing specific pain nerve fibers to prevent pain signals from reaching the brain.[14–16]

Descartes' *specificity theory* was further developed by physician Charles Bell in his influential essay, the *Idea of a New Anatomy of the Brain*, which ultimately led to the discovery of the central nervous system (CNS).[15] The CNS provides a direct relationship between a stimulus and the sensation of pain via sensory receptors known as "nociceptors." Nociceptive pain reception occurs when noxious stimuli are sensed by pain receptors, or nociceptors, located in the skin and then transmitted via electric signals to higher brain centers for processing.[12,15,17,18]

The relationship between nociception and pain is complex because the inputs involved are beyond biological nociception. Opposition of Descartes' specificity theory of pain has led to other historical pain conceptualizations, including the *intensity theory of pain* and the *pattern theory of pain*. The intensity theory of pain hypothesizes that the experience of pain is the result of a significant intensity or threshold being reached.[14] This led neurologists and physiologists in the 1800s to formulate the theory that the intensity of pain is directly related to the amount of associated tissue injury.[15] After a certain threshold, an increased painful sensory input would summate and transmit in the spinal cord (i.e., CNS) and then to the brain.[15] Researchers during this time theorized that this central summation generated impulse sensations that were interpreted as pain for the individual only when the number of intense responding fibers and their discharge frequency exceeded a certain threshold that then determined the perceptual response to the nociceptive (sensory) input.[12,14,15,19–21]

Modern theories of pain foretold the most utilized theoretical perspective to date, the biopsychosocial model. The *gate control theory* sought to combine and support the main principles of the specificity, intensity, and pattern theories of pain.[17] Melzack and Wall theorized that there is a mechanistic gate in the spinal cord, specifically in the dorsal horn, that controls the transmission of sensory information in the spinal cord and to the brain. This mechanism is controlled by the activity in the large and small fibers. Large fibers inhibit or close the gate, whereas small fibers enable or open the gate. When nociceptive pain, tissue injury, or pain information reaches a certain threshold that exceeds the inhibition of the gate, this opens the gate and activates the pathways that lead to the experience of pain and pain-related behaviors (e.g., taking hand away from fire).[15] Therefore this theory provided a neural basis and reconciled the earlier biomedical models of pain (i.e., specificity, intensity, and pattern theories of pain). This also laid the foundation for pain research and pain mechanisms in the 20th century.[12] However, Melzack and Wall (1965) acknowledged that a more comprehensive model was needed to consider the emotional and cognitive effects of pain and their effects on pain-related behavior when an individual is experiencing pain.[12,17,22]

The need for a more comprehensive pain model led Melzack to create the neuromatrix theory of pain, which attempted to explain the nature of pain, and is based on prominent pain biomedical models. Melzack (in 2001) proposed that pain is a complex experience that is shaped by unique neurosignatures within the brain's neural network, which he coined as the body-self neuromatrix.[23,24] This network assimilates cognitive evaluation, sensory-discriminative, and motivational-affective networks and posits that the output patterns of the neuromatrix engage perceptual, behavioral, and homeostatic systems within the body and mind in response to an injury and/or chronic physical and cognitive stress.[23–25] Melzack's theory was formulated on pain syndromes that had no organic injury such as phantom limb pain and nonspecific low-back pain. Preceding biomedical models dating back to Descartes did not hold true to the assumption that there must be tissue damage in order for pain to occur. Similarly, according to Melzack's neuromatrix model, pain could have no correlation with tissue damage and can be the product of multiple parts of the CNS working together to generate a painful experience (e.g., fibromyalgia).[23] This theory provided a comprehensive explanation of pain by integrating tenets from the *specificity theory* with affective and pattern-response theories to formulate the *neuromatrix theory of pain*, with the experience of pain being the result of an interplay of these various neural networks.[26] Melzack and Casey encouraged medical professionals to move away from a sensory-dominant approach (e.g., surgical, pharmacologic) and treat chronic pain with a more multidisciplinary/multimodal (including pharmacologic and nonpharmacologic approaches) biopsychosocial approach.[12,27,28] This multimodal theory contributed to a biopsychosocial model for evaluating and treating pain.[12]

Recent movement toward a biopsychosocial approach for treating chronic pain views an individual as an integrated "whole person" whose mind and body are interconnected and manifest dynamic interactions between biological, psychologic, and social components of their painful experience.[26] The biopsychosocial model of pain is well supported by research and has expanded upon the biological mediators of chronic pain, elucidating the role of maladaptive stress responses via the hypothalamic-pituitary-adrenal (HPA) axis.[29-32] Chronic pain dysregulates the HPA axis activity, and thus cortisol levels, which in turn is associated with differences in pain intensity, pain thresholds, and anxiety levels.[33]

Pain, Cognitions, and Affect

Psychological components of the pain experience, such as pain catastrophizing ("an exaggerated negative mental set brought to bear during actual or anticipated painful experience"[34]), fear-avoidance, and negative affect, have been recognized as common aspects of the chronic pain experience within the fear-avoidance model of pain.[35,36] Social factors such as solicitous and punishing responses from marital partners, lower perceived level of social support, and lower socioeconomic status negatively impact self-reported pain intensity and disability level.[37-41] Moreover, there are cultural norms surrounding appropriate expressions of pain, and they may influence pain tolerance and the perceived pain intensity ratings of others.[42] Lethem and colleagues contended that ultimately there are two options when experiencing a fear: "confrontation" or "avoidance." The central premise of the fear-avoidance model is that confrontation diminishes fear over time, whereas avoidance maintains or exacerbates the fear response.[43]

Mood affects how individuals view pain and is considered an integral component of the fear-avoidance

model.[36] A review of the literature paints a picture indicating chronic pain comorbidity should be expected within clinical settings.[44] Depression and anxiety disorders, PTSD, substance abuse, suicidality, and sexual abuse have all been linked to chronic pain.[44] Prevalence rates of depressive disorders vary by chronic pain disorder, with 4%−12% prevalence rates among those with neuropathic disorders and 21%−83% prevalence rates among those with fibromyalgia.[44] Temporomandibular joint (TMJ) disorder prevalence rates for comorbid depressive disorders are also notably high: 16%−65%.[44] Anxiety disorders, when including PTSD, are as high as 65% for TMJ, 60% for fibromyalgia, 51% for abdominal pain, and 45% for migraine headache.[44] Examining PTSD specifically, nearly a quarter of individuals with chronic pain have comorbid PTSD.[44] Fibromyalgia also appears to have the highest range of prevalence rates for substance use disorders (up to 25%), with spinal chronic pain up to 14%, and arthritis up to 12%.[44] Opioid use disorder, specifically, has been reported in up to 43% with chronic pain.[44]

Mental health comorbidities associated with chronic pain not only affect mood and exacerbation of pain-related disability[35,36] but also the perception of pain. A meta-analysis examining depression and pain perception showed that, overall, individuals with depression have a higher pain threshold (i.e., the moment pain is felt).[45,46] However, the method by which pain is induced is also predictive, with ischemic methods resulting in lower pain threshold.[45] No overall differences emerged in pain tolerance or pain ratings across those with and without depression.[45] Finally, comorbid PTSD and chronic pain has higher pain thresholds and pain sensitivity (i.e., the same stimuli feel more painful for those with comorbid chronic pain and PTSD).[47-50] Anxiety, depression, and other mood disorders have the potential to affect how one experiences pain, linking these psychosocial processes to the pain experience. Viewing pain as a problem only related to physical symptoms with an organic cause does not fully capture the pain phenomenon. Thus, treatments only focusing on pain sensations have limited effectiveness.

Treating Chronic Pain

Taking a biopsychosocial perspective is increasingly shown to be essential in effectively treating and managing chronic pain.[51] The primary aim of biopsychosocial treatment is not to reduce pain intensity, but instead to focus on restoring and optimizing an individual's ability to function in their daily lives while reducing long-term reliance on pharmacologic interventions.[52] Biopsychosocial pain management can involve medication, psychotherapeutic interventions, physical therapy, stimulatory analgesia and neuromodulation, interventional procedures and surgery, and functional restoration programs. Within the biopsychosocial perspective, the emphasis of chronic pain treatment shifts from efforts to cure the pain or symptoms to efforts of improving functioning and quality of life through better management.[53] This perspective allows for the implementation of an interdisciplinary approach toward the treatment of chronic pain, wherein the treatment team consists of a coordinating multidisciplinary group of individuals who are treating the patient under one treatment plan.[54] This collaborative group may consist of a physician, nurse, psychologist, physical therapist, and occupational therapist.[54] Within this team, each member has a specific role.[54] These roles include (but are not limited to) the following: physicians are in charge of the medical aspects of treatment; nurses monitor the patient after treatments; psychologists provide cognitive behavioral psychosocial interventions; physical therapists engage the patient in treatment focused on movement; and occupational therapists engage the patient around work-related factors.[54] By using an interdisciplinary approach, the entirety of the person is treated. For patients, much of the time may be spent in psychosocial interventions, which include a variety of interventions and techniques.

Psychological treatments for chronic pain often consist of several components. Many chronic pain interventions utilize cognitive behavioral techniques that improve pain-related outcomes.[55,56] Cognitive behavior therapies (CBTs) focus on modifying problematic thoughts (e.g., automatic thoughts related to self-efficacy), emotions (e.g., an irrational fear of re-injury), and behaviors (e.g., sedentary behaviors) to reduce pain-related disability and intensity. A more recent iteration of CBT is acceptance and commitment therapy (ACT), which Hayes et al.[57] explain as focusing on mindfulness, valued actions, and acceptance of difficult thoughts, emotions, and/or circumstances.[58] ACT and other acceptance-based interventions, such as mindfulness, is efficacious in treating chronic pain, with randomized controlled trials (RCTs) of acceptance-based interventions for pain resulting in significant improvements in pain and physical well-being.[59,60] However, when mindfulness and mindfulness-based stress reduction (MBSR) were systematically examined, mixed results emerged. An early meta-analysis examining MBSR to active controls showed a medium and statistically significant effect size for mental health variables.[61] A meta-analysis showed that MBSR for chronic pain, compared to usual care, resulted in significant differences in the

short term, but not long term, regarding pain intensity, and also showed nonsignificant effects when comparing MBSR to active treatment groups in both the short term and long term.[62] Short-term effects of MBSR, compared to usual care, on pain-related disability approached significance but was nonsignificant regarding long-term effects. Short-term effects and long-term effects of MBSR compared to active treatment were nonsignificant.[62] Another meta-analysis that looked at both mindfulness and MBSR interventions also showed nonsignificant effects for mindfulness-based cognitive therapy and MBSR (although the MBSR effect size approached significance) and significant effects for other mindfulness interventions.[63] Taking publication bias into consideration, the authors state that effects of mindfulness meditation are "low overall for both short and long term."[63] Discrepant results may be due to the periods in which these meta-analyses were conducted, the heterogeneity of results leading to large confidence intervals, and/or how mindfulness was defined. Because mindfulness may support self-efficacy and can be taught in a relatively brief time-frame, the available research, although equivocal, supports the use of mindfulness-based interventions for chronic pain.

EXPLAINING THE CHRONIC PAIN AND POSTTRAUMATIC STRESS DISORDER COMORBIDITY

As far back as 2001, researchers have attempted to coalesce the available research in order to explain the relationship between chronic pain and PTSD. During this time, the *shared vulnerability* and *mutual maintenance* models of comorbidity[64,65] began their ascent as prominent heuristics through which to view the co-occurring disorders. Both acknowledge the role of psychological and social variables, while not ignoring the biological contributions, through the biopsychosocial model. Nevertheless, there is a great deal that has yet to be determined about how these disorders are linked.[66]

SHARED VULNERABILITY: ANXIETY SENSITIVITY

One of the earliest models of pain and PTSD comorbidity was based on observations of hypervigilance associated with both conditions that created a mutual vulnerability for the comorbidity. Viewing chronic pain and PTSD from a shared vulnerability perspective highlights a diathesis related to anxiety sensitivity (AS) and genetic predispositions. AS refers to how people think about their bodily sensations, as they relate to how manageable the thoughts are (e.g., "It is an impossibility to control my thoughts about my disorders."), whether the sensations have potential social consequences (e.g., "I may be unwelcome if people see me limping."), and whether the sensations have potential physical consequences (e.g., "If this pain continues, my leg will probably be amputated.").[67,68] Separate lines of research show that individuals with chronic pain and PTSD symptoms have increased levels of AS.[64] Within a chronic pain context, AS predicts increased opioid dependence, severity, and misuse,[69] stress,[70] and disordered eating.[71] Within a PTSD context, AS is implicated in emotion dysregulation,[72] symptoms of obsessive-compulsive disorder[72a], and decreased distress tolerance.[73] Sensations within the body prime mental representations of what may occur; when these mental representations occur within a comorbid context (such as chronic pain and PTSD), they may have compounding detrimental consequences. In other words, among those who have comorbid PTSD and chronic pain, any reminder of physical pain or trauma may be associated with increased levels of anxiety and attention to the symptoms compared with those who have one or none of the disorders.

Among a comorbid PTSD and chronic pain population, AS plays an important role in symptom manifestation and evidence supports its inclusion within a stress-diathesis model of chronic pain and PTSD.[74,75] Among those with musculoskeletal pain, AS was elevated if they had been through a traumatic experience and exhibited symptoms of PTSD, compared with those who did not exhibit these symptoms.[76] Separately, AS and PTSD symptoms predict emotional distress and interact with each other, whereby emotional distress worsens among those with musculoskeletal pain.[76] This suggests that heightened anxiety around physical symptoms may worsen the effect of PTSD on one's physical pain-related distress. Among those with chronic pain, AS is a significant predictor of PTSD symptoms above and beyond one's history of trauma,[77] highlighting how thoughts related to the pain experience and bodily sensations may play a role in PTSD.

Hyperarousal symptoms of PTSD are often characterized via their physiologic manifestations, relating this symptom cluster to AS. Indeed, both hyperarousal and numbing symptoms are significantly related to AS among individuals diagnosed with chronic musculoskeletal back pain.[78] Among prisoners of war, hyperarousal longitudinally mediates the relationship between captivity and AS and between captivity and pain catastrophizing.[79] Nevertheless, the long-term implications of AS are unclear, as AS predicts initial, but not later, neuropathic pain among those who received treatment in a trauma center.[80]

SHARED VULNERABILITY: GENETIC CAUSE

Within the shared vulnerability model, genetic vulnerabilities play a prominent role, highlighting the biological component of the biopsychosocial model. Decades of research on the stress-vulnerability model shows that genetic predispositions play a role in both physical and mental health. Approximately 30%–40% of the variance in PTSD is heritable.[81] Much of the genetic architecture underlying the risk for PTSD appears to overlap with vulnerabilities for depression and anxiety.[82] It is quite possible that there are multiple genetic architectures underlying PTSD, which may explain the difficulties in the replication of findings by genome-wide association studies.[83]

At this time, there are few well-supported genetic markers of both PTSD and chronic pain. However, the current research of genetic markers of stress (HPA axis) and inflammation for PTSD and chronic pain supports overlap of these disorders. FK506 binding protein 5 (FKBP5) polymorphisms provide one of the most promising gene candidates for PTSD vulnerability. High expression of FKBP5 is linked to greater glucocorticoid receptor sensitivity and lower basal cortisol levels, and low basal cortisol levels are thought to be a vulnerability factor for developing PTSD after a traumatic event.[84] In an epigenetic study, Blacker and colleagues[85] found that FKBP5 methylation increased in nonresponders to PTSD treatment and decreased in responders to treatment. The direction of methylation related to PTSD appears to be allele-specific, with the methylation or demethylation associated with greater severity of PTSD dependent on the exact allele being modified.[86]

There is even less known about genetic and epigenetic involvement in chronic pain. Variants of the FKBP5 gene are associated with chronic pain development after trauma exposure,[87] and the stress response microRNA (miRNA) 320a is linked to the development of chronic pain after car accidents.[88]

Both the HPA axis and the immune system are involved in PTSD and chronic pain,[89] further substantiating a fundamental biological link between the two conditions. Expression of immune system genes is associated with the presence of PTSD[90] and upregulation of immune system genes is associated with greater intrusion symptoms of PTSD.[91] Polymorphisms of immune system genes have been implicated as vulnerabilities for PTSD.[92,93] Studies of stress hormones and inflammatory markers support genetic findings of altered immune and HPA axis regulation in PTSD.[94–96] Interestingly, many of the miRNAs associated with PTSD are involved in the regulation of stress and proinflammatory responses implicated in chronic pain.[97] Indeed, there are several miRNAs associated with pain sensitization, inflammation, and stress responses.[98,99] Further studies are still needed to conclusively elucidate specific shared markers for underlying vulnerability.

MUTUAL MAINTENANCE MODEL

The mutual maintenance model[64] of the chronic pain and PTSD comorbidity incorporates all three factors of the tripartite biopsychosocial model, weaving an intricate tale of biological predispositions, affective and cognitive components, and social aspects of the pain experience into one explanatory model. The model hypothesizes that the unique comorbidity associated with chronic pain and PTSD is due to each disorder influencing the other (i.e., mutually maintaining). The mutual maintenance model highlights seven different cognitive and emotional processes that form a shared mechanism of comorbidity: attentional biases, AS, reminders of traumatic experiences, avoidance, negative affect and decreased physical activity, negative perceptions of illness, and the inability to use effective coping strategies. Despite the considerable attention paid to the chronic pain and PTSD comorbidity, research has marginally progressed from its original formulation of nearly 20 years ago.

Attentional Biases

As established earlier in this chapter, those with chronic pain are prone toward hypervigilance related to pain sensations, similar to how those with PTSD are prone toward hypervigilance related to potentially dangerous internal or external stimuli related to their traumatic experiences.[64] These attentional biases are often measured in a laboratory setting utilizing a Stroop task, an experimental paradigm whereby participants are presented with a word in a specific color.[100] The more time an individual takes to name the color of the word, the more attention is being placed on the word itself.[100] For instance, it would be expected that those with chronic pain would take longer to name a color of the word "pain" versus "chair." Similarly, reasoning biases are biases related to probability—for instance, believing it is more probable than it actually is to experience pain and/or a traumatic experience.[100] More recent research suggests that those with chronic pain and PTSD become

more focused on pain and trauma-related cues than those with chronic pain but without PTSD, providing evidence that it does not matter if the stimulus is pain- or trauma-related.[101] Indeed, there may be a generalization of hypervigilance occurring within this comorbidity. Individuals with chronic pain are acutely aware of pain sensations that occur, and those with PTSD are threatened by reminders of the trauma. When both disorders play a significant role, hypervigilance then becomes focused on both trauma reminders and pain sensations.

Intrusive Reminders

Intrusive reminders of the traumatic experience have long been hypothesized to play an important role in maintaining the chronic pain/PTSD comorbidity.[64,100] Those with pain are more likely to endorse a PTSD diagnosis,[102] and PTSD-related negative cognitions are associated with pain severity above and beyond PTSD symptoms and alcohol use among veterans with comorbid PTSD and alcohol use disorder.[103] When individuals experience a pain sensation, this may result in intrusive thoughts about the traumatic experience, thus serving as a reminder for both the pain and the trauma.[64] Conversely, reminders of the trauma may result in individuals becoming focused on the body part(s) associated with the trauma, thus provoking a physical pain response. When the pain sensations or reminders of the traumatic events come to mind, engagement in activities that promote wellness and recovery decreases.[64] The interplay between the experience of pain and PTSD symptoms results in experiences that individuals with PTSD and chronic pain want to avoid. Of course, avoidance of thoughts, emotions, and behaviors comes with its own complications.

Avoidance

Avoidance is considered one of the main contributors to the onset and exacerbation of chronic pain[35] and PTSD.[104] It has been linked to increased pain-related disability and PTSD symptoms and is considered a driving force behind the chronic pain and PTSD comorbidity.[35,64,105] Individuals with chronic pain prefer to avoid painful experiences, and individuals with PTSD prefer to avoid reminders of trauma, cues that may be internal or external. When facial expressions are used as stimuli, veterans with chronic pain show an attentional bias away from painful expressions and toward happy faces, compared to controls.[106] Nevertheless, little has been done to qualitatively define the purpose of pain-related avoidance, and research designed to better understand these goals is needed.[100] Theoretic and empirical perspectives point toward focusing on goal cognitions and better understanding what is most meaningful to an individual.[107,108] Avoidance of emotionally or physically painful stimuli may eventually result in decreased engagement with one's community and social activities, resulting in adverse clinical outcomes, because these activities are mechanisms by which individuals maintain their identity (i.e., Who am I?) and sense of self-worth. Consequences of decreased engagement in meaningful activities within this comorbidity have yet to be fully explored.

Negative Affect and Decreased Physical Activity

Negative affect is common in those with comorbid chronic pain and PTSD.[64] Research shows how symptoms of depression mediate the relationship between PTSD symptoms and pain,[109] indicating the depressive experience, whether endogenous or from inactivity, is associated with increased pain in the context of PTSD. Social isolation and a lack of desire for increased activity levels (both putative mechanisms for poor outcomes in chronic pain and PTSD) have been linked to depression.[110,111] Although negative affect has long been hypothesized as an influencing component of chronic pain,[35] it has only recently been established as an integral part of PTSD symptomology.[6]

Anxiety Sensitivity and Negative Perceptions of Illness

AS (which has already been discussed as part of the shared vulnerability perspective of the chronic pain and PTSD comorbidity) and perceptions of pain are closely linked, and both play a role within the mutual maintenance model.[64] Perception of one's pain refers to how sensitive individuals are to the experience of pain.[64] Although pain sensitivity has been proposed as a mutually maintaining component of the PTSD and chronic pain comorbidity,[64] research around this assertion is still developing. For patients with chronic pain and those with comorbid PTSD, there is an increase in one's pain threshold and pain sensitivity.[47-49] Interestingly, those with PTSD and without chronic pain exhibit decreased pain sensitivity,[50,112] although these results may be due to the differences in pain thresholds among those with PTSD.[47] More research within the comorbid population is indicated.[47]

Coping Strategies

Finally, Sharp and Harvey[64] implicate (in)effective coping strategies as a mutually maintaining factor of the comorbidity, explaining that cognitive processes, such as pain catastrophizing, prevent individuals from effectively coping with their chronic pain. Increased pain catastrophizing and decreased self-efficacy is endorsed among those with comorbid PTSD and chronic pain, compared with those with chronic pain only.[113] Among military personnel with chronic pain, PTSD symptoms are associated with decreased pain acceptance, increased fear avoidance, and increased catastrophizing.[114] Moreover, those with comorbid chronic pain and PTSD experience increased healthcare utilization compared with those with just one of the disorders,[115] indicating that the coping strategies being used are ineffective and/or do not lead to decreased need for medical care and pharmacological and non-pharmacological pain management treatment.

COMMON PHARMACOLOGIC TARGETS OF CHRONIC PAIN/POSTTRAUMATIC STRESS DISORDER COMORBIDITY

There is some overlap between the pharmacological interventions recommended for chronic pain and PTSD, further substantiating an underlying process that may mutually maintain both conditions. Common treatments for chronic pain include acetaminophen, nonsteroidal antiinflammatory drugs, tricyclic antidepressants, serotonin and norepinephrine reuptake inhibitors (SNRIs), anticonvulsants, opioids, and muscle relaxants. A couple selective serotonin reuptake inhibitors (SSRIs) are approved by the US Food and Drug Administration (FDA) for PTSD, but research shows mixed effectiveness of SSRIs for PTSD symptoms. Research indicates that an SNRI, venlafaxine, may be more effective in reducing symptoms of PTSD compared with SSRIs.[116] There is also evidence that noradrenaline, which is increased by SNRIs, has anti-inflammatory and neuroprotective roles in chronic pain.[117]

Medications for PTSD may or may not be prescribed directly after a traumatic experience. There is some research indicating that glucocorticoids used immediately after a traumatic event reduce the risk of developing PTSD.[118] Holbrook and colleagues found postinjury use of opioids was linked to lower rates of PTSD after severe injuries; however, the exact mechanisms for lower PTSD rates (whether biological or psychological) are unknown. Although benzodiazepines are frequently prescribed to individuals with PTSD, they may increase the risk of suppressed breathing when taken with opioids. Concurrent use of benzodiazepines and opioids predicts problematic opioid use.[119,120]

Although controversial, there is increasing interest in cannabinoid compounds (including cannabidiol

[CBD] and Δ^9-tetrahydrocannabinol [THC]), because these compounds have accumulated some support for benefit in separate studies of chronic pain and PTSD. Indeed, the endocannabinoid system is currently under investigation for both chronic pain and PTSD and the pain and PTSD comorbidity. In an observational study of self-administered cannabis, investigators identified a 3-point decrease in pain using a 0–10 visual analogue scale after cannabis use.[121] Unfortunately, the outcomes of the study were limited (e.g., the duration of reduced pain was not reported) and more work is needed to substantiate a benefit of causal cannabis use for pain. The author did specify, however, that THC potency, not CBD potency, was the strongest predictor of pain reduction. Cannabinoids have been shown to enhance fear extinction, exhibit anxiolytic effects, and reduce inflammation, all of which are potentially relevant to both PTSD and chronic pain.[122] Much more information is needed to endorse cannabinoids as the recommended treatment for either condition, and both CBD and THC derivatives are regulated by the FDA in the United States. Epidiolex (a form of CBD), Marinol (a form of THC), Syndros (a form of THC), and Cesamet (structurally similar to THC) have limited approved treatment uses. To date, there are no FDA-approved cannabinoids for the treatment of chronic pain,[123] and there is still a lack of high-quality research regarding safety and effectiveness of cannabinoids.[124]

NONPHARMACOLOGICAL TARGETS OF CHRONIC PAIN AND POSTTRAUMATIC STRESS DISORDER COMORBIDITY

Nonpharmacological treatment approaches for addressing the chronic pain and PTSD comorbidity are still in their infancy, with only a handful of clinical trials providing a guideline for clinicians. Overall, treatment recommendations include the following: psychoeducation related to PTSD and chronic pain symptoms, treatments related to how these symptoms are associated with each other, decreasing avoidance, decreasing attentional biases and arousal, and increasing positive mood and acceptance.[125]

The most common treatments for chronic pain and PTSD, separately, are built upon the foundations of CBT techniques and the biopsychosocial model. In PTSD treatment, avoidance[126] and maladaptive thinking patterns[127] are often targeted. Similarly, maladaptive coping strategies (e.g., pain nonacceptance and catastrophizing) are often targeted in chronic pain treatment using an integrated biopsychosocial model.[54]

Current treatments designed to decrease symptoms within the chronic pain and PTSD comorbidity often pull from these approaches. When treatments do not necessarily target the chronic pain and PTSD comorbidity but assess outcomes related to both disorders, moderate effects for PTSD and small effects for pain outcomes emerge,[128] which shows psychological interventions can provide benefit for both of these comorbid conditions. ACT is a third-wave CBT intervention that focuses on valued actions, acceptance, and cognitive flexibility.[129] A recent meta-analysis revealed that ACT for chronic pain results in small effect sizes for improvements in functioning, quality of life, and pain intensity. It found a moderate effect size for anxiety and large effect sizes for pain acceptance and comorbid depression. Another meta-analysis found similar results with a smaller effect size for depression when ACT was used for chronic pain.[59] In veterans with chronic pain and PTSD, clinically significant reductions in PTSD symptoms and improved pain outcomes were observed after treatment with ACT.[130]

Targeting the chronic pain and PTSD comorbidity, Otis et al.[131] developed a treatment that included elements from cognitive processing therapy and CBT for pain, producing mixed results. The treatment included goal-setting, meaning-making, and exposure. Although the small trial (of six total individuals) resulted in three individuals dropping out of treatment, those who stayed in treatment endorsed a decrease in pain-related disability and PTSD symptoms. In a study focused on chronic PTSD symptoms, Beck et al.[132] implemented a CBT group therapy protocol, wherein 80% of individuals endorsed chronic pain in the sample. Although the sample size was small, medium to large effect sizes were found after treatment for PTSD and pain-related disability. Nevertheless, one-third of the sample subjects dropped out, and only 29% of the treatment group endorsed what the authors called "high end-state functioning," defined as minimal PTSD and depression scores. Finally, a trauma-focused CBT intervention, which included psychoeducation, exposure, cognitive restructuring, and relaxation techniques, resulted in significant decreases in both PTSD and pain-related disability in the treatment group compared with the waitlist control.[133]

With such a complicated population, wherein treatments for even one of the two disorders remain to be completely understood, nontraditional approaches offer a compelling and holistic alternative that has been tested with some success. Somatic reexperiencing, which focuses on bodily sensations related to traumatic experiences, combined with exercise, was implemented in a RCT for comorbid chronic pain and PTSD.[134] Although the treatment resulted in a decrease in PTSD symptoms, pain-related disability remained unchanged, indicating more was needed to address the symptoms of pain. Other treatments have been more successful in concurrently treating pain symptoms and PTSD, including eye movement desensitization and reprocessing (EMDR) therapy[135] and accelerated response therapy, a therapy that utilizes eye movements, along with imaginal exposure and rescripting.[136]

MODIFICATION OF PAIN MANAGEMENT DELIVERY PATHWAYS

Chronic pain and PTSD are notably complex, and both clinicians and researchers confronting this problem understand that the strongest treatments are likely to include multiple modalities. Indeed, some of the strongest work in chronic pain management focuses on interdisciplinary models of care that include medical, physical, and psychological interventions meaningfully integrated into a unified conceptual model of care (see Functional Restoration).[54] Complex PTSD also responds well to intensive outpatient treatment that mimics interdisciplinary pain management through a strong focus on both functional and psychologic treatments (see Massed Prolonged Exposure).[126] Although effective, these high-intensity treatments are notoriously difficult to implement, so large medical systems have begun to explore care systems designed to organize different treatments for pain and PTSD using existing but disconnected clinical resources. By organizing existing treatments and increasing communication between providers, health systems hope to better address the comorbid pain and PTSD complexity and obtain better outcomes. For example, the Department of Veterans' Affairs has established a stepped care model of pain management that encourages routine assessment of PTSD and recommendations for referral to evidence-based care for pain-suffering veterans who screen positive for PTSD.[113] The Defense Health Agency (DHA) has begun to implement a comprehensive pain management pathway that includes components for both pain and PTSD treatment organized under a comprehensive system of care. Research on pain and PTSD comorbidity has begun to shift toward pragmatic studies of these integrated systems, offering perhaps the strongest potential for effectively addressing this comorbidity. Future studies should capitalize on nascent health systems and clinical informatics resources to enhance this endeavor.

FUTURE DIRECTIONS

Research on interventions for either chronic pain or PTSD has grown for decades, and more needs to be done to strengthen and refine interventions for each of these conditions. Unfortunately, few studies have examined treatments designed to effectively address both conditions concordantly. This lack of research attention is particularly disturbing in light of the growing recognition of high comorbidity rates between these conditions and the well-demonstrated complexity of the pain-PTSD phenotype. Initial models explaining the chronic pain and PTSD comorbidity have provided invaluable insight toward better understanding how and why these disorders seem to be so difficult to treat. For one, treating PTSD or chronic pain alone comes with its own problems: attrition rates are high;[137] individuals fail to respond to treatment;[138] and, each disorder has a multifaceted symptom profile affecting many aspects of individuals' lives (e.g., social and physical functioning). In one sense, the comorbidity is like any other, wherein common thoughts, emotions, and behaviors maintain the disorders. In a more complicated sense, each disorder challenges patients in finding alternative *ways of being* in the world. One's assumptions about a fair and just world are disrupted;[139] interpretations of bodily sensations that once seemed harmless are now terrifying; enjoyable and meaningful activities may no longer be possible; and the feedback received from others that imply acceptance and commonality may now be altered. If a more thorough understanding is to be attained and treatments are to be improved, methodological considerations and novel mechanisms will need to be addressed.

Methodological Considerations

Much emphasis has been placed on the "mutually maintaining" components of this comorbidity. For instance, intrusive thoughts related to a traumatic experience may trigger thoughts of pain, increasing pain severity. Certainly, analyses comparing those with comorbid chronic pain and PTSD with other groups are able to show between-group effects of certain symptom profiles. Although these studies provide insight into these symptoms, they fail to show causality and leave other confounding variables as possible explanations. In addition, cross-sectional studies provide data at one time point, essentially providing a snapshot of symptoms with little context. Even longitudinal designs, including RCTs, often measure participants using self-report data at only a few time points, resulting in insufficient data for truly understanding the causal moment-by-moment symptom presentations that are hypothesized to maintain the comorbidity.

Ecological momentary assessment (EMA) offers a potentially more informative way to understand pain and PTSD comorbidity (compared with longitudinal RCTs). EMA is a technologic advancement within the field of longitudinal research, whereby participants receive a notification on an electronic device (e.g., a smartphone) instructing them to answer several items about their symptoms, condition, or functioning at that moment. This can be done at several points during the day, providing rich data on momentary emotional and physical states. Despite the hypothesized role of mutually maintaining symptoms, only one study using these methods within this population has been published. Pacella et al.[139a] assessed 67 individuals who were admitted into an emergency room for various types of injuries (e.g., motor vehicle accident or fall). Each day, they received five text messages asking them about PTSD symptoms, pain, and social support. EMA was carried out for 14 days, wherein pain severity significantly decreased across the time of the study. Moreover, daily changes in hyperarousal (and, to a marginal degree, avoidance) were predictive of pain severity. Studies such as this would provide ecological data related to a variety of psychosocial variables known to be associated with the chronic pain and PTSD comorbidity. New technology may also provide biological data on a moment-by-moment basis.

Technology allowing for wearable devices to monitor biomarkers of pain and PTSD have skyrocketed in recent years. Activity trackers, such as Fitbit or Apple Watch, are able to monitor heart rate and the number of steps an individual has taken, including the intensity of those steps. Use of wearable devices has grown, in part, through improvements in sensor design resulting in strong reliability and validity for biomarkers such as activity and heart rate. Smart shirts are available that measure heart rate, temperature, blood pressure, and respiration[140] and have the potential to provide a clearer picture of CNS responses to life stressors compared with what could be gleaned from wristwatch devices. Knowing the HPA axis is a primary common factor between PTSD and chronic pain,[89] gathering real-time biological data associated with pain severity may be highly impactful. Research could focus on attaining pain severity levels when there is evidence of an increase in heart rate or respiration. Causal directionality could be assessed, and interventions could target these moments in an attempt to shape behavior and internal responses to external stimuli. For instance, it may be that a trauma reminder results in a response from the sympathetic nervous system, whereby one's heart rate increases, and thoughts of the reminder become acutely salient. Awareness of these moments, made possible due to wearable technology and real-time data, provides feedback to patients that now is the time they should use mindfulness techniques, breathing exercises, or another skill learned in therapy.

The Role of Identity

The biopsychosocial model attempts to incorporate most or all aspects of an individual into treatment. Yet somehow the self and issues related to identity, changing social roles, and other losses are often left out of consideration. Nevertheless, theoretical work has shown how issues of identity play a role in pain-related disability and a focus on valued goals may be an important pathway toward patient improvement.[107,140a] Among individuals with pain, tension related to met and/or unmet goals has been associated with fear of pain and pain severity.[141,142] Individuals with chronic pain struggle to meet the demands of community and social engagements, behaviors that provide individuals with a sense of meaning and purpose. Similarly, those who recover from PTSD engage in social activities and are an active member of their family,[143] both of which provide individuals with a coherent sense of self, identity, and sense of meaning and purpose.

A recent advancement in the PTSD literature is the study of moral injury, which essentially amounts to an injury to the sense of self. Moral injury is defined as the effect of participating in an event or events that is incompatible with one's internal moral code:[144] values, worldviews, and culturally derived beliefs have somehow not been maintained. Moral injury may occur, for example, when a member of the armed services is forced to harm someone else for survival, thus acting outside the realm of previously held ethical boundaries.[144] These values and ethics are the more tangible manifestations of one's identity, and when these are disrupted, negative consequences can emerge.

A patient with comorbid PTSD and chronic pain struggles on two fronts: an identity that has been disrupted and limited resources to engage in behaviors and cognitions that enable a coherent identity to reemerge. A coherent identity has been linked to a bevy of positive outcomes, including less emotional distress, avoidance, depression and anxiety symptoms and social anxiety,[145–148] and serves as a means to buffer against existential concerns.[149,150]

However, current treatments for the chronic pain and PTSD comorbidity do not adequately focus on developing a coherent sense of self or cultivating a "true self" that is always there despite changing social roles and physical abilities. Although ACT may touch on these subjects,[129] the focus of ACT consists of defining one's values *already in place* and acting on them. Individuals with comorbid chronic pain and PTSD have experienced abrupt changes in multiple aspects of their lives, and additional work may be needed in order to answer the question of "Who am I?" Future treatments that specifically target identity disturbances may be beneficial to many patients, particularly those who struggle to complete traditional treatments that target avoidance, such as cognitive processing therapy or prolonged exposure therapy.

Researchers may find it beneficial to examine treatment approaches outside the confines of trauma and chronic pain. For instance, dialectical behavior therapy (DBT),[151] a third-wave CBT that incorporates mindfulness and cognitive dialectics, is highly effective for the treatment of borderline personality disorder, a disorder characterized, in part, by an unstable sense of self.[6] Indeed, research implicates identity disturbances as a factor of opioid misuse above and beyond pain severity and interference within a chronic pain sample.[152] Incorporating elements of DBT into a treatment approach for this comorbidity may be highly beneficial for reducing opioid misuse and pain-related disability.

Identity is but one component of the sociocultural buffer that prevents existential concerns from becoming an issue.[149] When a traumatic event occurs, those with increased PTSD symptoms endorse increased death thoughts and death anxiety, an inability to utilize self-affirmation strategies, and negative biases in coping strategies.[153–155] Traumatic events disrupt cognitions that allow individuals to believe that the world is a just, safe, trustworthy, and meaningful place (e.g., just-world theory).[139,156,157] It is not a far leap to assume that similar internal events happen in those with chronic pain. Indeed, existential concerns appear to play a unique role within chronic pain populations, in whom these concerns have broad implications related to pain intensity, pain disability, life satisfaction, and depression.[158] Treatment with an existential focus has been shown to be effective in decreasing pain-related disability, especially for those with higher spirituality/religiosity.[108] Treatment approaches that target moral injury, identity, meaning, and valued goals, when combined with other CBT techniques and pharmacotherapy, may be particularly beneficial in reducing disability, as well as symptoms of PTSD. It remains to be seen not only if patients would find these treatments more rewarding and beneficial, but also whether they can be readily translated into short-term treatments implemented as adjunct therapies within primary care or pain clinics.

CONCLUSION

This chapter characterized the epidemiology, cause, maintaining factors, current treatments, and future directions of the unique comorbidity between chronic pain and PTSD. Within either a chronic pain or PTSD sample, rates of having the other disorder are high, particularly in military personnel and those who are more vulnerable at developing this comorbid condition. Various genetic, cognitive, and emotional components appear to play a role in how these disorders are developed and maintained. The shared vulnerability model posits that AS and genetic predispositions (particularly as they relate to the HPA axis and stress response) make it more likely that certain individuals will develop this comorbidity. Similarly, it appears these disorders are mutually maintained by individuals avoiding physical and psychological pain, being more attuned to their experiences as they relate to chronic pain and PTSD, having negative affective and cognitive responses to these experiences, being constantly reminded of the pain and/or traumatic event, and being unable to effectively cope with the pain and/or PTSD symptoms. Since these theoretical models have been introduced, little progress has been made in how to best understand and treat this comorbidity. Recent technological advances have allowed for the possibility to gain causal and moment-by-moment knowledge (e.g., EMA) of how these disorders interact. Finally, the role of identity within this comorbidity has yet to be fully explored and offers a promising novel target of change that encompasses many aspects of both the shared vulnerability and mutual maintenance models.

REFERENCES

1. Interagency Pain Research Coordinating Committee. *National Pain Strategy: A Comprehensive Population Health-Level Strategy for Pain*; 2016. https://www.iprcc.nih.gov/sites/default/files/HHSNational_Pain_Strategy.pdf.
2. Dahlhamer JM, Lucas J, Zelaya C, et al. Prevalence of chronic pain and high-impact chronic pain among adults — United States, 2016. *Morb Mortal Wkly Rep*. 2018;67(36):1001–1006. https://doi.org/10.15585/mmwr.mm6736a2.
3. Giummarra MJ, Casey SL, Devlin A, et al. Co-occurrence of posttraumatic stress symptoms, pain, and disability 12 months after traumatic injury. *Pain Rep*. 2017;2(5):1–12. https://doi.org/10.1097/PR9.0000000000000622.
4. Fallon M, Giusti R, Aielli F, et al. Management of cancer pain in adult patients: ESMO Clinical Practice Guidelines. *Ann Oncol*. 2018;29:iv166–iv191. https://doi.org/10.1093/annonc/mdy152.
5. Andersen TE, Karstoft KI, Brink O, Elklit A. Pain-catastrophizing and fear-avoidance beliefs as mediators between post-traumatic stress symptoms and pain following whiplash injury — a prospective cohort study.

Eur J Pain. 2016;20(8):1241−1252. https://doi.org/10.1002/ejp.848.

6. American Psychiatric Association. *Diagnostic and Statistical Manual.* 5th ed. Washington, DC: American Psychiatric Association; 2013.

7. Gaskin DJ, Richard P. The economic costs of pain in the United States. *J Pain.* 2012;13(8):715−724.

8. Gallagher RMC, Sandbrink F. The socioeconomic burden of pain from war. *Am J Publ Health.* 2019;109(1):41−45. https://doi.org/10.2105/AJPH.2018.304744.

9. Olenick M, Flowers M, Diaz V. US veterans and their unique issues: enhancing health care professional awareness. *Adv Med Educ Pract.* 2015:635. https://doi.org/10.2147/amep.s89479.

10. Clark ME, Bair MJ, Buckenmaier CC, Gironda RJ, Walker RL. Pain and combat injuries in soldiers returning from operations enduring freedom and Iraqi freedom: implications for research and practice. *J Rehabil Res Dev.* 2007;44(2):179−193. https://doi.org/10.1682/JRRD.2006.05.0057.

11. Duncan G. Mind-body dualism and the biopsychosocial model of pain: what did descartes really say? *J Med Philos.* 2000;25(4):485−513. https://doi.org/10.1076/0360-5310(200008)25:4;1-a;ft485.

12. Gatchel RJ, Bo Peng Y, Peters ML, Fuchs PN, Turk DC. Biopsychosocial approach to chronic pain: scientific advances and future directions. *Psychol Bull.* 2007;133(4):581−624. https://rc.library.uta.edu/uta-ir/bitstream/handle/10106/5000/BIOPSYCHO2006-0750-R-Final-single 701.pdf?sequence=1.

13. Burmistr I. Theories of pain, up to descartes and after neuromatrix: what role do they have to develop future paradigms? *Pain Med.* 2018;3(1):6−12. https://www.practicalpainmanagement.com/pain/history-pain-brief-overview-17th-18th-centuries.

14. Chen J. History of pain theories. *Neurosci Bull.* 2011;27(5):343−350. https://doi.org/10.1007/s12264-011-0139-0.

15. Moayedi M, Davis KD. Theories of pain: from specificity to gate control. *J Neurophysiol.* 2013;109(1):5−12. https://doi.org/10.1152/jn.00457.2012.

16. Olsen K. History of pain: a brief overview of the 17th and 18th centuries. *Pract Pain Manag.* 2015;13(6):5−12.

17. Melzack R, Wall PD. Pain Mechanisms: a new theory. *Science.* 1965;150(3699):971−979.

18. Perl ER. Pain mechanisms: a commentary on concepts and issues. *Prog Neurobiol.* 2011;94(1):20−38. https://doi.org/10.1016/j.pneurobio.2011.03.001.

19. Nafe JP. The pressure, pain, and temperature senses. In: Murchison C, ed. *International University Series in Psychology. A Handbook of General Experimental Psychology.* Worcester, MA: Clark University Press; 1934:037−1087. https://doi.org/10.1037/11374-019.

20. Weddell G. Somesthesis and the chemical senses. *Annu Rev Psychol.* 1955;6(1):119−136. https://doi.org/10.1146/annurev.ps.06.020155.001003.

21. Mendell LM. Constructing and deconstructing the gate theory of pain. *Pain.* 2014;155(2):210−216. https://doi.org/10.1016/j.pain.2013.12.010.

22. Melzack R. From the gate to the neuromatrix. *Pain.* 1999;82(Suppl 1). https://doi.org/10.1016/S0304-3959(99)00145-1.

23. Melzack R. Pain and the neuromatrix in the brain. *J Dent Educ.* 2001;65(12):1378−1382.

24. Melzack R. Evolution of the neuromatrix theory of pain. The Prithvi Raj lecture: presented at the Third World Congress of World Institute of Pain, Barcelona 2004. *Pain Pract.* 2005;5(2):85−94. https://doi.org/10.1111/j.1533-2500.2005.05203.x.

25. Melzack R, Casey K. Sensory, motivational, and central control determinants of pain. In: Kenshalo DR, ed. *The Skin Senses : Proceedings. Springfield (Illinois): Ski Senses Proc First Int Symp Ski Senses.* December 1968:423−443.

26. Bevers K, Watts L, Kishino ND, Gatchel RJ. The Biopsychosocial model of the assessment, prevention, and treatment of chronic pain. *US Neurol.* 2016;12(2):98−104. https://doi.org/10.17925/USN.2016.12.02.98.

27. Ospina M, Harstall C. *Multidisciplinary Pain Programs for Chronic Pain: Evidence from Systematic Reviews HTA 30: Series A Health Technology Assessment Alberta Heritage Foundation for Medical Research.* Edmonton, Canada: Alberta Heritage Foundation for Medical Research; 2003. https://s3.amazonaws.com/academia.edu.documents/39376893/Multidisciplinary_Pain_Programs_for_Chro20151023-24675-1qlhgl5.pdf?AWSAccessKeyId=AKIAIWOWYYGZ2Y53UL3A&Expires=1550404617&Signature=r0oUSLiItS2kMOYsyhVt5t%2Basig%3D&response-content-disposition=inli.

28. Gatchel RJ, Okifuji A. Evidence-based scientific data documenting the treatment and cost-effectiveness of comprehensive pain programs for chronic nonmalignant pain. *J Pain.* 2006;7(11):779−793. https://doi.org/10.1016/j.jpain.2006.08.005.

29. Turk DC, Monarch ES. Biopsychosocial perspective on chronic pain. In: *Psychological Approaches to Pain Management: A Practitioner's Handbook.* 1996:3−32.

30. Parker AJR, Wessely S, Cleare AJ. The neuroendocrinology of chronic fatigue syndrome. *Psychol Med.* 2001;31:1331−1345. https://doi.org/10.1017/S0033291701004664.

31. Walker JG, Littlejohn GO, McMurray NE, Cutolo M. Stress system response and rheumatoid arthritis: a multilevel approach. *Rheumatology.* 1999;38(11):1050−1057. https://doi.org/10.1093/rheumatology/38.11.1050.

32. Wippert PM, Wiebking C. Stress and alterations in the pain matrix: a biopsychosocial perspective on back pain and its prevention and treatment. *Int J Environ Res Publ Health.* 2018;15(4). https://doi.org/10.3390/ijerph15040785.

33. Nees F, Löffler M, Usai K, Flor H. Hypothalamic-pituitary-adrenal axis feedback sensitivity in different states of back pain. *Psychoneuroendocrinology.* 2019;101:60−66. https://doi.org/10.1016/j.psyneuen.2018.10.026.

34. Sullivan MJ, Thorn B, Haythornthwaite JA, et al. Theoretical perspectives on the relation between catastrophizing and pain. *Clin J Pain.* 2001;17:52−64.

35. Vlaeyen JWS, Linton SJ. Fear-avoidance and its consequences in chronic musculoskeletal pain: a state of the art. *Pain*. 2000;85(3):317−332. https://doi.org/10.1016/S0304-3959(99)00242-0.

36. Vlaeyen JWS, Linton SJ. Fear-avoidance model of chronic musculoskeletal pain: 12 years on. *Pain*. 2012;153(6):1144−1147. https://doi.org/10.1016/j.pain.2011.12.009.

37. Green CR, Hart-Johnson T. The association between race and neighborhood socioeconomic status in younger black and white adults with chronic pain. *J Pain*. 2012;13(2):176−186. https://doi.org/10.1016/j.jpain.2011.10.008.

38. López-Martínez AE, Esteve-Zarazaga R, Ramírez-Maestre C. Perceived social support and coping responses are independent variables explaining pain adjustment among chronic pain patients. *J Pain*. 2008;9(4):373−379. https://doi.org/10.1016/j.jpain.2007.12.002.

39. McCracken LM. Social context and acceptance of chronic pain: the role of solicitous and punishing responses. *Pain*. 2005;113(1−2):155−159. https://doi.org/10.1016/j.pain.2004.10.004.

40. Romano JM, Jensen MP, Turner JA, Good AB, Hops H. Chronic pain patient-partner interactions: further support for a behavioral model of chronic pain. *Behav Ther*. 2000;31(3):415−440. https://doi.org/10.1016/S0005-7894(00)80023-4.

41. Schwartz L, Slater MA, Birchler GR. Interpersonal stress and pain behaviors in patients with chronic pain. *J Consult Clin Psychol*. 1994;62(4):861−864. https://doi.org/10.1037/0022-006X.62.4.861.

42. Nayak S, Shiflett SC, Eshun S, Levine FM. Culture and gender effects in pain beliefs and the prediction of pain tolerance. *Cross Cult Res*. 2000;34(2):135−151. https://doi.org/10.1177/106939710003400203.

43. Lethem J, Slade PD, Troup JDG, Bentley G. Outline of a fear-avoidance model of exaggerated pain perception-I. *Behav Res Ther*. 1983;21(4):401−408. https://doi.org/10.1016/0005-7967(83)90009-8.

44. Hooten WM. Chronic pain and mental health disorders: shared neural mechanisms, epidemiology, and treatment. *Mayo Clin Proc*. 2016;91(7):955−970. https://doi.org/10.1016/j.mayocp.2016.04.029.

45. Thompson T, Correll CU, Gallop K, Vancampfort D, Stubbs B. Is pain perception altered in people with depression? A systematic review and meta-analysis of experimental pain research. *J Pain*. 2016;17(12):1257−1272. https://doi.org/10.1016/j.jpain.2016.08.007.

46. García-blanco A, González-valls P, Iranzo-tatay C, et al. Hypoesthesia in generalised anxiety disorder and major depression disorder hypoesthesia in generalised anxiety disorder and major depression disorder. *Int J Psychiatr Clin Pract*. 2018;22(4):310−313. https://doi.org/10.1080/13651501.2017.1417441.

47. Defrin R, Ginzburg K, Solomon Z, et al. Quantitative testing of pain perception in subjects with PTSD - implications for the mechanism of the coexistence between PTSD and chronic pain. *Pain*. 2008;138(2):450−459. https://doi.org/10.1016/j.pain.2008.05.006.

48. Vaegter HB, Andersen TE, Harvold M, Andersen PG, Graven-Nielsen T. Increased pain sensitivity in accident-related chronic pain patients with comorbid posttraumatic stress. *Clin J Pain*. 2018;34(4):313−321. https://doi.org/10.1097/AJP.0000000000000543.

49. Tuna T, Van Obbergh L, Van Cutsem N, Engelman E. Usefulness of the pain sensitivity questionnaire to discriminate the pain behaviour of chronic pain patients. *Br J Anaesth*. 2018;121(3):616−622. https://doi.org/10.1016/j.bja.2018.04.042.

50. Geuze E, Westenberg HGM, Jochims A, et al. Altered pain processing in veterans with posttraumatic stress disorder. *Arch Gen Psychiatr*. 2007;64(1):76−85. https://doi.org/10.1001/archpsyc.64.1.76.

51. Gatchel RJ. *Clinical Essentials of Pain Management*. Washington, DC, US: American Psychological Association; 2005.

52. Blackburn JP. The diagnosis and management of chronic pain. *Medicine*. 2018;46(12):786−791. https://doi.org/10.1016/j.mpmed.2018.09.001.

53. Gatchel RJ, Howard K, Haggard R. Pain: the biopsychosocial perspective. In: Contrada R, Baum A, eds. *The Handbook of Stress Science: Biology, Psychology, and Health*. New York, NY: Springer Publishing; 2011:461−473.

54. Gatchel RJ, McGeary DD, McGeary CA, Lippe B. Interdisciplinary chronic pain management. *Am Psychol*. 2014;69(2):119−130. https://doi.org/10.1037/a0035514.

55. Hoffman BM, Papas RK, Chatkoff DK, Kerns RD. Meta-analysis of psychological interventions for chronic low back pain. *Health Psychol*. 2007;26(1):1−9. https://doi.org/10.1037/0278-6133.26.1.1.

56. Morley S, Eccleston C, Williams A. Systematic review and meta-analysis of randomized controlled trials of cognitive behaviour therapy and behaviour therapy for chronic pain in adults, excluding headache. *Pain*. 1999;80:1−13. https://doi.org/10.1016/S0304-3959(98)00255-3.

57. Hayes SC, Strosahk KD, Wilson KG. *Acceptance and Commitment Therapy: The Process and Practice of Mindful Change*. 2nd ed. New York: Guilford Press; 2012.

58. Vowles KE, Sowden G, Ashworth J. A comprehensive examination of the model underlying acceptance and commitment therapy for chronic pain. *Behav Ther*. 2014;45(3):390−401. https://doi.org/10.1016/j.beth.2013.12.009.

59. Veehof MM, Oskam MJ, Schreurs KMG, Bohlmeijer ET. Acceptance-based interventions for the treatment of chronic pain: a systematic review and meta-analysis. *Pain*. 2011;152(3):533−542. https://doi.org/10.1016/j.pain.2010.11.002.

60. McCracken LM, Sato A, Taylor GJ. A trial of a brief group-based form of acceptance and commitment therapy (ACT) for chronic pain in general practice: pilot outcome and process results. *J Pain*. 2013;14(11):1398−1406. https://doi.org/10.1016/j.jpain.2013.06.011.

61. Grossman P, Niemann L, Schmidt S, Walach H. Mindfulness-based stress reduction and health benefits:

a meta-analysis. *J Psychosom Res.* 2004;57(1):35–43. https://doi.org/10.1016/S0022-3999(03)00573-7.

62. Anheyer D, Haller H, Jurgen B, Lauche R, Dobos G. Mindfulness-based stress reduction for treating low back pain: a systematic review and meta-analysis. *Ann Intern Med.* 2017;166:799–807. https://doi.org/10.7326/M16-1997.

63. Hilton L, Hempel S, Ewing BA, et al. Mindfulness meditation for chronic pain: systematic review and meta-analysis. *Ann Behav Med.* 2017;51(2):199–213. https://doi.org/10.1007/s12160-016-9844-2.

64. Sharp TJ, Harvey AG. Chronic pain and posttraumatic stress disorder: mutual maintenance? *Clin Psychol Rev.* 2001;21(6):857–877. https://doi.org/10.1016/S0272-7358(00)00071-4.

65. Asmundson GJG, Coons MJ, Taylor S, Katz J. PTSD and the experience of pain: research and clinical implications of shared vulnerability and mutual maintenance models. *Can J Psychiatr.* 2002;47(10):930–937. https://doi.org/10.1177/070674370204701004.

66. Brennstuhl MJ, Tarquinio C, Montel S. Chronic pain and PTSD: evolving views on their comorbidity. *Perspect Psychiatr Care.* 2015;51(4):295–304. https://doi.org/10.1111/ppc.12093.

67. Taylor S, Zvolensky MJ, Cox BJ, et al. Robust dimensions of anxiety sensitivity: development and initial validation of the anxiety sensitivity index-3. *Psychol Assess.* 2007;19(2):176–188. https://doi.org/10.1037/1040-3590.19.2.176.

68. Taylor S. Treating anxiety sensitivity in adults with anxiety and related disorders. In: Smits JAJ, Otto MW, Powers MB, Baird S, eds. *The Clinician's Guide to Anxiety Sensitivity Treatment and Assessment.* Academic Press; 2019:55–75. https://doi.org/10.1016/B978-0-12-813495-5.00004-8.

69. Rogers AH, Kauffman BY, Bakhshaie J, McHugh RK, Ditre JW, Zvolensky MJ. Anxiety sensitivity and opioid misuse among opioid-using adults with chronic pain. *Am J Drug Alcohol Abuse.* 2019;45(5):470–478. https://doi.org/10.1080/00952990.2019.1569670.

70. Rice DB, Mehta S, Serrato J, et al. Stress in patients diagnosed with rheumatoid arthritis compared to chronic pain. *Rehabil Psychol.* 2017;62(4):571–579. https://doi.org/10.1037/rep0000103.

71. Janke EA, Jones E, Hopkins CM, Ruggieri M, Hruska A. Catastrophizing and anxiety sensitivity mediate the relationship between persistent pain and emotional eating. *Appetite.* 2016;103:64–71. https://doi.org/10.1016/j.appet.2016.03.022.

72. Paltell KC, Bing-Canar H, Ranney RM, Tran JK, Berenz EC, Vujanovic AA. Anxiety sensitivity moderates the effect of posttraumatic stress disorder symptoms on emotion dysregulation among trauma-exposed firefighters. *J Psychopathol Behav Assess.* 2019:524–535. https://doi.org/10.1007/s10862-019-09731-4.

72a Aldea MA, Michael K, Alexander K, Kison S. Obsessive-compulsive tendencies in a sample of veterans with post traumatic stress disorder. *J Cogn Psychother [Internet].* 2019;33(1):33–45. Available from: http://connect.

springerpub.com/lookup/doi/10.1891/0889-8391.33.1.33.

73. Overstreet C, Brown E, Berenz EC, et al. Anxiety sensitivity and distress tolerance typologies and relations to posttraumatic stress disorder: a cluster analytic approach. *Mil Psychol.* 2018;30(6):547–556. https://doi.org/10.1080/08995605.2018.1521682.

74. Asmundson GJG, Carleton RN. Fear of pain is elevated in adults with Co-Occurring Trauma-Related stress and social anxiety symptoms. *Cognit Behav Ther.* 2005;34(4):248–255. https://doi.org/10.1080/16506070510011557.

75. Martin AL, Halket E, Asmundson GJG, Flora DB, Katz J. Posttraumatic stress symptoms and the diathesis-stress model of chronic pain and disability in patients undergoing major surgery. *Clin J Pain.* 2010;26(6):518–527. https://doi.org/10.1097/AJP.0b013e3181e15b98.

76. Ruiz-Párraga GT, López-Martínez AE. The contribution of posttraumatic stress symptoms to chronic pain adjustment. *Health Psychol.* 2014;33(9):958–967. https://doi.org/10.1037/hea0000040.

77. Lies J, Lau ST, Jones LE, Jensen MP, Tan G. Predictors and moderators of post-traumatic stress disorder: an investigation of anxiety sensitivity and resilience in individuals with chronic pain. *Ann Acad Med Singapore.* 2017;46(3):102–110.

78. López-Martínez AE, Ramírez-Maestre C, Esteve R. An examination of the structural link between post-traumatic stress symptoms and chronic pain in the framework of fear avoidance models. *Eur J Pain.* 2014;18(8):1129–1138. https://doi.org/10.1002/j.1532-2149.2014.00459.x.

79. Tsur N, Defrin R, Lahav Y, Solomon Z. The traumatized body: long-term PTSD and its implications for the orientation towards bodily signals. *Psychiatr Res.* 2018;261:281–289. https://doi.org/10.1016/j.psychres.2017.12.083.

80. Rosenbloom BN, Katz J, Chin KYW, et al. Predicting pain outcomes after traumatic musculoskeletal injury. *Pain.* 2016;157(8):1733–1743. https://doi.org/10.1097/j.pain.0000000000000580.

81. Almli LM, Fani N, Smith AK, Ressler KJ. Genetic approaches to understanding post-traumatic stress disorder. *Int J Neuropsychopharmacol.* 2014;17(2):355–370. https://doi.org/10.1017/S1461145713001090.

82. Banerjee SB, Morrison FG, Ressler KJ. Genetic approaches for the study of PTSD: advances and challenges. *Neurosci Lett.* 2017;649:139–146. 10.1016/j.neulet.2017.02.058.

83. Nievergelt CM, Ashley-Koch AE, Dalvie S, et al. Genomic approaches to posttraumatic stress disorder: the psychiatric genomic consortium initiative. *Biol Psychiatr.* 2018;83(10):831–839. https://doi.org/10.1016/j.biopsych.2018.01.020.

84. Hawn SE, Sheerin CM, Lind MJ, et al. GxE effects of FKBP5 and traumatic life events on PTSD: a meta analysis. *J Affect Disord.* 2019;243:455–462. https://doi.org/10.1016/j.jad.2018.09.058.

85. Blacker CJ, Frye MA, Morava E, Kozicz T, Veldic M. A review of epigenetics of PTSD in comorbid psychiatric

conditions. *Genes.* 2019;10(2):1–15. https://doi.org/10.3390/genes10020140.

86. Kang JI, Kim TY, Choi JH, So HS, Kim SJ. Allele-specific DNA methylation level of FKBP5 is associated with post-traumatic stress disorder. *Psychoneuroendocrinology.* 2019;103:1–7. https://doi.org/10.1016/j.psyneuen.2018.12.226.

87. Linnstaedt SD, Riker KD, Rueckeis CA, et al. A functional riboSNitch in the 3′ untranslated region of FKBP5 alters MicroRNA-320a binding efficiency and mediates vulnerability to chronic post-traumatic pain. *J Neurosci.* 2018;38(39):8407–8420. https://doi.org/10.1523/JNEUROSCI.3458-17.2018.

88. Linnstaedt SD, Riker KD, Walker MG, et al. MicroRNA 320a predicts chronic axial and widespread pain development following motor vehicle collision in a stress-dependent manner. *J Orthop Sports Phys Ther.* 2016;46(10):911–919. https://doi.org/10.2519/jospt.2016.6944.

89. Hammamieh R, Chakraborty N, Gautam A, et al. Whole-genome DNA methylation status associated with clinical PTSD measures of OIF/OEF veterans. *Transl Psychiatry.* 2017;7(7):e1169. https://doi.org/10.1038/tp.2017.129.

90. Mehta D, Voisey J, Bruenig D, et al. Transcriptome analysis reveals novel genes and immune networks dysregulated in veterans with PTSD. *Brain Behav Immun.* 2018;74:133–142. https://doi.org/10.1016/j.bbi.2018.08.014.

91. Rusch HL, Robinson J, Yun S, et al. Gene expression differences in PTSD are uniquely related to the intrusion symptom cluster: a transcriptome-wide analysis in military service members. *Brain Behav Immun.* 2019;80:904–908. https://doi.org/10.1016/j.bbi.2019.04.030.

92. Katrinli S, Lori A, Kilaru V, et al. Association of HLA locus alleles with posttraumatic stress disorder. *Brain Behav Immun.* 2019;81:655–658. https://doi.org/10.1016/j.bbi.2019.07.016.

93. Wang Y, Karstoft K-I, Nievergelt CM, et al. Post-traumatic stress following military deployment: genetic associations and cross-disorder genetic correlations. *J Affect Disord.* 2019;252:350–357. https://doi.org/10.1016/j.jad.2019.04.070.

94. Morrison FG, Miller MW, Logue MW, Assef M, Wolf EJ. DNA methylation correlates of PTSD: recent findings and technical challenges. *Prog Neuro-Psychopharmacol Biol Psychiatry.* 2019;90:223–234. https://doi.org/10.1016/j.pnpbp.2018.11.011.

95. Dunlop BW, Wong A. The hypothalamic-pituitary-adrenal axis in PTSD: pathophysiology and treatment interventions. *Prog Neuro-Psychopharmacol Biol Psychiatry.* 2019;89:361–379. https://doi.org/10.1016/j.pnpbp.2018.10.010.

96. Pape JC, Carrillo-Roa T, Rothbaum BO, et al. DNA methylation levels are associated with CRF 1 receptor antagonist treatment outcome in women with post-traumatic stress disorder. *Clin Epigenet.* 2018;10(1):1–11. https://doi.org/10.1186/s13148-018-0569-x.

97. Descalzi G, Ikegami D, Ushijima T, Nestler EJ, Zachariou V, Narita M. Epigenetic mechanisms of chronic pain. *Trends Neurosci.* 2015;38(4):237–246. https://doi.org/10.1016/j.tins.2015.02.001.

98. Polli A, Ickmans K, Godderis L, Nijs J. When environment meets genetics: a clinical review of the epigenetics of pain, psychological factors, and physical activity. *Arch Phys Med Rehabil.* 2019;100(6):1153–1161. https://doi.org/10.1016/j.apmr.2018.09.118.

99. López-González MJ, Landry M, Favereaux A. MicroRNA and chronic pain: from mechanisms to therapeutic potential. *Pharmacol Ther.* 2017;180:1–15. https://doi.org/10.1016/j.pharmthera.2017.06.001.

100. Beck JG, Clapp JD. A different kind of comorbidity: understanding posttraumatic stress disorder and chronic pain. *Psychol Trauma.* 2011;3(2):101–108. https://doi.org/10.1037/a0021263.

101. Harvold M, MacLeod C, Vaegter HB. Attentional avoidance is associated with increased pain sensitivity in patients with chronic posttraumatic pain and comorbid posttraumatic stress. *Clin J Pain.* 2018;34(1):22–29. https://doi.org/10.1097/AJP.0000000000000505.

102. Herrera-Escobar JP, Apoj M, Weed C, et al. Association of pain after trauma with long-term functional and mental health outcomes. *J Trauma Acute Care Surg.* 2018;85(4):773–779. https://doi.org/10.1097/TA.0000000000002017.

103. Curry I, Malaktaris AL, Lyons R, Herbert MS, Norman SB. The association between negative trauma-related cognitions and pain-related functional status among veterans with posttraumatic stress disorder and alcohol use disorder. *J Trauma Stress.* 2019;32(2):317–322. https://doi.org/10.1002/jts.22394.

104. Foa EB, Kozak MJ. Emotional processing of fear. Exposure to corrective information. *Psychol Bull.* 1986;99(1):20–35. https://doi.org/10.1037/0033-2909.99.1.20.

105. Foa EB, Steketee G, Rothbaum BO. Behavioral/cognitive conceptualizations of post-traumatic stress disorder. *Behav Ther.* 1989;20(2):155–176. https://doi.org/10.1016/S0005-7894(89)80067-X.

106. Mazidi M, Vig K, Ranjbar S, Ebrahimi M-R, Khatibi A. Attentional bias and its temporal dynamics among war veterans suffering from chronic pain: investigating the contribution of post-traumatic stress symptoms. *J Anxiety Disord.* 2019;66:102115. https://doi.org/10.1016/j.janxdis.2019.102115.

107. Crombez G, Eccleston C, Van Damme S, Vlaeyen JWS, Karoly P. Fear-avoidance model of chronic pain: the next generation. *Clin J Pain.* 2012;28(6):475–483. https://doi.org/10.1097/AJP.0b013e3182385392.

108. Gebler FA, Maercker A. Effects of including an existential perspective in a cognitive-behavioral group program for chronic pain: a clinical trial with 6 months follow-up. *Humanist Psychol.* 2014;42(2):155–171. https://doi.org/10.1080/08873267.2013.865188.

109. Irwin KC, Konnert C, Wong M, O'Neill TA. PTSD symptoms and pain in Canadian military veterans: the mediating roles of anxiety, depression, and alcohol use. *J Trauma Stress.* 2014;27:175–181. https://doi.org/10.1002/jts.21897.

110. Seng EK, Kuka AJ, Mayson SJ, Smitherman TA, Buse DC. Acceptance, psychiatric symptoms, and migraine

disability: an observational study in a headache center. *Headache*. 2018;58(6):859−872. https://doi.org/10.1111/head.13325.

111. Smith TO, Dainty JR, Williamson E, Martin KR. Association between musculoskeletal pain with social isolation and loneliness: analysis of the English Longitudinal Study of Ageing. *Br J Pain*. 2019;13(2):82−90. https://doi.org/10.1177/2049463718802868.

112. Kraus A, Geuze E, Schmahl C, et al. Differentiation of pain ratings in combat-related posttraumatic stress disorder. *Pain*. 2009;143(3):179−185. https://doi.org/10.1016/j.pain.2008.12.018.

113. Outcalt SD, Kroenke K, Krebs EE, et al. Chronic pain and comorbid mental health conditions: independent associations of posttraumatic stress disorder and depression with pain, disability, and quality of life. *J Behav Med*. 2015;38(3):535−543. https://doi.org/10.1007/s10865-015-9628-3.

114. Moreno JL, Nabity PS, Kanzler KE, Bryan CJ, McGeary CA, McGeary DD. Negative life events (NLEs) contributing to psychological distress, pain, and disability in a U.S. military sample. *Mil Med*. 2019;184(1−2):E148−E155. https://doi.org/10.1093/milmed/usy259.

115. Outcalt SD, Yu Z, Hoen HM, Pennington TM, Krebs EE. Health care utilization among veterans with pain and posttraumatic stress symptoms. *Pain Med*. 2014;15(11):1872−1879. https://doi.org/10.1111/pme.12045.

116. Bernardy NC, Friedman MJ. Pharmacological management of posttraumatic stress disorder. *Curr Opin Psychol*. 2017;14:116−121. https://doi.org/10.1016/j.copsyc.2017.01.003.

117. Caraci F, Merlo S, Drago F, Caruso G, Parenti C, Sortino MA. Rescue of noradrenergic system as a novel pharmacological strategy in the treatment of chronic pain: focus on microglia activation. *Front Pharmacol*. 2019;10:1−8. https://doi.org/10.3389/fphar.2019.01024.

118. Birur B, Math SB, Fargason RE. A review of psychopharmacological interventions post-disaster to prevent psychiatric sequelae. *Psychopharmacol Bull*. 2017;47(1):8−26.

119. Holbrook TL, Galarneau MR, Dye JL, Quinn K, Dougherty AL. Morphine use after combat injury in Iraq and post-traumatic stress disorder. *N Engl J Med*. 2010;362(2):110−117. https://doi.org/10.1056/NEJMoa0903326.

120. Sutherland AM, Nicholls J, Bao J, Clarke H. Overlaps in pharmacology for the treatment of chronic pain and mental health disorders. *Prog Neuro-Psychopharmacol Biol Psychiatry*. 2018;87:290−297. https://doi.org/10.1016/j.pnpbp.2018.07.017.

121. Li X, Vigil JM, Stith SS, Brockelman F, Keeling K, Hall B. The effectiveness of self-directed medical cannabis treatment for pain. *Compl Ther Med*. 2019;46(July):123−130. https://doi.org/10.1016/j.ctim.2019.07.022.

122. Ney LJ, Matthews A, Bruno R, Felmingham KL. Progress in neuropsychopharmacology & biological Psychiatry cannabinoid interventions for PTSD: where to next ? *Prog Neuro-Psychopharmacol Biol Psychiatry*. 2019;93:124−140. https://doi.org/10.1016/j.pnpbp.2019.03.017.

123. FDA. FDA Regulation of Cannabis and Cannabis-Derived Products, Including Cannabidiol (CBD). U.S Food & Drug Administration.

124. Mallick-Searle T, St. Marie B. Cannabinoids in pain treatment: an overview. *Pain Manag Nurs*. 2019;20(2):107−112. https://doi.org/10.1016/j.pmn.2018.12.006.

125. Bosco MA, Gallinati JL, Clark ME. Conceptualizing and treating comorbid chronic pain and PTSD. *Pain Res Treat*. 2013;2013. https://doi.org/10.1155/2013/174728.

126. Foa EB, McLean CP, Zang Y, et al. Effect of prolonged exposure therapy delivered over 2 weeks vs 8 weeks vs present-centered therapy on PTSD symptom severity in military personnel A randomized clinical trial. *J Am Med Assoc*. 2018;319(4):354−364. https://doi.org/10.1001/jama.2017.21242.

127. Resick PA, Wachen JS, Mintz J, et al. A randomized clinical trial of group cognitive processing therapy compared with group present-centered therapy for PTSD among active duty military personnel. *J Consult Clin Psychol*. 2015;83(6):1058−1068. https://doi.org/10.1037/ccp0000016.

128. Goldstein E, Mcdonnell C, Atchley R, et al. The impact of psychological interventions on posttraumatic stress disorder and pain symptoms: a systematic review and meta-analysis. *Clin J Pain*. 2019;35(8):703−712. https://doi.org/10.1097/AJP.0000000000000730.

129. Hayes SC, Levin ME, Plumb-Vilardaga J, Villatte JL, Pistorello J. Acceptance and commitment therapy and contextual behavioral science: examining the progress of a Distinctive model of behavioral and cognitive therapy. *Behav Ther*. 2013;44(2):180−198. https://doi.org/10.1016/j.beth.2009.08.002.

130. Herbert MS, Malaktaris AL, Dochat C, Thomas ML, Wetherell JL, Afari N. Acceptance and commitment therapy for chronic pain: does post-traumatic stress disorder influence treatment outcomes? *Pain Med*. 2019;20(9):1728−1736. https://doi.org/10.1093/pm/pny272.

131. Otis JD, Keane TM, Kerns RD, Monson C, Scioli E. The development of an integrated treatment for veterans with comorbid chronic pain and posttraumatic stress disorder. *Pain Med*. 2009;10(7):1300−1311. https://doi.org/10.1111/j.1526-4637.2009.00715.x.

132. Beck JG, Coffey SF, Foy DW, Keane TM, Blanchard EB. Group cognitive behavior therapy for chronic posttraumatic stress disorder: an initial randomized Pilot study. *Behav Ther*. 2009;40(1):82−92. https://doi.org/10.1016/j.beth.2008.01.003.

133. Dunne RL, Kenardy J, Sterling M. A randomized controlled trial of cognitive-behavioral therapy for the treatment of PTSD in the context of chronic whiplash. *Clin J Pain*. 2012;28(9):755−765. https://doi.org/10.1097/AJP.0b013e318243e16b.

134. Andersen TE, Lahav Y, Ellegaard H, Manniche C. A randomized controlled trial of brief somatic experiencing for chronic low back pain and comorbid post-traumatic stress disorder symptoms. *Eur J Psychotraumatol*. 2017;8(1). https://doi.org/10.1080/20008198.2017.1331108.

135. Tesarz J, Gerhardt A, Leisner S, et al. Effects of eye movement desensitization and reprocessing (EMDR) on non-specific chronic back pain: a randomized controlled trial with additional exploration of the underlying mechanisms. *BMC Muscoskel Disord*. 2013;14:1−8. https://doi.org/10.1186/1471-2474-14-256.

136. Kip KE, Rosenzweig L, Hernandez DF, et al. Accelerated resolution therapy for treatment of pain secondary to symptoms of combat-related posttraumatic stress disorder. *Eur J Psychotraumatol.* 2014;5(Suppl). https://doi.org/10.3402/ejpt.v5.24066.

137. Straud CL, Siev J, Messer S, Zalta AK. Examining military population and trauma type as moderators of treatment outcome for first-line psychotherapies for PTSD: a meta-analysis. *J Anxiety Disord.* 2019;67:102133. https://doi.org/10.1016/j.janxdis.2019.102133.

138. Dewar M, Paradis A, Fortin CA. Identifying trajectories and predictors of response to psychotherapy for post-traumatic stress disorder in adults: a systematic review of literature. *Can J Psychiatr.* 2019. https://doi.org/10.1177/0706743719875602.

139. Janoff-Bulman R. *Shattered Assumptions: Toward a New Psychology of Trauma.* New York: The Free Press; 1992.

139a Pacella ML, Girard JM, Wright AGC, Suffoletto B, Callaway CW. The Association Between Daily Posttraumatic Stress Symptoms and Pain Over the First 14 Days After Injury: An Experience Sampling Study. *Acad Emerg Med.* 2018;25(8):844−855.

140. Zhang ZB, Shen YH, Wang WD, Wang BQ, Zheng JW. Design and implementation of sensing shirt for ambulatory cardiopulmonary monitoring. *J Med Biol Eng.* 2011; 31(3):207−216.

140a Morley S. Psychology of pain. *Br J Anaesth.* 2008;101(1): 25−31. https://doi.org/10.1093/bja/aen123.

141. Karoly P, Okun MA, Ruehlman LS, Pugliese JA. The impact of goal cognition and pain severity on disability and depression in adults with chronic pain: an examination of direct effects and mediated effects via pain-induced fear. *Cognit Ther Res.* 2008;32(3):418−433. https://doi.org/10.1007/s10608-007-9136-z.

142. Hardy JK, Crofford LJ, Segerstrom SC. Goal conflict, distress, and pain in women with fibromyalgia: a daily diary study. *J Psychosom Res.* 2011;70(6):534−540. https://doi.org/10.1016/j.jpsychores.2010.10.013.

143. Ajdukovic D, Ajdukovic D, Bogic M, et al. Recovery from posttraumatic stress symptoms: a qualitative study of attributions in survivors of war. *PloS One.* 2013;8(8). https://doi.org/10.1371/journal.pone.0070579.

144. Drescher KD, Foy DW, Kelly C, Leshner A, Schutz K, Litz B. An exploration of the viability and usefulness of the construct of moral injury in war veterans. *Traumatology.* 2011;17(1):8−13. https://doi.org/10.1177/1534765610395615.

145. Butzer B, Kuiper NA. Relationships between the frequency of social comparisons and self-concept clarity, intolerance of uncertainty, anxiety, and depression. *Pers Indiv Differ.* 2006;41:167−176. https://doi.org/10.1016/j.paid.2005.12.017.

146. Kindermans HPJ, Huijnen IPJ, Goossens MEJB, Roelofs J, Verbunt JA, Vlaeyen JWS. "Being" in pain: the role of self-discrepancies in the emotional experience and activity patterns of patients with chronic low back pain. *Pain.* 2011;152(2): 403−409. https://doi.org/10.1016/j.pain.2010.11.009.

147. Schwartz SJ, Klimstra TA, Luyckx K, et al. Daily dynamics of personal identity and self-concept clarity. 2011;385: 373−385. https://doi.org/10.1002/per.798.

148. Gregory B, Peters L. *Unique Relationships Between Self-Related Constructs, Social Anxiety, and Depression in a Non-Clinical Sample.* vol. 34(2). 2017:117−133. https://doi.org/10.1017/bec.2017.9.

149. Koole SL, Greenberg J, Pyszczynski T. Introducing science to the psychology of the soul: experimental existential psychology. *Curr Dir Psychol Sci.* 2006;15(5):212−217.

150. Landau MJ, Greenberg J, Sullivan D, Routledge C, Arndt J. The protective identity: evidence that mortality salience heightens the clarity and coherence of the self-concept. *J Exp Soc Psychol.* 2009;45(4):796−807. https://doi.org/10.1016/j.jesp.2009.05.013.

151. Linehan M. *Cognitive-Behavioral Treatment of Borderline Personality Disorder.* New York, NY: The Guilford Press; 1993.

152. Reynolds CJ, Vest N, Tragesser SL. Borderline personality disorder features and risk for prescription opioid misuse IN a chronic pain sample : roles for identity disturbances and impulsivity. *J Pers Disord.* 2019:1−18.

153. Pyszczynski T, Kesebir P. Anxiety buffer disruption theory: a terror management account of posttraumatic stress disorder. *Hist Philos Logic.* 2011;24(1):3−26. https://doi.org/10.1080/10615806.2010.517524.

154. Vail KE, Morgan A, Kahle L. Self-affirmation attenuates death-thought accessibility after mortality salience, but not among a high post-traumatic stress sample. *Psychol Trauma.* 2018;10(1):112−120. https://doi.org/10.1037/tra0000304.

155. Vail III KE, Reed II DE, Goncy EA, Cornelius T, Edmondson D. Anxiety buffer disruption: self-evaluation, death anxiety, and stressor appraisals among low and high posttraumatic stress symptom samples. *J Soc Clin Psychol.*

156. Lerner MJ. *The Belief in a Just World.* Boston, MA: Springer; 1980.

157. Edmondson D, Chaudoir SR, Mills MA, Park CL, Holub J, Bartkowiak JM. From shattered assumptions to weakened worldviews: trauma symptoms signal anxiety buffer disruption. *J Loss Trauma.* 2011;16(4):358−385. https://doi.org/10.1080/15325024.2011.572030.

158. Dezutter J, Offenbaecher M, Vallejo MA, Vanhooren S, Thauvoye E, Toussaint L. Chronic pain care: the importance of a biopsychosocial-existential approach. *Int J Psychiatr Med.* 2016;51(6):563−575. https://doi.org/10.1177/0091217417696738.

CHAPTER 16

Opioids in Pain

AMEET S. NAGPAL, MD, MS, MED • BRIAN BOIES, MD • NATHAN CLEMENTS, MD •
DARRELL VYDRA, MD

INTRODUCTION/GENERAL CONSIDERATIONS

Opium and its derivatives have been described and used for analgesia for thousands of years, making it one of the oldest medicinal plants. In 3500 BC, the opium plant was often called "joy plant" by the Sumerians. Other ancient cultures also document the use of opium for treatment of pain, crying, and sleep. Morphine is the first alkaloid isolated from opium by Friedrich Wilhelm Adam Sertürner in 1817. By the 1830s, morphine became a very commonly used analgesic during the American Civil War. The use of morphine became so widespread at that time that the term "soldier disease" was used to describe those who had become dependent on morphine. Since that time, many additional derivatives have become common practice in managing acute, chronic, and terminal pain.

From 1999 to 2014, the sale of prescription opioid medications quadrupled.[1-4] This increase in prescription writing has been accompanied by concordant rise in opioid use disorder (OUD), increased mortality, overdose, sexual dysfunction, fractures, myocardial infarction, constipation, and sleep-disordered breathing, leading many to question their utility and labeling this rise an epidemic,[5,6] particularly with regard to the management of chronic, nonterminal pain given lack of high-quality research examining long-term effects. It is important to note that evidence supports short-term (<12 weeks) efficacy of opioids for reducing pain and improving function in noncancer nociceptive and neuropathic pain and for the use in terminal pain management.[7-12] Thus, careful patient screening and monitoring is paramount in the safe management of pain with opioid medications.

In this chapter, we will examine the pharmacology, side effects, indications, and recommendations for monitoring in the clinical setting.

OPIOID RECEPTORS

Many pain modulating systems are found in the human body; the most widely studied is that of the endogenous opioid system. The first endogenous opioid, enkephalin, was discovered in 1975.[5] Since then, several have been described, including endorphins and enkephalins (Table 16.1). To date, four opioid receptor systems have been characterized at cellular, molecular, and pharmacological levels.[6] These include the three classical receptors: μ-, κ-, and δ-, while the opioid receptor-like receptor-1 (ORL-1), cloned in 1994,[7] represents the most recently discovered of the opioid receptor family.[6] The International Union of Pharmacology (IUPHAR) has renamed μ, κ, δ, and ORL-1 receptors to MOR, KOP, DOP, and nociceptin opioid peptide receptor (NOP), respectively.[8] Multiple additional subtypes within each of these receptor systems have since been proposed.[9]

Opioid receptors are found abundantly in the central nervous system (CNS), with highest concentrations in the thalamus, the periaqueductal gray matter, and the dorsal horn of the spinal cord,[10] as well as in peripheral organs, such as heart, lungs, liver, and gastrointestinal (GI) and reproductive tracts.[11] Most of the spinal μ receptor binding sites are located presynaptically on the terminals of primary afferent nociceptors.[12] It is the μ receptor that is most strongly correlated with the analgesic and addiction properties of opioid drugs.[13] An important factor of δ and κ receptor activation is the production of spinal analgesia without concomitant respiratory depression, while the ORL-1 receptor appears to be free of abuse potential.[14] Physiological properties of each receptor type can be seen in Table 16.2.

Opioid receptors are G protein-coupled receptors and consist of an extracellular amino acid N-terminus, seven transmembrane loops, and an intracellular carboxyl C-terminus. There is significant structural

Pain Care Essentials and Innovations. https://doi.org/10.1016/B978-0-323-72216-2.00016-8

TABLE 16.1
Endogenous Opioid Receptors and Preferred Receptors.

Endogenous Opioid	Receptor
Enkephalin	μ
Endorphin	Δ
Dynorphin	K
Nociceptin/orphanin FQ	NOP/ORL
Endomorphins	μ
Morphiceptin	μ

Adapted from Feng Y, He X, Yang Y, Chao D, Lazarus LH, Xia Y. Current research on opioid receptor function. *Curr Drug Targets.* 2012;13(2):230–246.

TABLE 16.2
Physiological Effects of Opioid Receptors' Binding.

Opioid Receptor	Physiological Effect
Mu (μ)	Nociception, respiration, cardiovascular functions, intestinal transit, feeding, learning and memory, locomotor activity, thermoregulation, hormone secretion, immune function
μ_1	Supraspinal analgesia, spinal analgesia, respiratory depression, slowing of gastrointestinal motility and secretions
μ_2	Pruritus, nausea, vomiting, majority of cardiovascular effects, physical dependence, euphoria
Kappa (K)	Nociception, diuresis, hyperphagia, immune function, neuroendocrine function
K^1	Spinal analgesia, diuresis (via inhibition of ADH release), sedation, miosis
K^2	Minimal abuse potential for abuse, appetite
K^3	Supraspinal analgesia
Delta (δ)	Analgesia, motor integration, cognitive function, mood-driven behavior, gastrointestinal motility, olfaction, respiration
ORL-1	Instinctive and emotional behaviors, nociception

homology between the three classic opioid receptors. Each receptor demonstrates a binding preference for endogenous opioids, though significant overlap does exist. The μ receptor is 66% identical to the δ receptor and 68% identical to the κ receptor and binds to endorphins more so than enkephalins.[15] While the δ and κ receptors have 58% identical amino acid sequences,[15] the δ receptors prefer binding to enkephalins, and the κ receptors potently bind to dynorphins. Nociceptin/orphanin FQ (N/OFQ or nociceptin) binds to the ORL-1 (NOP receptor).

Distribution, Metabolism, and Excretion

Opioid distribution is dependent on the lipophilicity of the parent compound and metabolites. The more lipophilic, the greater potential to reach the target tissue. The most lipophilic opioids are fentanyl and methadone.

Opioids differ with respect to the means by which they are metabolized, and patients differ in their ability to metabolize individual opioids. With this in mind, most opioids observe similar patterns of metabolism. The majority undergo first-pass metabolism in the liver via cytochrome enzymes,[16] which reduces the bioavailability of the opioid (see Table 16.3). These enzymes promote two forms of metabolism: phase 1 metabolism (modification reactions) and phase 2 metabolism (conjugation reactions).[16] The purpose of this metabolism is to produce a hydrophilic drug in order to facilitate its excretion in the urine. The opioids that undergo phase 2 reaction have less potential for drug-drug interactions due to the glucuronidation by the enzyme uridine diphosphate glucuronosyltransferase (UGT), which produces molecules that are highly hydrophilic and therefore easily excreted.[17] Morphine, oxymorphone, tapentadol, and hydromorphone are each metabolized by phase 2 glucuronidation and are less prone to drug interactions than those eliminated using the CYP450 pathways.[18]

A byproduct of metabolism is the formation of metabolites. Metabolites produced are typically less active than the parent compound with a few exceptions. Examples are that of morphine, whose metabolite, M6G, is substantially more potent than that of morphine itself and that of codeine, in which 10% is metabolized into morphine.[19] Additionally, some metabolites are responsible for the toxic side effects produced by opioids. The morphine metabolite, morphine-3-glucuornide (M3G), is found to have antianalgesic, allodynic, and neuroexcitatory effects.[20] Since the majority of opioid metabolites are excreted via the kidney, accumulation and side effect risk occurs in patients with renal failure.

TABLE 16.3
Metabolic Pathways/Enzyme Involvement.

Opioid	Phase 1 Metabolism	Phase 2 Metabolism	Comments
Morphine	None	Glucuronidation via UGT2B7	
Codeine	CYP2D6	None	
Hydrocodone	CYP2D6	None	One of the metabolites of hydrocodone is hydromorphone, which undergoes phase 2 glucuronidation
Oxycodone	CYP3A4, CYP2D6	None	Oxycodone produces a small amount of oxymorphone, which undergoes glucuronidation
Methadone	CYP3A4[†], CYP2D6, CYP2B6[†], CYP2C8, CYP2C19, CYP2C9	None	
Tramadol	CYP3A4, CYP2D6	None	
Fentanyl	CYP3A4	None	
Hydromorphone	None	Glucuronidation via UGT2B7	
Oxymorphone	None	Glucuronidation via UGT2B7	

CYP, cytochrome P450; *UGT2B7*, uridine diphosphate glucuronosyltransferase 2B7; †, primary enzymes involved in methadone metabolism.
Adapted from Smith HS. Opioid metabolism. *Mayo Clin Proc*. 2009. https://doi.org/10.1016/S0025-6196(1160750-7).

Due to their varied metabolism, opioids demonstrate varied absorption rates from the GI tract. Absorption is reduced as one ages, and recent literature suggests that genetic polymorphism is responsible for a varied interindividual response to the same doses of an opioid.[5]

Certain diseases play a major role in opioid metabolism, namely liver and renal disease. Because the liver is the main site for most of opioid metabolism, hepatic impairment can significantly alter the bioavailability of an opioid and its metabolites. Liver disease, such as cirrhosis, can significantly affect opioids metabolism through the CYP450 system as well as through impaired glucuronidation.[2] Dose reductions for most opioids may be necessary for patients with hepatic impairment. In the case of methadone, higher doses may be required to offset the lack of liver capacity to store and release methadone.[19]

Current data indicate that in those with renal impairment, morphine and codeine administration should be used with caution due to metabolite accumulation. Oxycodone should be used with caution with careful monitoring, while hydromorphone, methadone, and fentanyl are safest (Table 16.4). In those on dialysis, methadone and fentanyl are the safest opioids because they are not

dialyzed and therefore do not require dose adjustments, and the major route of excretion is fecal.[21] Fentanyl appears be the safest for short-term pain relief due to inactive metabolites. Of note, fentanyl can adsorb onto a CT 190 dialyzer membrane filter; therefore, if a CT 190 filter is used during dialysis, rotation to methadone is recommended.[22]

OPIOID SIDE EFFECTS

Opioid use for the management of pain has received widespread scrutiny due to the high risk of abuse, misuse, addiction, and potentially fatal adverse effects. The most commonly encountered side effects include constipation, nausea, vomiting, central sedation, and respiratory suppression (Table 16.5). Tolerance and physical dependency are also commonly encountered and often confused with addiction.[27]

Constipation is the most common side effect of opioid administration. This occurs due to opioid receptors distributed throughout the tract in GI tract smooth muscle and particularly in high concentrations throughout the antrum of the stomach and the proximal small bowel. As a result, opioids inhibit relaxation of the lower esophageal sphincter, decrease propulsion

TABLE 16.4
Opioid Use in Renal Failure.

Recommendation of Use	Comment
RECOMMENDED	
• Fentanyl	
• Methadone	Biliary excretion increases as renal excretion decreases. Methadone appears to be safe in renal failure, and no dose recommendations are necessary.
• Hydromorphone	Well tolerated in dialysis patients; toxic metabolites may accumulate in stage 5 CKD, therefore manage conservatively.
USE WITH CAUTION	
• Tramadol	Maximum dose of 200 mg daily, associated with lower seizure threshold.
AVOID	
• Morphine	Should be avoided in patients in severe renal failure (GFR <30 mL/min) due to accumulation of M3G.
• Codeine	Absorption effect, distribution, and metabolism of codeine are unknown, and it has reduced excretion.
INSUFFICIENT EVIDENCE	
• Oxycodone	Oxycodone is recommended only if alternative opioids are not available. The metabolites are thought to be less neurotoxic than those of morphine and hydromorphone.

CKD, chronic kidney disease; *M3G*, morphine-3-glucuornide
Adapted from Goldstein N.E and Morrison S.E. Which opioids are safest and most effective in renal failure? In: Gelfman LP CE, ed. *Evidence-Based Practice of Palliative Medicine*. 1st ed. Elsevier Health; 2013:28–33.

of smooth muscles in the small and large intestines, increase pyloric and anal sphincter tone, delay gastric emptying, and enhance absorption of fluids from intestinal contents.[28] This can lead to significant constipation and ileus if not properly managed.

Nausea is seen in up to 40% of patients after opioid administration. The exact mechanism is unclear but three mechanisms are often described: 1. Stimulation of the μ and δ receptors in the chemoreceptor trigger zone (CTZ),[29] 2. Increased vestibular sensitivity which activates the medullary vomiting center,[30] and 3. decreased GI motility due to activation of the μ receptors throughout the GI tract.[31]

Respiratory depression is the most feared complication of opioid therapy (OT). It occurs due to direct μ receptor depression in the brainstem centers that mediate respiratory drive. The effects of opioids impact respiratory rate, minute volume, and decreases the body's response to carbon dioxide by shifting the carbon dioxide response curve to the right.[27–32] Combining OT with other sedative drugs is strongly discouraged. In recent years, naloxone, a selective opioid receptor antagonist, has been used widely in the management of opioid-induced respiratory depression.

Sedation is common in opioid naïve patients and those undergoing dose adjustments. Sedation secondary to opioids is generally temporary and has been shown in studies in cancer patients to resolve over 1 week.[33] However, it has been documented that up to 81% of those on long-term OT demonstrate memory deficits and up to 10% demonstrate chronic fatigue.[34] If sedation persists, it is important to evaluate for other sedative medications and metabolic abnormalities (decreased clearance), and switching to a new agent may be indicated.[27]

Opioid-induced hyperalgesia (OIH) is a state of nociceptive sensitization whereby patients who are on chronic OT experience increased pain. The pain may be the same or of new type as the pain for which they were originally treated. The mechanism by which this paradoxical response occurs is not well defined but is thought to be the result of neuroplastic changes in the central and peripheral nervous system. Clinicians should suspect OIH when opioid treatment effects wane despite the lack of disease progression, development of diffuse allodynia that is different from original pain, evidence of a true hyperalgesic state demonstrated on pinprick testing, or symptom worsening with increasing opioid use.[35,36] Initial diagnosis and treatment should include reduction of current opioid dosage which has been shown to decrease symptoms.[37] Other interventions include ketamine, dextromethorphan, nonsteroidal antiinflammatory drugs (NSAIDs), opioid switching, amantadine, buprenorphine, alpha 2 agonists, and methadone.[31,38]

Immunomodulatory effects have also been reported and studied with opioids. The mechanism by which this occurs is not well defined but is thought to occur by interaction of opioids with receptors in the CNS and

TABLE 16.5
Opioid Side Effects and Management.

Common Side Effects	Comments and Management
Sedation	Mostly resolves after 3–4 days. Consider decreasing opioid dose by 10%–25% or increasing frequency of administration with decreased dose. May consider adding a neurostimulant (e.g., caffeine, methylphenidate).
Constipation	Patient do not develop tolerance to this opioid effect and require prophylactic treatment. Begin a scheduled stimulant when opioid therapy is initiated (e.g., bisacodyl, senna). If constipation continues with monotherapy, an osmotic laxative should be then initiated (e.g., lactulose, polyethylene glycol, milk of magnesia, magnesium citrate). For those who do not respond to initial bowel program, consider using a peripherally acting mu-opioid receptor antagonist.
Nausea and vomiting	Typically resolves in 3–5 days, though can reemerge with titration of opioid dose. Antiemetics (especially those that bind to dopaminergic receptors, such as haloperidol, metoclopramide, and prochlorperazine) are most effective.
Less Common side effects	
Pruritus	Due to histamine release versus neuraxial induced [23] (less understood and challenging to treat). Treat with a nonsedating antihistamine (e.g., loratadine). Consider opioid dose decrease or opioid rotation.
Urinary retention	Reduce opioid dose by 10%–25%. In males, rule out postobstructive causes. Consider opioid rotation.
Myoclonic jerks	Often misdiagnosed and therefore under appreciated. Rotation to different opioid often helpful. Benzodiazepine is the primary symptomatic treatment. May consider baclofen.
Rare side effects	
Respiratory depression	Rare in chronic, stable use. More common in acute use. Thorough education with the patient and family members should be done prior to initiation and have a plan in place that family members can initiate if encountered. Prescribe naloxone rescue kits that either the patient or family members are familiar with and can administer.
Opioid allergy	Do not use the opioid that results in allergy. Most common are codeine, morphine, and meperidine. Codeine is the one opioid in which allergy is not uncommon.
Opioid-induced Hyperalgesia	Most commonly seen with low dose morphine or intraoperative remifentanil.[24,25] Decreasing the opioid dose (40%–50%) and adding adjuvants or a low dose of methadone can be used to treat opioid-induced hyperalgesia.[26] Ketamine has proven effective.[25] Other possible treatment regimens include dextromethorphan, and nonsteroidal antiinflammatory drugs (NSAIDs), opioid switching, amantadine, buprenorphine, alpha 2 agonists, and methadone.

TABLE 16.6

DSM-V Criteria for OUD: A Problematic Pattern of Opioid Use Leading to Clinically Significant Impairment and Stress and at Least Two of the Following Observed Within a 12-Month Period.[47]

1. Opioids taken in larger amounts or over a longer period than was intended.
2. There is a persistent desire or unsuccessful efforts to cut down or control opioid use.
3. A great deal of time is spent in activities necessary to obtain the opioid, use the opioid, or recover from its effects.
4. Craving or a strong desire or urge to use opioids.
5. Recurrent opioid use resulting in a failure to fulfill major role obligations at work, school, or home.
6. Continued opioid use despite having persistent or recurrent social or interpersonal problems caused or exacerbated by the effects of opioids.
7. Important social, occupational, or recreational activities are given up or reduced because of opioid use.
8. Recurrent opioid use in situations in which it is physically hazardous.
9. Continued opioid use despite knowledge of having a persistent or recurrent physical or psychological problem that is likely to have been caused or exacerbated by the substance.
10. Exhibits tolerance.
11. Exhibits withdrawal.

TABLE 16.7

IV Opioid Morphine Milligram Equivalent (MME) Table[127,128]

Opioid	Routes of administration	Equianalgesic dose (mg)	Onset of analgesia (mins)	Half life (hr)	Dose interval (h)
Morphine	IV	10	5–10	3–4 h	4
Hydromorphone	IV	1.5	15–30	2.3 h	3–4
Fentanyl (mcg)	IV	0.1	1–2	2–4 h	1–2
Tapentadol	Oral	0.4	30	4 h	4–6
Remifentanil	IV	N/A	1–3	3–10 min	

peripherally. Opioids have been shown to affect the innate and adaptive immune systems by interfering with phagocytic activity, inhibit T- and B-cell antibody response, and interference with chemotaxis of immune cells, but this effect varies depending on opioid type as with a 2019 study by Maher et al. showing suppression of natural killer cell cytotoxicity with μ and κ receptor agonists but not δ receptor agonists.[39,40]

Opioid tolerance is used to describe the phenomenon where increasing opioid doses are required for analgesia due to prolonged drug administration. Higher opioid doses are associated with increased risk of adverse events (for which tolerance develops slower or not at all), and thus, patients should be monitored closely.[41]

Physical dependence is defined as the physiologic state and constellation of symptoms that occur when a medication is abruptly stopped. Withdrawal occurs in the setting of abrupt discontinuation or when an antagonist is given. Opioid withdrawal symptoms include irritability, anxiety, tachypnea, mydriasis,

insomnia, yawning, lacrimation, diaphoresis, and other symptoms of a hyperadrenergic state if not treated. This state of withdrawal is generally self-limiting and uncomfortable but not typically life-threatening. Treatment is supportive in nature.[42]

OUD or opioid addiction is characterized by opioid use that results in physical, psychological, or social dysfunction and continued use despite the dysfunction.[27] See Table 16.6 for current DSM V criteria for OUD. Addiction is commonly reported in those who were initially prescribed opioids for legitimate reasons.[43] These risks are much higher in those with concurrent use of other substances including alcohol, tobacco, and benzodiazepines.[44] The risk of developing OUD is highest in those aged 18–30 with one study by Edlund et al. finding that patients 18- to 30-year old carried 11 times the odds of OUD and overdose.[45,46] In 2017, there were 47,600 drug overdose deaths involving opioids—primarily synthetic opioids. Due to these risks, careful screening for concurrent

TABLE 16.8
Opioid Morphine Milligram Equivalent (MME) Table [8,121-126]

Opioid	Routes of administration	MME Factor	Onset of analgesia (mins)	Half life (hr)	Dose interval (h)
Codeine	Oral	0.15	30–60	2.9 h	4
Tramadol	Oral	0.1	60	5.1 h	4–6
Hydrocodone	Oral	1	10–20	4.0 h	4–6
Hydrocodone SR	Oral	1	N/A	7–9 h	12 (capsule) 24 (tablet)
Oxycodone	Oral	1.5	15–30	4.5 h	4–6
Oxycodone SR	Oral	1.5	60		12
Morphine	Oral	1	30	2–3 h	4
Morphine SR	Oral	1	20–40		8–12
Oxymorphone	Oral	3	15–30	9 h	4–6
Hydromorphone	Oral	4	15–30	2.3 h	3–4
Hydromorphone SR	Oral		N/A		24
Fentanyl	Oral-buccal or SL tablets, or lozenge/troche (mcg)	0.2–0.4	5–15 (transmucosal)		1–2
Fentanyl	Patch (in mcg/hr)	2.4	12–24 (h)		72
Tapentadol	Oral	0.4	30	4 h	4–6

OME, oral morphine equivalent.

substance use disorders (SUDs) and other risk factors should be performed prior to prescribing.

OPIOID-RELATED TREATMENT OUTCOMES

Acute Pain

Pain is the most common reason for seeking care in the emergency department. This includes exacerbations of chronic pain and acute traumatic pain. Opioids have been reported to be the most commonly administered pain medications for a broad range of symptoms. Large studies have found small reductions in pain intensity but high patient satisfaction.[48,49] A 2017 randomized controlled trial (RCT) including 411 patients in the ED found no statistically or clinically significant differences in pain reduction when comparing ibuprofen and acetaminophen with 3 different opioid and acetaminophen combination medications.[50] Another study found that the addition of hydrocodone-acetaminophen combination to naproxen alone for the treatment of acute low back pain did not improve functional or pain outcomes at 1 week follow-up.[51] Similar results are seen in the management of acute renal colic in patients with no contraindications to NSAIDs.[52]

On the other hand, opioids have been shown to be efficacious for the treatment of acute pancreatitis[53] and sickle cell vaso-occlusive crisis.[54]

Acute/Postoperative Pain

Adequate control of postoperative pain is essential in promoting recovery, improving quality of life, and decreasing duration of hospital stays.[55,56] Both intensity and duration of postoperative pain have been shown to lead to development of chronic pain syndromes.[57,58] OT as part of a multimodal pain treatment plan is considered by many to be the mainstay treatment for the management of severe acute postoperative pain.[57,59-61] Opioids in the acute postoperative period have been shown to provide improved pain control and improve function with medications administered via oral, transdermal, and intravenous formulations. Interestingly, oral oxycodone has been shown to provide similar analgesia to IV pain medications, decrease the need for rescue analgesics and potential less opioid consumption overall in acute postoperative pain, and may be an alternative to IV opioids.[62] Postoperative opioid overprescribing is well documented in the literature; therefore, guidelines have been established for the recommended duration of treatment in this period.[63,64] It is recommended that patients undergoing surgical intervention such as simple tooth extractions, laparoscopic surgeries of the abdomen, carpal tunnel repair, biopsies and other procedures where rapid recovery is expected that no more than 3 days of opioids be prescribed. For surgeries expecting a medium duration recovery, no more than 7 days of opioids should be prescribed; and the Center for Disease Control & Prevention (CDC) states that rarely more than 7 days will be required. If exceptional circumstances arise, it is recommended that opioid tapering should take place by 6 weeks postoperative. More extensive surgeries, such as total joint replacement, invasive abdominal surgeries, among others, may require up to 14 days of OT; again, if additional medications are needed, these should be evaluated regularly and tapering commenced within 6 weeks of surgery.[65] Hydrocodone and oxycodone are among the most commonly prescribed opioids in the acute setting and have also been shown to be the most common in opioid-related overdose deaths[66] and patients receiving opioid prescriptions after short-stay surgeries have a 44% increased risk of long-term opioid use,[67] OUD, and overdose.

Chronic Nonmalignant Pain
Osteoarthritis
Results from large studies and systematic reviews examining the effectiveness of opioids are mixed. However, more recent studies, including 2014 systematic review inclusive of 8275 patients who underwent treatment with various nontramadol opioids for osteoarthritis of the hip and knee, found that opioids resulted in small improvements in pain and function scores when compared with placebo. Importantly, it was also noted that these small benefits were decreased further as treatment duration increased to >4 weeks.[68] Given the relatively small improvements in pain and function, lack of evidence via high-quality long-term studies, and concomitant rise in risks of opioid-related complications, opioid use for the treatment of chronic osteoarthritis pain is discouraged.[69,70]

Low back pain
Recommendations and outcomes in the literature for the treatment of chronic low back pain are mixed.[71] Many high-quality reviews have found greater efficacy in the short-term management of low back pain.[72,73] However, opioids have been shown to decrease efficacy over time despite escalating doses due to the development of tolerance.[74] Despite the modest reported benefits in pain control, there is lack of evidence supporting improvement in function and quality of life.[75] Thus,

there is lack of high-quality evidence supporting the use of OT for the treatment of chronic low back pain and thus opioids are not recommended at this time.[76,77]

Headaches
The role of OT in the management of headaches and migraines is controversial. Studies have shown opioids to be efficacious as treatment for acute, severe, refractory headaches.[78] However, the use of chronic opioids has been shown to contribute to medication overuse headaches and may impair prophylactic measures.[79,80] Studies have shown that in select patients with intolerance or contraindications for preferred agents OT may be effective though opioids should be considered as a last resort in the treatment of chronic headaches.[81,82]

Fibromyalgia
Despite previous widespread use, there is no evidence available in the literature to support the use of opioids for the treatment of chronic pain related to fibromyalgia with regard to pain control and function/quality of life. In fact, studies have shown that patients treated with opioids for fibromyalgia have worse outcomes with regard to pain control and risk of dependence and OUD.[83,84]

Opioids in Cancer-Related Pain
Opioid medications are the cornerstone treatment of moderate to severe cancer pain. The World Health Organization (WHO) pain ladder recommends the use of opioids for the management of moderate to severe pain.[85] Morphine is often considered the gold standard given its prolonged history of use despite studies suggesting that morphine may contribute to angiogenesis and metastasis due to immunosuppressive, proinflammatory, and proangiogenetic properties discussed previously.[86] It is recommended that pain medications should be given as scheduled medications for basal pain relief and additional as needed medications for breakthrough pain.

Large studies and systematic reviews have been conducted and support the use of opioids. Oral morphine[87] and transdermal fentanyl in particular have shown to be the most efficacious treatment options with a high percentage of patients reporting only mild pain within 2 weeks of initiation.[88−90] Oxycodone has also been studied extensively and has shown similar efficacy and side effect profiles.[91] Methadone's pharmacokinetics have also been evaluated as an effective treatment options but must be initiated and monitored by experienced physicians due to its long half life, difficulty converting between other opioids, and the concern for QTc prolongation.[92]

Opioids for Neuropathic Pain

The use of opioids for the management of neuropathic pain is controversial due to concerns of efficacy and fear of side effects, dependence, and addiction associated with opioid pain medications. Studies have also shown mixed results, a 2003 study identified opioids as first line for management of neuropathic pain.[93] A 2013 metaanalysis found mixed results with regard to efficacy for short-term management of neuropathic pain; however, when intermediate term studies were assessed, the metaanalysis found that the number of patients in groups achieving at least 33% and at least 50% pain relief, respectively, was higher in the opioid treatment group when compared with placebo. Secondary outcomes including function and quality of life were not significantly different.[94]

Several head to head studies have compared the efficacy of various opioids versus more commonly accepted neuropathic pain agents with relatively few showing superiority to opioids.[95,96] However, as discussed previously, the risk of opioid-related side effects, addiction, and tolerance should weigh heavily on medication choice as neuropathic medications have shown similar efficacy with less side effects and dramatically lower risk of addiction, misuse, and abuse.[97]

Individual studies vary on specific opioid choice. One small study of 18 patients with a variety of neuropathic pain syndromes found that methadone 20 mg daily resulted in statistically significant improvements in pain.[98] Tramadol, a weak opioid agonist and serotonin and norepinephrine reuptake inhibitor, has been shown in several studies to provide effective pain relief.[97] Oxycodone has also been found to be effective in treatment of acute neuropathic pain secondary to herpes zoster.[99]

Overall, the literature varies with regard to recommendations for the use of opioids for neuropathic pain. Fillerup et al. grade the evidence for the use of tramadol and stronger opioids as weak when evaluated using the GRADE criteria and recommend their use as second or third line. Close monitoring is always strongly recommended when opioids are utilized.[97]

OPIOID PRESCRIBING OUTCOMES IN PEDIATRICS

Chronic noncancer pain is defined as pain of 3 months or more in duration from a nonmalignant origin. Such conditions resulting in chronic pain include HIV/AIDS, sickle-cell disease, burns, trauma, and phantom limb pain.[2] Cooper et al. performed a Cochrane review to assess the analgesic efficacy and adverse events of opioids used to treat chronic noncancer pain in children and adolescents aged between birth and 17 years.

Similar to cancer pain in adults, there was no evidence from RCTs to support or refute the use of opioids to treat chronic noncancer pain in children and adolescents.[1] Therefore, no conclusions can be made about efficacy or harm in the use of opioids to treat chronic noncancer pain in children and adolescents. The WHO states that there is no class of medicines other than opioids that is effective in the treatment of moderate and severe pain.[2] Unfortunately, fear and lack of knowledge about the use of opioids in children is often a barrier to the relief of pain. Indirect evidence from adult, chronic, noncancer pain RCTs demonstrates that opioids, such as morphine and codeine, may be beneficial in certain instances. The WHO provides a strong recommendation, with a very low quality of evidence, for morphine as the first-line strong opioid for the treatment of chronic noncancer moderate to severe pain in children. Without robust RCTs to guide opioid use in chronic noncancer pain for the pediatric population, current treatment is based on clinical experience and advice from respected authorities.[100,101]

PEDIATRIC CANCER PAIN OUTCOMES

Pediatric cancer is one of the leading causes of mortality and morbidity for children and adolescents in the world today. Cancer pain in infants, children, and adolescents is primarily nociceptive pain with negative long-term effects. OT is the cornerstone in the management of severe chronic pain in the field of cancer patients. The amount and quality of evidence around the use of opioids for treating cancer pain in the pediatric population is low. Wiffen et al. performed a Cochrane review of those between birth and 17 years of age assessing opioid efficacy and adverse events to treat cancer-related pain. This review found that there are no RCTs with evidence to support or refute the use of opioids to treat cancer-related pain in children and adolescents. Therefore, no conclusions can be drawn about efficacy or harm in the use of opioids to treat cancer-related pain in children and adolescents.[1] Additionally, there are no RTCs, and only one study overall, to assess the management of breakthrough pain in children with cancer. Friedrichsdorf and Postier revealed that younger children (7–12 years of age) had a significantly higher risk of experiencing breakthrough pain compared with teenagers, and the most effective treatment of an episode of breakthrough pain was a patient-controlled analgesia opioid bolus dose in those > 6 years old.[2] This means that, at present, treatment is based on clinical experience and advice from respected authorities.[102,103]

RATIONAL PRESCRIBING

Recognizing chronic pain as a public health crisis, the CDC released guidelines for prescribing opioids for chronic pain to assist providers with clinical decision-making with regard to chronic OT including validated scales for detecting risk for opioid misuse prior to initiation therapy such as the Opioid Risk Tool (ORT),[104] Screener and Opioid Assessment for Patients with Pain (SOAPP-R),[105] and during treatment such as the Current Opioid Misuse Measure (COMM).[106] Guidelines have also been established by the American Society of Interventional Spine Physicians (ASIPP),[107-109] American Academy of Pain Medicine (AAPM), American Pain Society (APS),[110] American Academy of Physical Medicine and Rehabilitation,[111] and the Veterans Affairs (VA)/Department of Defense (DOD)[112] to name a few.

The seriousness of the risks of opioid-related side effects, dependence, addiction, and overdose cannot be overstated. However, as discussed previously, opioids are recommended for the treatment of cancer-related pain. In the setting of noncancer pain if opioids are chosen, it is essential that appropriate patient screening, education, and monitoring are implemented to reduce the risk of severe complications.

PATIENT SELECTION

Before initiation of OT, providers should perform a thorough history and physical examination including assessment of chronic medical conditions, current medications, history of substance abuse, misuse or addiction, pain, functional goals, and any psychological factors. Risks and benefits of OT should be discussed at initial visit and each visit thereafter.[70,107,109,112,113]

INFORMED CONSENT/OPIOID MANAGEMENT PLAN

When starting OT, informed consent should be obtained with each patient and a management plan including realistic goals of therapy, education on opioid administration, requirements/expectations for follow-up, potential indications for tapering/discontinuation of opioids, and termination of controlled substance agreement. It is often considered helpful to have family members and caregivers present for such discussion if patient is agreeable.[108,113-115]

INITIATION AND TITRATION OF CHRONIC OPIOID THERAPY

OT should be initiated at the lowest therapeutic dose and titrated slowly to appropriate response. Specific opioid selection should be individualized, and it is generally accepted that short-acting opioids are probably safer for initial therapy due to their shorter half life and therefore lower theoretical risk of overdose, although there is lack of data in the literature to support short-acting versus long-acting therapy.[115-117] Commonly used first-line opioid agents include hydrocodone, oxycodone, codeine, and tramadol, among others. Dosing intervals should be determined on a case-by-case basis. The CDC guidelines recommend careful reassessment of individual benefits and risks when increasing daily dosage to >50 morphine milligram equivalents (MME)/day and should avoid increasing dosage to > 90 MME/day unless carefully considered after extensive discussion with patients (Tables 16.7 and 16.8).[113,118] Per the VA DOD guidelines, dose escalation beyond 20-50 MME/day has not been shown to improve function.[112]

MONITORING

Prior to each visit, data from respective states prescription drug monitoring program (PDMP) data should be reviewed. Urine testing should be performed at least annually, and should be considered more frequently if there is any concern of diversion or misuse.[119] Ongoing assessment of the risk of opioid-related harms should be explored and appropriate interventions prescribed.[113,114] The next section will discuss recommended monitoring policies in detail.

TAPERING/TREATMENT ENDPOINTS

Determining treatment endpoints for OT are challenging due to the subjectivity of pain rating. Many recommend utilizing function as a more effective gauge of treatment effectiveness as improved pain control should theoretically improve function.[120] Clinicians should continually reassess the risks and benefits of OT and discuss with patients at each visit. When risks are determined to outweigh the benefits, tapering of opioids to reduced dose or discontinuation is recommended. Rate of taper should be determined on an individual basis with the patient. Taper regimens range from dose reductions of 5%-20% every 1-4 weeks. Opioids should be discontinued immediately if there is concern for diversion or misuse of opioid prescriptions.

CLINICAL MONITORING

The use of opioids for pain management has been broadly accepted by regulatory bodies, professional organizations, and practitioners. The magnitude of prescription opioid abuse has grown over the last decade, leading the CDC to classify prescription opioid analgesic abuse as an epidemic.[113] This appears to be due in large part to individuals using a prescription drug nonmedically, most often an opioid analgesic. Drug-induced deaths have rapidly risen and continue to be one of the leading causes of death in Americans. Patients often do not voluntarily report prescription drug misuse or illicit substance use,[129] and some may feign symptoms to obtain opioids for diversion,[130] which necessitates objective assessments such as drug monitoring.[113] Compliance monitoring is viewed as necessary for safe opioid prescribing, and chronic opioid prescribing includes "contracts" or treatment agreements, periodic urine drug monitoring (UDM), and random pill counts.

Over time, multiple guidelines from professional societies and organizations and regulatory bodies have evolved to include standard practices of assessing risk and documenting responsible care in a systematic way. In general, there is agreement that urine drug testing (UDT) is recommended before the initiation of treatment with opioids and during therapy.[129–132] Currently, three main types of UDT are used in clinical settings: immunoassay, gas chromatography-mass spectrometry (GCMS) confirmatory testing, and liquid chromatography-mass spectrometry (LCMS) confirmatory testing. Immunoassay screening is inexpensive, fast, and widely available. It does, however, have a higher potential for false positives and negatives as well as lack of specificity of the actual opiate or benzodiazepine being tested. GCMS is highly sensitive and specific; however, it is expensive and time consuming. LCMS is less expensive than GCMS but more expensive than immunoassay. It can provide confirmation for a large number of medications, substances, and drugs at one time and may be helpful to many patients at initiation of OT, periodically during OT, and following cessation of OT if SUD is a possibility.[132] For those whom are anuric, serum or plasma is an acceptable alternate matrix for the detection of relevant over-the-counter medications, prescribed and nonprescribed drugs, and illicit substances in pain management patients. For dialysis patients, the blood (serum/plasma) should be collected prior to dialysis.[131]

The American Association of Clinical Chemistry (AACC) and American Academy of Pain Medicine (AAPM) cosponsored peer-reviewed guidelines to help providers monitor drug therapy in pain management patients.[131] It is recommended that baseline drug testing be performed prior to initiation of acute or chronic controlled substance therapy. Random drug testing should be performed at a minimum of one to two times a year for low-risk patients (based on history of past substance abuse/addiction, aberrant behaviors, and opioid risk screening criteria), with increased frequency for higher-risk patients prescribed controlled substances.[131]

The American Pain Society and American Academy of Pain Medicine also teamed up to develop the landmark APS/AAPM 2009 Guidelines (http://americanpainsociety.org/uploads/education/guidelines/chronic-opioid-therapy-cncp.pdf accessed 07/14/2017), which include examination of various aspects of UDT and recommend pretreatment and concurrent monitoring of patients. For those on methadone, electrocardiogram (EKG) should be monitored before initiation and 4–7 days after starting methadone and after any dose adjustments and periodically monitor an EKG in those with chronic stable use.[109,133]

Federal regulatory agencies have also developed guidelines and policies that support compliance testing. These include the Veterans Administration/Department of Defense VA/DoD Clinical Practice Guidelines for COT: Management of Opioid Therapy for Chronic Pain, May 2010 (http://www.healthquality.va.gov/guidelines/Pain/cot/COT_312_Full-er.pdf accessed October 07, 2019), which recommends using LCMS confirmatory testing over immunoassay or GCMS confirmatory testing for UDM.

In 2016, the CDC introduced the CDC Guidelines for Prescribing Opioids for Chronic Pain—United States for primary care physicians, which has similar recommendations for opioid prescription monitoring.[113] Random urine drug screening (UDS) is preferred to schedule UDS because patients receive advanced notice with scheduled tests and can therefore plan procedures to defeat the reliability of the tests.

Recently, the Centers for Medicare & Medicaid Services (CMS) released new guidance to states to promote proper use of prescription opioids by updating standard requirements for the Medicaid Drug Utilization Review (DUR) program. This will help states implement drug use review procedures newly required under the Substance Use-Disorder Prevention that Promotes Opioid Recovery and Treatment for Patients and Communities Act (the SUPPORT Act), so state Medicaid programs can better monitor opioid prescribing and dispensing patterns, including new requirements for states to implement electronic notifications, also known as safety edits. The full guideline can be seen at https://www.medicaid.gov/federal-policy-guidance/downloads/cib080519-1004.pdf. All states have specific opioid monitoring guidelines, and clinicians are encouraged to consult the state's PDMP before initiating opioids for pain and during ongoing therapy.

SUMMARY

Opium and its derivatives have been used as analgesics for hundreds of years. The potent analgesic effects of opioid pain medications have made them a popular choice historically for the management of acute and chronic pain. However, recent increases in the number of opioid prescriptions and subsequently the identification of significant side effects, tolerance development, and OUD and potentially catastrophic overdoses have led many to question their utility in the management of chronic pain. Many subsequent studies have found opioids to be a poor choice for the management of chronic noncancer pain and recommend alternative treatments. In the setting of acute pain secondary to trauma or surgical interventions, a short course of opioids is generally sufficient.

When opioid pain medications are prescribed, it is important that careful patient screening both before and during treatment is recommended and includes frequent PDMPs, pain contracts, urine drug screens, and frequent follow-up.

REFERENCES

1. Schiff PL. Opium and its alkaloids. *Am J Pharm Educ.* 2002;66:186−194.
2. Brownstein MJ. A brief history of opiates, opioid peptides, and opioid receptors. *Proc Natl Acad Sci.* 1993. https://doi.org/10.1073/pnas.90.12.5391.
3. Dewick PM. *Medicinal Natural Products: A Biosynthetic Approach.* 3rd ed. 2009. https://doi.org/10.1002/9780470742761.
4. Benyamin R, Trescot AM, Datta S, et al. Opioid complications and side effects. *Pain Physician.* 2008.
5. Hughes J, Smith TW, Kosterlitz HW, Fothergill LA, Morgan BA, Morris HR. Identification of two related pentapeptides from the brain with potent opiate agonist activity. *Nature.* 1975. https://doi.org/10.1038/258577a0.
6. Al-Hasani R, Bruchas MR. Molecular mechanisms of opioid receptor-dependent signaling and behavior. *Anesthesiology.* 2011. https://doi.org/10.1097/ALN.0b013e318238bba6.
7. Mollereau C, Parmentier M, Mailleux P, et al. ORL1, a novel member of the opioid receptor family. Cloning, functional expression and localization. *FEBS Lett.* 1994. https://doi.org/10.1016/0014-5793(94)80235-1.
8. Pathan H, Williams J. Basic opioid pharmacology: an update. *Br J Pain.* 2012. https://doi.org/10.1177/2049463712438493.
9. Dietis N, Rowbotham DJ, Lambert DG. Opioid receptor subtypes: fact or artifact? *Br J Anaesth.* 2011. https://doi.org/10.1093/bja/aer115.
10. Mansour A, Fox CA, Akil H, Watson SJ. Opioid-receptor mRNA expression in the rat CNS: anatomical and functional implications. *Trends Neurosci.* 1995. https://doi.org/10.1016/0166-2236(95)93946-U.
11. Wittert G, Hope P, Pyle D. Tissue distribution of opioid receptor gene expression in the rat. *Biochem Biophys Res Commun.* 1996. https://doi.org/10.1006/bbrc.1996.0156.
12. Besse D, Lombard MC, Zajac JM, Roques BP, Besson JM. Pre- and postsynaptic distribution of μ, δ and κ opioid receptors in the superficial layers of the cervical dorsal horn of the rat spinal cord. *Brain Res.* 1990. https://doi.org/10.1016/0006-8993(90)91519-M.
13. Emmerson PJ, Liu MR, Woods JH, Medzihradsky F. Binding affinity and selectivity of opioids at mu, delta and kappa receptors in monkey brain membranes. *J Pharmacol Exp Therapeut.* 1994;271(3):1630−1637.
14. Bovill JG. Update on opioid and analgesic pharmacology. *Anesth Analg.* 2001. https://doi.org/10.1097/00000539-200103001-00001.
15. Lord JAH, Waterfield AA, Hughes J, Kosterlitz HW. Endogenous opioid peptides: multiple agonists and receptors. *Nature.* 1977. https://doi.org/10.1038/267495a0.
16. Smith HS. Opioid metabolism. *Mayo Clin Proc.* 2009. https://doi.org/10.1016/S0025-6196(11)60750-7.
17. Gudin J. Opioid therapies and cytochrome P450 interactions. *J Pain Symptom Manag.* 2012. https://doi.org/10.1016/j.jpainsymman.2012.08.013.
18. Adams M, Pieniaszek HJ, Gammaitoni AR, Ahdieh H. Oxymorphone extended release does not affect CYP2C9 or CYP3A4 metabolic pathways. *J Clin Pharmacol.* 2005. https://doi.org/10.1177/0091270004271969.
19. Smith HS. The metabolism of opioid agents and the clinical impact of their active metabolites. *Clin J Pain.* 2011. https://doi.org/10.1097/AJP.0b013e31821d8ac1.
20. Lötsch J. Opioid metabolites. *J Pain Symptom Manag.* 2005. https://doi.org/10.1016/j.jpainsymman.2005.01.004.
21. Furlan V, Hafi A, Dessalles MC, Bouchez J, Charpentier B, Taburet AM. Methadone is poorly removed by haemodialysis [17]. *Nephrol Dial Transplant.* 1999. https://doi.org/10.1093/ndt/14.1.254.
22. Joh J, Sila MK, Bastani B. Nondialyzability of fentanyl with high-efficiency and high-flux membranes. *Anesth Analg.* 1998. https://doi.org/10.1097/00000539-199802000-00049.
23. Kumar K, Singh SI. Neuraxial opioid-induced pruritus: an update. *J Anaesthesiol Clin Pharmacol.* 2013;29(3):303−307. https://doi.org/10.4103/0970-9185.117045.
24. Angst MS, Clark JD. Opioid-induced hyperalgesia: a qualitative systematic review. *Anesthesiology.* 2006. https://doi.org/10.1097/00000542-200603000-00025.
25. Joly V, Richebe P, Guignard B, et al. Remifentanil-induced postoperative hyperalgesia and its prevention with small-dose ketamine. *Anesthesiology.* 2005. https://doi.org/10.1097/00000542-200507000-00022.
26. Vorobeychik Y, Chen L, Bush MC, Mao J. Improved opioid analgesic effect following opioid dose

reduction. *Pain Med.* 2008. https://doi.org/10.1111/j.1526-4637.2008.00501.x.

27. Benzon HT, Rathmell JP, Wu CL, Turk DC, Argoff CE. *Raj's Practical Management of Pain.* 2008. https://doi.org/10.1016/B978-0-323-04184-3.X5001-8.

28. Sobczak M, Sałaga M, Storr MA, Fichna J. Physiology, signaling, and pharmacology of opioid receptors and their ligands in the gastrointestinal tract: current concepts and future perspectives. *J Gastroenterol.* 2014. https://doi.org/10.1007/s00535-013-0753-x.

29. Coluzzi F, Pappagallo M. Opioid therapy for chronic noncancer pain: practice guidelines for initiation and maintenance of therapy. *Minerva Anestesiol.* 2005.

30. Herndon CM, Jackson KC, Hallin PA. Management of opioid-induced gastrointestinal effects in patients receiving palliative care. *Pharmacotherapy.* 2002. https://doi.org/10.1592/phco.22.3.240.33552.

31. Mallick-Searle T, Fillman M. The pathophysiology, incidence, impact, and treatment of opioid-induced nausea and vomiting. *J Am Assoc Nurse Pract.* 2017. https://doi.org/10.1002/2327-6924.12532.

32. Kriegler JS. The Massachusetts general hospital handbook of pain management. *Neurology.* 2012. https://doi.org/10.1212/wnl.48.2.560-b.

33. Bruera E, Macmillan K, Hanson J, MacDonald RN. The cognitive effects of the administration of narcotic analgesics in patients with cancer pain. *Pain.* 1989. https://doi.org/10.1016/0304-3959(89)90169-3.

34. Dhingra L, Ahmed E, Shin J, Scharaga E, Magun M. Cognitive effects and sedation. *Pain Med.* 2015. https://doi.org/10.1111/pme.12912.

35. St??len T, Chamari K, Castagna C, Wisl??ff U. Physiology of Soccer. *Sports Med.* 2005. https://doi.org/10.2165/00007256-200535060-00004.

36. Velayudhan A. Opioid-induced hyperalgesia. In: *The Essence of Analgesia Analgesics.* 2010. https://doi.org/10.1017/CBO9780511841378.038.

37. Tompkins DA, Campbell CM. Opioid-induced hyperalgesia: clinically relevant or extraneous research phenomenon? *Curr Pain Headache Rep.* 2011;15(2):129–136. https://doi.org/10.1007/s11916-010-0171-1.

38. Ramasubbu C, Gupta A. Pharmacological treatment of opioid-induced hyperalgesia: a review of the evidence. *J Pain Palliat Care Pharmacother.* 2011. https://doi.org/10.3109/15360288.2011.589490.

39. Odunayo A, Dodam JR, Kerl ME, DeClue AE. Immunomodulatory effects of opioids. *J Vet Emerg Crit Care.* 2010. https://doi.org/10.1111/j.1476-4431.2010.00561.x.

40. Maher DP, Walia D, Heller NM. Suppression of human natural killer cells by different classes of opioids. *Anesth Analg.* 2019;128(5):1013–1021. https://doi.org/10.1213/ANE.0000000000004058.

41. Morgan MM, Christie MJ. Analysis of opioid efficacy, tolerance, addiction and dependence from cell culture to human. *Br J Pharmacol.* 2011;164(4):1322–1334. https://doi.org/10.1111/j.1476-5381.2011.01335.x.

42. Kosten TR, George TP. The neurobiology of opioid dependence: implications for treatment. *Sci Pract Perspect.* 2002;1(1):13–20. http://www.ncbi.nlm.nih.gov/pubmed/18567959.

43. Miech R, Johnston L, O'Malley PM, Keyes KM, Heard K. Prescription opioids in adolescence and future opioid misuse. *Pediatrics.* 2015. https://doi.org/10.1542/peds.2015-1364.

44. Turner BJ, Liang Y. Drug overdose in a retrospective cohort with non-cancer pain treated with opioids, antidepressants, and/or sedative-hypnotics: interactions with mental health disorders. *J Gen Intern Med.* 2015. https://doi.org/10.1007/s11606-015-3199-4.

45. Edlund MJ, Martin BC, Russo JE, Devries A, Braden JB, Sullivan MD. The role of opioid prescription in incident opioid abuse and dependence among individuals with chronic noncancer pain: the role of opioid prescription. *Clin J Pain.* 2014. https://doi.org/10.1097/AJP.0000000000000021.

46. Bohnert ASB, Valenstein M, Bair MJ, et al. Association between opioid prescribing patterns and opioid overdose-related deaths. *J Am Med Assoc.* 2011. https://doi.org/10.1001/jama.2011.370.

47. Earle WJ. DSM-5. *Philos Forum.* 2014. https://doi.org/10.1111/phil.12034.

48. Todd KH. A review of current and emerging approaches to pain management in the emergency department. *Pain Ther.* 2017;6(2):193–202. https://doi.org/10.1007/s40122-017-0090-5.

49. Cisewski DH, Motov SM. Essential pharmacologic options for acute pain management in the emergency setting. *Turkish J Emerg Med.* 2019;19(1):1–11. https://doi.org/10.1016/j.tjem.2018.11.003.

50. Chang AK, Bijur PE, Esses D, Barnaby DP, Baer J. Effect of a single dose of oral opioid and nonopioid analgesics on acute extremity pain in the emergency department: a randomized clinical trial. *J Am Med Assoc.* 2017. https://doi.org/10.1001/jama.2017.16190.

51. Friedman BW, Dym AA, Davitt M, et al. Naproxen with cyclobenzaprine, oxycodone/acetaminophen, or placebo for treating acute low back pain: a randomized clinical trial. *J Am Med Assoc.* 2015;314(15):1572–1580. https://doi.org/10.1001/jama.2015.13043.

52. Pathan SA, Mitra B, Cameron PA. A systematic review and meta-analysis comparing the efficacy of nonsteroidal anti-inflammatory drugs, opioids, and paracetamol in the treatment of acute renal colic. *Eur Urol.* 2018. https://doi.org/10.1016/j.eururo.2017.11.001.

53. Basurto Ona X, Rigau Comas D, Urrútia G. Opioids for acute pancreatitis pain. *Cochrane Database Syst Rev.* 2013. https://doi.org/10.1002/14651858.CD009179.pub2.

54. Lovett PB, Sule HP, Lopez BL. Sickle cell disease in the emergency department. *Hematol Oncol Clin N Am.* 2017. https://doi.org/10.1016/j.hoc.2017.08.009.

55. Pavlin DJ, Chen C, Penaloza DA, Polissar NL, Buckley FP. Pain as a factor complicating recovery and discharge after

ambulatory surgery. *Anesth Analg.* 2002. https://doi.org/10.1213/00000539-200209000-00025.

56. Wu CL, Naqibuddin M, Rowlingson AJ, Lietman SA, Jermyn RM, Fleisher LA. The effect of pain on health-related quality of life in the immediate postoperative period. *Anesth Analg.* 2003. https://doi.org/10.1213/01.ANE.0000081722.09164.D5.

57. Lovich-Sapola J, Smith CE, Brandt CP. Postoperative pain control. *Surg Clin N Am.* 2015. https://doi.org/10.1016/j.suc.2014.10.002.

58. Brummett CM, Waljee JF, Goesling J, et al. New persistent opioid use after minor and major surgical procedures in us adults. *JAMA Surg.* 2017. https://doi.org/10.1001/jamasurg.2017.0504.

59. Wu CL, Raja SN. Treatment of acute postoperative pain. *Lancet.* 2011. https://doi.org/10.1016/S0140-6736(11)60245-6.

60. Kehlet H, Wilmore DW. Evidence-based surgical care and the evolution of fast-track surgery. *Ann Surg.* 2008. https://doi.org/10.1097/SLA.0b013e31817f2c1a.

61. Lamplot JD, Wagner ER, Manning DW. Multimodal pain management in total knee arthroplasty. a prospective randomized controlled trial. *J Arthroplasty.* 2014. https://doi.org/10.1016/j.arth.2013.06.005.

62. Cheung CW, Wong SSC, Qiu Q, Wang X. Oral oxycodone for acute postoperative pain: a review of clinical trials. *Pain Physician.* 2017.

63. Han B, Compton WM, Blanco C, Crane E, Lee J, Jones CM. Prescription opioid use, misuse, and use disorders in U.S. adults: 2015 national survey on drug use and health. *Ann Intern Med.* 2017. https://doi.org/10.7326/M17-0865.

64. Hill MV, Mcmahon ML, Stucke RS, Barth RJ. Wide variation and excessive dosage of opioid prescriptions for common general surgical procedures. *Ann Surg.* 2017. https://doi.org/10.1097/SLA.0000000000001993.

65. Scully RE, Schoenfeld AJ, Jiang W, et al. Defining optimal length of opioid pain medication prescription after common surgical procedures. *JAMA Surg.* 2018. https://doi.org/10.1001/jamasurg.2017.3132.

66. Rudd RA, Aleshire N, Zibbell JE, Gladden RM. Increases in drug and opioid overdose deaths — United States, 2000—2014. *Morb Mortal Wkly Rep.* 2015. https://doi.org/10.15585/mmwr.mm6450a3.

67. Alam A, Gomes T, Zheng H, Mamdani MM, Juurlink DN, Bell CM. Long-term analgesic use after low-risk surgery: a retrospective cohort study. *Arch Intern Med.* 2012. https://doi.org/10.1001/archinternmed.2011.1827.

68. da Costa B, Nuesch E, Kasteler R, et al. Oral or transdermal opiods for osteoarthritis of the knee or hip (review). *Cochrane Database Syst Rev.* 2014.

69. Chou R, Turner JA, Devine EB, et al. The effectiveness and risks of long-term opioid therapy for chronic pain: a systematic review for a national institutes of health pathways to prevention workshop. *Ann Intern Med.* 2015. https://doi.org/10.7326/M14-2559.

70. Evidence D, Practice B. Clinical practice guideline management of opioid therapy for chronic pain VA/DoD evidence based practice. *Management.* 2010.

71. Deyo RA, Von Korff M, Duhrkoop D. Opioids for low back pain. *BMJ.* 2015. https://doi.org/10.1136/bmj.g6380.

72. Chaparro LE, Furlan AD, Deshpande A, Mailis-Gagnon A, Atlas S, Turk DC. Opioids compared to placebo or other treatments for chronic low-back pain. *Cochrane Database Syst Rev.* 2013. https://doi.org/10.1002/14651858.CD004959.pub4.

73. Chou R, Huffman LH, American Pain Society, American College of Physicians. Medications for acute and chronic low back pain: a review of the evidence for an American Pain Society/American College of Physicians Clinical Practice Guideline. *Ann Intern Med.* 2007;147(7):505—514. https://doi.org/10.7326/0003-4819-147-7-200710020-00008.

74. Ballantyne JC, Shin NS. Efficacy of opioids for chronic pain: a review of the evidence. *Clin J Pain.* 2008. https://doi.org/10.1097/AJP.0b013e31816b2f26.

75. Eriksen J, Sjøgren P, Bruera E, Ekholm O, Rasmussen NK. Critical issues on opioids in chronic non-cancer pain: an epidemiological study. *Pain.* 2006. https://doi.org/10.1016/j.pain.2006.06.009.

76. Shaheed CA, Mathieson S, Day RO, et al. What is the evidence for opioid analgesia for low back pain? *Med Today.* 2017.

77. Waljee JF, Brummett CM. Opioid prescribing for low back pain: what is the role of payers? *JAMA Netw open.* 2018. https://doi.org/10.1001/jamanetworkopen.2018.0236.

78. Von Seggern RL, Adelman JU. Oral narcotic protocol to reduce narcotic injections in refractory migraine patients. *Headache.* 1997. https://doi.org/10.1046/j.1526-4610.1997.3706341.x.

79. IHS (Headache Classification Committee of the International Headache Society). The International Classification of Headache Disorders, 3rd edition. *Cephalalgia.* 2018. https://doi.org/10.1177/0333102417738202.

80. Mathew NT. Transformed migraine, analgesic rebound, and other chronic daily headaches. *Neurol Clin.* 1997. https://doi.org/10.1016/S0733-8619(05)70302-9.

81. Saper JR, Lake AE, Hamel RL, et al. Daily scheduled opioids for intractable head pain: long term observations of a treatment program. *Neurology.* 2004. https://doi.org/10.1212/01.WNL.0000125189.17830.02.

82. Saper JR, Lake AE. Continuous opioid therapy (COT) is rarely advisable for refractory chronic daily headache: limited efficacy, risks, and proposed guidelines. *Headache.* 2008. https://doi.org/10.1111/j.1526-4610.2008.01153.x.

83. Goldenberg DL, Clauw DJ, Palmer RE, Clair AG. Opioid use in fibromyalgia a cautionary tale. *Mayo Clin Proc.* 2016. https://doi.org/10.1016/j.mayocp.2016.02.002.

84. Borchers AT, Gershwin ME. Fibromyalgia: acritical and comprehensive review. *Clin Rev Allergy Immunol.* 2015. https://doi.org/10.1007/s12016-015-8509-4.

85. WHO. *WHO's Cancer Pain Ladder for Adults*. World Health Organanisation; 2016.

86. Grandhi RK, Lee S, Abd-Elsayed A. Does opioid use cause angiogenesis and metastasis? *Pain Med*. 2017. https://doi.org/10.1093/pm/pnw132.

87. Klepstad P, Kaasa S, Borchgrevink PC. Start of oral morphine to cancer patients: effective serum morphine concentrations and contribution from morphine-6-glucuronide to the analgesia produced by morphine. *Eur J Clin Pharmacol*. 2000. https://doi.org/10.1007/s002280050003.

88. Wiffen PJ, Wee B, Moore RA. Oral morphine for cancer pain. *Cochrane Database Syst Rev*. 2016. https://doi.org/10.1002/14651858.CD003868.pub4.

89. Hadley G, Derry S, Moore RA, Wiffen PJ. Transdermal fentanyl for cancer pain. *Cochrane Database Syst Rev*. 2013;10:CD010270. https://doi.org/10.1002/14651858.CD010270.pub2.

90. Moore RA, Straube S, Aldington D. Pain measures and cut-offs - "no worse than mild pain" as a simple, universal outcome. *Anaesthesia*. 2013. https://doi.org/10.1111/anae.12148.

91. Schmidt-Hansen M, Bennett MI, Arnold S, Bromham N, Hilgart JS. Oxycodone for cancer-related pain. *Cochrane Database Syst Rev*. 2017. https://doi.org/10.1002/14651858.CD003870.pub6.

92. Bao YJ, Hou W, Kong XY, et al. Hydromorphone for cancer pain. *Cochrane Database Syst Rev*. 2016. https://doi.org/10.1002/14651858.CD011108.pub2.

93. Dworkin RH, Backonja M, Rowbotham MC, et al. Advances in neuropathic pain: diagnosis, mechanisms, and treatment recommendations. *Arch Neurol*. 2003. https://doi.org/10.1001/archneur.60.11.1524.

94. McNicol ED, Midbari A, Eisenberg E. Opioids for neuropathic pain. *Cochrane Database Syst Rev*. 2013;8:CD006146. https://doi.org/10.1002/14651858.CD006146.pub2.

95. Zin CS, Nissen LM, O'Callaghan JP, Duffull SB, Smith MT, Moore BJ. A randomized, controlled trial of oxycodone versus placebo in patients with PostHerpetic neuralgia and painful diabetic neuropathy treated with pregabalin. *J Pain*. 2010. https://doi.org/10.1016/j.jpain.2009.09.003.

96. Raja SN, Wu CL, Agarwal S, et al. Morphine versus mexiletine for treatment of postamputation pain: a randomized, placebo-controlled, crossover trial. *Anesthesiology*. 2008. https://doi.org/10.1097/ALN.0b013e31817f4523.

97. Finnerup NB, Attal N, Haroutounian S, et al. Pharmacotherapy for neuropathic pain in adults: systematic review, meta-analysis and updated NeuPSig recommendations. *Lancet Neurol*. 2015. https://doi.org/10.1016/S1474-4422(14)70251-0.

98. Morley JS, Bridson J, Nash TP, Miles JB, White S, Makin MK. Low-dose methadone has an analgesic effect in neuropathic pain: a double-blind randomized controlled crossover trial. *Palliat Med*. 2003. https://doi.org/10.1191/0269216303pm815oa.

99. Dworkin RH, Barbano RL, Tyring SK, et al. A randomized, placebo-controlled trial of oxycodone and of gabapentin for acute pain in herpes zoster. *Pain*. 2009. https://doi.org/10.1016/j.pain.2008.12.022.

100. Cooper TE, Fisher E, Gray AL, et al. Opioids for chronic non-cancer pain in children and adolescents. *Cochrane Database Syst Rev*. 2017. https://doi.org/10.1002/14651858.CD012538.pub2.

101. World Health Organisation (WHO). *Guidelines on the Pharmacological Treatment of Persisting Pain in Children with Medical Illnesses*. 2012.

102. Wiffen PJ, Cooper TE, Anderson AK, et al. Opioids for cancer-related pain in children and adolescents. *Cochrane Database Syst Rev*. 2017. https://doi.org/10.1002/14651858.CD012564.

103. Friedrichsdorf SJ, Postier A. Management of breakthrough pain in children with cancer. *J Pain Res*. 2014. https://doi.org/10.2147/JPR.S58862.

104. Institute on Drug Abuse N. Opioid risk Tool. *Pain Med*. 2005.

105. Butler SF, Fernandez K, Benoit C, Budman SH, Jamison RN. Validation of the revised screener and opioid assessment for patients with pain (SOAPP-R). *J Pain*. 2008. https://doi.org/10.1016/j.jpain.2007.11.014.

106. Current T, Misuse O, Comm T, et al. *Current Opioid Misuse Measure (COMM)* [TM]. 2008. Heal (San Fr).

107. Trescot AM, Helm S, Hansen H, et al. Opioids in the management of chronic non-cancer pain: an update of American society of the interventional pain physicians' (ASIPP) guidelines. *Pain Physician*. 2008.

108. Manchikanti L, Abdi S, Atluri S, et al. American Society of Interventional Pain Physicians (ASIPP) guidelines for responsible opioid prescribing in chronic non-cancer pain: Part 2—guidance. *Pain Physician*. 2012.

109. Manchikanti L, Kaye AM, Knezevic NN, et al. Responsible, safe, and effective prescription of opioids for chronic non-cancer pain: American Society Of Interventional Pain Physicians (ASIPP) Guidelines. *Pain Physician*. 2017.

110. Chou R. 2009 Clinical Guidelines from the American Pain Society and the American Academy of Pain Medicine on the use of chronic opioid therapy in chronic non-cancer pain: what are the key messages for clinical practice? *Pol Arch Med Wewn*. 2009.

111. Shaw E, Braza DW, Cheng DS, et al. American academy of physical medicine and rehabilitation position statement on opioid prescribing. *PM R*. 2018. https://doi.org/10.1016/j.pmrj.2018.05.004.

112. Rosenberg JM, Bilka BM, Wilson SM, Spevak C. Opioid therapy for chronic pain: overview of the 2017 us department of veterans affairs and us department of defense clinical practice guideline. *Pain Med*. 2018. https://doi.org/10.1093/pm/pnx203.

113. Dowell D, Haegerich TM, Chou R. CDC guideline for prescribing opioids for chronic pain-United States, 2016. *J Am Med Assoc*. 2016. https://doi.org/10.1001/jama.2016.1464.

114. Chou R, Fanciullo GJ, Fine PG, et al. Clinical guidelines for the use of chronic opioid therapy in chronic non-cancer pain. *J Pain*. 2009. https://doi.org/10.1016/j.jpain.2008.10.008.

115. Gourlay DL, Heit HA, Almahrezi A. Universal precautions in pain medicine: a rational approach to the treatment of chronic pain. *Pain Med.* 2005. https://doi.org/10.1111/j.1526-4637.2005.05031.x.

116. Wilson PR. Responsible opioid prescribing. A clinician's guide, second edition revised &expanded. *Pain Med.* 2015. https://doi.org/10.1111/pme.12711.

117. Chou R, Clark E, Helfand M. Comparative efficacy and safety of long-acting oral opioids for chronic non-cancer pain: a systematic review. *J Pain Symptom Manag.* 2003;26(5):1026–1048. http://www.ncbi.nlm.nih.gov/pubmed/14585554.

118. Cdc. *Drug Overdose in the United States: Fact Sheet.* Centers for Disease Control Prevention; 2013.

119. Owen GT, Burton AW, Schade CM, Passik S. Urine drug testing: current recommendations and best practices. *Pain Physician.* 2012.

120. Model policy for the use of controlled substances for the treatment of pain. *J Pain Palliat Care Pharmacother.* 2008. https://doi.org/10.1300/j354v19n02_14.

121. Grond S, Sablotzki A. Clinical pharmacology of tramadol. *Clin Pharmacokinet.* 2004. https://doi.org/10.2165/00003088-200443130-00004.

122. Inturrisi CE, Jamison RN. Clinical pharmacology of opioids for pain. *Clin J Pain.* 2002. https://doi.org/10.1097/00002508-200207001-00002.

123. Franceschi F, Iacomini P, Marsiliani D, et al. Safety and efficacy of the combination acetaminophen-codeine in the treatment of pain of different origin. *Eur Rev Med Pharmacol Sci.* 2013.

124. Bravo L, Mico JA, Berrocoso E. Discovery and development of tramadol for the treatment of pain. *Expet Opin Drug Discov.* 2017. https://doi.org/10.1080/17460441.2017.1377697.

125. *Medicare C for M and. Opioid Oral Morphine Milligram Equivalent (MME) Conversion Factors.*

126. Singh D, Nag K, Shetti A, Krishnaveni N. Tapentadol hydrochloride: a novel analgesic. *Saudi J Anaesth.* 2013. https://doi.org/10.4103/1658-354x.115319.

127. Patanwala AE, Keim SM, Erstad BL. Intravenous opioids for severe acute pain in the emergency department. *Ann Pharmacother.* 2010. https://doi.org/10.1345/aph.1P438.

128. Barr J, Fraser GL, Puntillo K, et al. Clinical practice guidelines for the management of pain, agitation, and delirium in adult patients in the intensive care unit: executive summary. *Am J Health Pharm.* 2013.

129. Matteliano D, Chang YP. Describing prescription opioid adherence among individuals with chronic pain using urine drug testing. *Pain Manag Nurs.* 2015. https://doi.org/10.1016/j.pmn.2014.04.001.

130. Argoff CE, Alford DP, Fudin J, et al. Rational urine drug monitoring in patients receiving opioids for chronic pain: consensus recommendations. *Pain Med.* 2018. https://doi.org/10.1093/pm/pnx285.

131. Jannetto PJ, Langman LJ. Using clinical laboratory tests to monitor drug therapy in pain management patients. *J Appl Lab Med.* 2018. https://doi.org/10.1373/jalm.2017.025304.

132. Department of Veterans Affairs, Veterans Administration, Department of Defense. *VA/DoD Clinical Practice Guidelines for COT: Management of Opioid Therapy for Chronic Pain.* 2017.

133. Alinejad S, Kazemi T, Zamani N, Hoffman RS, Mehrpour O. A systematic review of the cardiotoxicity of methadone. *EXCLI J.* 2015. https://doi.org/10.17179/excli2014-553.

CHAPTER 17

Regenerative Medicine

GEORGE C. CHANG CHIEN, DO • AGNES STOGICZA, MD

Regenerative medicine (RM) encompasses an emerging field of medicine with the goal of replacing, engineering, or regenerating human cells, tissues, or organs lost or injured due to age, disease, or congenital defects to restore or establish normal function. Researcher scientists and medical practitioners are attempting to create new interventions to treat a variety of diseases that address every system in the body and treat chronic diseases such as diabetes, stroke, macular degeneration, congestive heart failure, and osteoarthritis. This chapter discusses the use of RM in the treatment of acute and chronic pain from painful musculoskeletal conditions.

RM therapies in the treatment of musculoskeletal conditions focus on promoting the body's innate healing capacity. Interventions include using prolotherapy principles to inject concentrated dextrose, platelet-rich plasma (PRP) injections, and adipose or bone marrow-derived stem cells. Significant evidence exists for the use of RM in the treatment of osteoarthritis, tendinopathy, and ligamentous pathology.[1−11] Importantly, the use of RM techniques is a shift in the treatment away from conventional destructive techniques such as corticosteroid and local anesthetic injections, and neurolysis. Numerous studies support that local anesthetic, corticosteroids, and contrast agents have deleterious effects on soft tissues including chondrocytes and tenocytes, the cells that constitute cartilage and tendons.[12−20]

While RM has capacity for healing various musculoskeletal disorders, it is important to recognize the limitations of these modalities and select patients and pathology that will best respond to these various techniques. Although RM is generally most effective for mild-to-moderate disease, some studies have demonstrated success with more severe disease states.[7,9,10,21] Even so, surgical management or alternative ablative techniques may be more appropriate for complete tears or end-stage, grade 4 osteoarthritis, and thus, preprocedural patient selection is key to intervention success. Additional patient characteristics that would impair the body's ability to heal or degrade its regenerative capacity include smoking cigarettes, uncontrolled blood glucose, immunosuppressed states, or active infections. Areas that lack adequate blood supply, such as eschars, avascular or necrotic limbs, are also unlikely to respond to RM techniques given their poor capacity to receive and utilize the necessary elements for healing.

THE HEALING CASCADE

The healing cascade lays the framework for RM and occurs over the course of weeks, with final tissue remodeling taking potentially many months before restoration of full tissue strength and integrity. Healing involves many of the same activating signals and growth factors released by platelets during degranulation. The process of wound healing can be subdivided into inflammation, proliferation, and maturation stages.

Differing models of the cascade may separate out the process of hemostasis (coagulation) as occurring to prior to the inflammation stage, while others include it. Despite the taxonomical variance, the entire process occurs as part of the spectrum of healing. After the formation of a fibrin mesh and a clot, cytokines and growth factors previously released during platelet degranulation stimulate the complement cascade and recruit leukocytes (primarily neutrophils), macrophages, and fibroblasts to the injured area. Local histamine release leads to increased capillary permeability via vasodilation and leakage, allowing migration of mesenchymal stem cells (MSCs) to the site. Neutrophils then lead the process of decontamination through bacterial lysis and scavenging of cellular debris. Monocytes previously activated by platelet growth factors also migrate to the area and may differentiate into macrophages. These macrophages play various important roles: bacterial phagocytosis, cytokine and collagenase secretion for tissue remodeling, and secretion of growth factors that contribute toward angiogenesis and formation of granulation tissue. Among the factors secreted by macrophages are many that are associated with bone repair, such as interleukins (ILs), tumor necrosis factor alpha (TNF-α), transforming growth factor beta (TGF-β), platelet-derived growth factor (PDGF), epidermal growth factor (EGF), and vascular endothelial growth factor (VEGF).[7,22]

The proliferation stage then begins with epithelialization by migratory epithelial progenitor cells as well as epithelial cells from the wound periphery. Angiogenesis takes place under the signals from previously released platelet growth factors. Fibroblasts drive the production of granulation tissue and collagen deposition around 4 days after an injury. MSCs are integral in coordinating the healing response, but can also be activated to begin differentiation down chondrogenic, osteogenic, or angiogenic pathways.[22]

During the final maturation or remodeling stage, a wound contract as collagen continues to be deposited by fibroblasts, granulation tissue compresses into smaller and newly formed scar tissue, and the strength of this new wound increases. This process is also driven by various growth factors that were present for the previous steps. Overall, while it is easier to comprehend all these steps linearly, in reality many of them overlap and occur simultaneously providing an onslaught of regeneration and remodeling.[22]

PROLOTHERAPY

Proliferant solutions vary in the mechanism by which they cause localized inflammation but, in general, they all act by causing localized tissue trauma or irritation which initiates an inflammatory response. Various injectates include osmotics (dextrose, glycerin), chemotactics (sodium morrhuate) neurolytics (phenol, dextrose), local irritants, and particulates (guaiacol, tannic acid, pumice), with the most commonly used solution being dextrose 15%–25%.

Dextrose 15%–25% is a hyperosmolar shock agent, which results in shrinking of the cell, lipid leakage, thus inflammation. Some cell death also occurs. This leads to the release of various cellular parts, proteins, and membrane fragments which are attractive for

granulocytes and macrophages, leading to stimulation of the healing cascade. Furthermore, the injection itself—especially with the "peppering technique"—causes tissue trauma, platelets activation, with release of bioactive cytokines and growth factors involved in the healing process.

The treatment regimen typically includes a series of injections to treat one injury. Many of the injection targets were traditionally described and injected based on landmark-guided technique. Some superficial structures-like supraspinous ligaments are still best targeted based on palpation; however, with the availability imaging, deeper anatomical structures are also precisely and safely injected with US or fluoroscopy guidance.[23]

PLATELET-RICH PLASMA

PRP is an autologous blood product defined as a volume of plasma that has a supraphysiologic platelet count. These platelets contain over 30 biologically active growth factors stored in alpha granules. Thus, increased platelet count is an ad hoc measurement of growth factor concentration which can be delivered to damaged tissues to promote healing. Growth factors include VEGF, PDGF, TGF, platelet-derived angiogenesis factor, epidermal growth factor (EGF), fibroblast growth factor, and connective tissue growth factor. PRP has been used for various indications including optimizing orthopedic and spine surgical outcomes, dentistry, wound care, tightening of the skin, and even hair growth. Factors that are important in the PRP extraction process include purity (reducing the red blood cells and white blood cells), concentration factor, and total amount of blood collected. The total amount of blood collected will directly correlate with the resultant total amount of platelets in your PRP fraction.[7–11]

Recent studies have demonstrated that higher platelet concentrations are ideal to promote healing of soft tissue. According to our current understanding, the ideal platelet concentration for tissue repair is 5–10× baseline, 1.5–3 million/μL.[23]

STEM CELLS

Stem cells are unspecialized cells distinguished by two unique characteristics: 1) they are capable of self-renewal through division and 2) under certain physiologic or experimental conditions, they can be nduced to become tissue- or organ-specific cells. Most organ systems of the body have a resident pool of somatic, tissue-specific stem cells, in many cases of traumatic injury or disease, the quantity and potency of endogenous stem cell populations are insufficient to regenerate compromised tissues.[24,25]

Embryonic stem cells (ESCs) are stem cells derived from the undifferentiated inner mass cells of a human embryo. ESCs are pluripotent, meaning they are able to grow (i.e., differentiate) into all derivatives of the three primary germ layers: ectoderm, endoderm, and mesoderm. These are currently only used for research purposes.[24–27]

MSCs have a narrower range of potential and can differentiate into a variety of cell types, including osteoblasts, chondrocytes, myocytes, and adipocytes. MSCs can be derived from a variety of sources, though the primary sites of extraction have been bone marrow and adipose tissue. Stem cells, in general are relatively scarce; they can be difficult to isolate; grow slowly; and do not differentiate well without appropriate peripheral cytokines. It can be further difficult to isolate sufficient amounts required for therapy, which is worse depending on the source.[24–27]

The therapeutic activity of MSCs is mediated by paracrine effects. Whereas the common misconception is that the stem cells will identify injured tissues and differentiate directly into those tissues by engraftment, it has been demonstrated that less than 1% of stem cells injected remain after as little as 7 days. MSCs respond to injured tissues and can coordinate a healing response via secretion of bioactive molecules, such as Ang-1, Ang-2, BMP, BDNF, IL-6, and VEGF.[24–27]

OSTEOARTHRITIS

A growing body of evidence has accumulated examining PRP and prolotherapy as a treatment of knee OA. Several studies now have demonstrated that intraarticular PRP injections are a safe and effective treatment to reduce pain and improve quality of life through increased function. The autologous nature of PRP and autologous stem cells theoretically reduces the risk of potential side effect associated with alternative injectates such as corticosteroids and hyaluronic acid (HA). A systematic review of all the studies comparing PRP to HA identified 12 studies, 10 of which were prospective randomized controlled studies, which found PRP to be superior to HA in reduction of pain, as well as demonstrating an improvement in functional outcome measures.[7]

Prolotherapy targets include knee stabilizing ligaments and intraarticular injections. Systematic review of 3 high quality RCTs, a total of 258 patients proved prolotherapy beneficial at 24 weeks, with one study following the patients up to a year and confirmed similarly better WOMAC and VAS scores.[28–33]

Dextrose prolotherapy has been also shown to benefit temporomandibular joint hypermobility and associated pain.[34]

TENDINOPATHY

Tendinopathies are the various conditions associated with tendon pain primarily caused by overuse. Tendinopathy is associated with histopathologic changes such as minimal inflammation, degeneration and disorganization of collagen fibers, and increased cellularity. Macroscopic changes include pain, tendon thickening, and the loss of structural integrity. Tendon overuse leads to an imbalance between the protective/regenerative changes of the tissue and pathologic responses from overuse, which results in pain, tearing, weakness, and degeneration. Tendons act as an interface between muscles and the skeletal structures. When tendons are exposed to supramaximal loading, injury occurs. A tendons' intrinsic low metabolic rate may also lead to delayed wound healing when injury does occur.[35–46]

With age, changes in collagen structure, such as a loss of water content, predispose tendons to damage. Vascularity also decreases with age, and tendon disease often occurs at these hypovascular areas. Instability or impingement leads to abnormal and excessive loading of the tendon which predisposes to injury. Collagen fibrils can rupture and these regions may together form intrasubstance tears. These intrasubstance tears may extend to the surface, eventually progressing to full thickness tears. Generally, degenerative changes occur before macroscopic tendon tears develop and as such, it is unusual for a tear to occur in a nondegenerated tendon.[35–47]

Level 1 evidence supports the use of PRP in the treatment of lateral epicondylopathy of the elbow (Tennis elbow) with superiority in pain relief and functional outcomes to corticosteroids up to 24-month follow-up. Evidence also supports the use of RM in the treatment of Achilles, patellar, and hamstring tendinopathy.[35–47]

LIGAMENT PATHOLOGY

Ligaments are dense connective tissue that connect bone to bone and provide stabilization to a joint. Though ligaments are functionally different from tendons as they connect bone to bone, they are structurally similar. The main differences are that ligaments have higher proteoglycan content, higher water content, lower in collagen content, and are less uniform. These structures are typically injured with supraphysiologic stretching, at the end range of motion for a joint. Acute trauma typically causes ligament abnormalities and is often marked by fluid surrounding the ligament, although chronic repetitive microtrauma may be a factor as with tendon injuries. Potential damage includes interstitial tearing of collagen fibers, partial tears that extend to the surface, and full thickness ligament ruptures. Over time, the ligament can become elongated and lax. Other evidence of injuries includes bone contusions, fractures, or joint effusion. After healing, the ligament may appear thickened, weakened, and prone to further damage. Common examples include the anterior talofibular ligament in ankle sprains and anterior cruciate ligament in knee injuries. There are limited studies investigating RM for ligamentous injuries, but there is evidence that PRP may promote the success rate of ACL repairs and provide pain relief in plantar fasciitis superior to corticosteroid.[44,45] Prolotherapy has been successfully used for sacroiliac joint related pain, low back pain, and coccydynia.[46–50]

ADJUNCT MEDICATIONS

Local anesthetics, corticosteroids, and contrast agents are routinely used during interventional orthopedic and pain management procedures for both diagnostic and therapeutic purposes. A growing body of literature suggests that these routinely used injectates promote catabolic processes including apoptosis which are thought to accelerate the disease process. It is therefore paramount to understand the effect of these agents on RM injectates, and on target tissues including tenocytes, chondrocytes, nucleus pulposus, and ligamentous tissue. Numerous studies have shown time- and dose-dependent chondrotoxicity of local anesthetics on

human and animal soft tissues, with ropivacain likely being the least toxic offender.[12–19]

Contrast agents are considered necessary for som procedures to confirm safe and accurate needle place ment. The use of contrast agents can be avoided b' basing accurate needle placement on radiographi imaging or utilizing alternative image guidance suc as ultrasound. Contrast agents exerted chondrotoxi effects in a dose- and type-dependent manner wit ionic contrasts being most detrimental. Nonioni demonstrated mild dose-dependent chondrotoxicit and were the least harmful of those studied.[51–53]

CONCLUSION

RM is an emerging field of medicine that demonstrate Level 1 evidence in the treatment of common musculo skeletal diseases. Further research is necessary t elucidate the parameters that optimize outcomes including patient selection, pre- and postinjectio protocols, and procurement of RM injectate.

High Yield Points

RM encompasses an emerging field medicine with th goal of replacing, engineering, or regenerating huma cells, tissues, or organs lost or injured due to age, dis ease, or congenital defects to restore or establish normal function.

Dextrose prolotherapy creates tissue injury an with that initiates the healing cascade, PRP itself i the start of the healing cascade with the degranulatio of the platelets. This inflammatory response by prolo therapy or PRP also attracts MSCs to further synchro nize healing, while there is also an option to directl inject MSCs with PRP acquired from bone marrow concentrate. Fig. 17.1.

PRP is an autologous blood product that concen trates platelets, which contain over 30 biologically active growth factors stored in alpha granules.

MSCs can be derived from a variety of sources though the primary sites of extraction have been bon marrow and adipose tissue.

Prolotherapy uses concentrated dextrose solutior and has Level 1 evidence for knee OA (Figs. 17.2–17.4)

Level 1 evidence supports the use of PRP in the treat ment of knee osteoarthritis and lateral epicondylopathy (Tennis elbow).

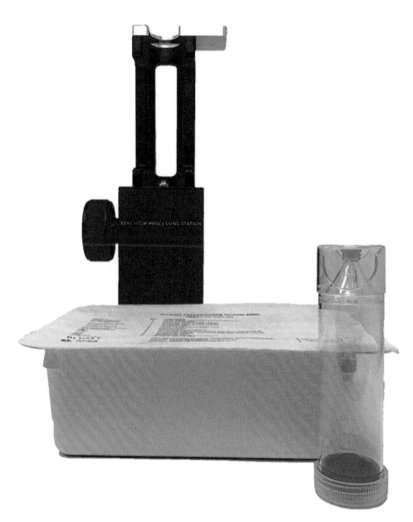

FIG. 17.1 Platelet-rich plasma (PRP) centrifugation system. The PRP collecting device is shown on the bottom right. The benchtop press used to extract the blood fractions is in the background of the image.

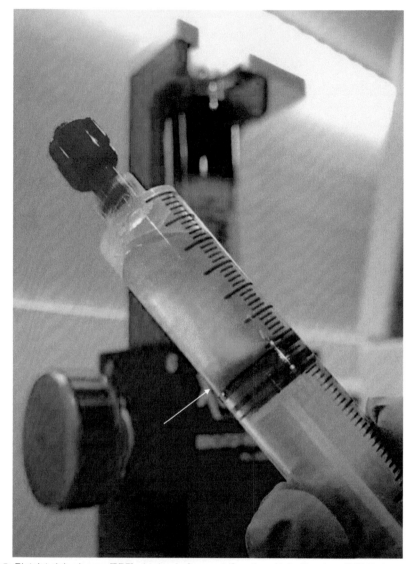

FIG. 17.2 Platelet-rich plasma (PRP) obtained after centrifugation. Note the clear PRP that was separated from red blood cell contaminant. The buffy coat (*white arrow*) which contains white blood cells and platelets is noticeable along the bottom portion of the syringe.

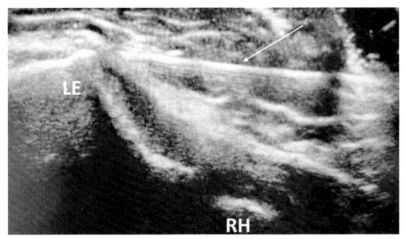

FIG. 17.3 Treatment of the common extensor tendon with platelet-rich plasma. Note the needle (*white arrow*) entry point through a gel bridge in the long axis parallel to the fibers of the tendon. The needle approaches the insertion point onto the most prominent point of the lateral epicondyle (LE) to treat the enthesopathy. *RH*, radial head.

REGENERATIVE MEDICINE & HEALING

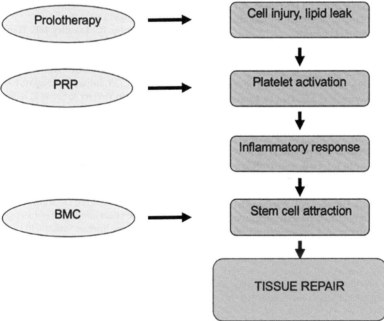

FIG. 17.4 Various regenerative medicine injectates feed into the healing cascade, initiating and resulting in tissue repair. *BMC*, bone marrow concentrate; *PRP*, platelet-rich plasma.

REFERENCES

1. Berdis AS, Veale K, Fleissner Jr PR. Outcomes of anterior cruciate ligament reconstruction using biologic augmentation in patients 21 Years of age and younger. *Arthroscopy.* 2019;35(11):3107–3113. https://doi.org/10.1016/j.arthro.2019.05.047.

2. Davenport KL, Campos JS, Nguyen J, Saboeiro G, Adler RS, Moley PJ. Ultrasound-guided intratendinous injections with platelet-rich plasma or autologous whole blood for treatment of proximal hamstring tendinopathy: a double-blind randomized controlled trial. *J Ultrasound Med.* 2015;34(8):1455–1463.

3. A Hamid MS, Mohamed Ali MR, Yusof A, George J, Lee LP. Platelet-rich plasma injections for the treatment of hamstring injuries: a randomized controlled trial. *Am J Sports Med.* 2014;42(10):2410–2418.

4. Lee JJ, Harrison JR, Boachie-Adjei K, Vargas E, Moley PJ. Platelet-rich Plasma Injections with needle tenotomy for gluteus medius tendinopathy: a registry study with prospective follow-up. *Orthop J Sports Med.* 2016;4(11), 2325967116671692.

5. Jacobson JA, Yablon CM, Henning PT, et al. Greater trochanteric pain syndrome: percutaneous tendon fenestration versus platelet-rich plasma injection for treatment of gluteal tendinosis. *J Ultrasound Med.* 2016;35(11): 2413–2420.

6. Wilson JJ, Lee KS, Chamberlain C, et al. Intratendinous injections of platelet-rich plasma: feasibility and effect on tendon morphology and mechanics. *J Exp Orthop.* 2015;2(5).

7. Chang Chien GC, Galang E, Rosenthal R, Calodney AK, *Intervent Pain Manag Rep;*1(1):63–69.

8. Lai LP, Stitik TP, Foye PM, Georgy JS, Patibanda V, Chen B. Use of platelet-rich plasma in intra-articular knee injections for osteoarthritis: a systematic review. *PM R.* 2015;7(6): 637–648. https://doi.org/10.1016/j.pmrj.2015.02.003.

9. Laver L, Marom N, Dnyanesh L, Mei-Dan O, Espregueira-Mendes J, Gobbi A. PRP for degenerative cartilage disease: a systematic review of clinical studies. *Cartilage.* 2016;8: 341–364. https://doi.org/10.1177/1947603516670709.

10. Jang S, Kim J, Cha S. Platelet-rich plasma (PRP) injections as an effective treatment for early osteoarthritis. *Eur J Orthop Surg Traumatol.* 2012;23:573–580. https://doi.org/10.1007/s00590-012-1037-5.

11. Moussa M, Lajeunesse D, Hilal G, et al. Platelet rich plasma (PRP) induces chondroprotection via increasing autophagy, anti-inflammatory markers, and decreasing apoptosis in human osteoarthritic cartilage. *Exp Cell Res.* 2017;352: 146–156. https://doi.org/10.1016/j.yexcr.2017.02.012.

12. B Scherb M, Han S-H, Courneya J-P, P Guyton G, Schon L. Effect of bupivacaine on cultured tenocytes. *Orthopedics.* 2009; 32:26. https://doi.org/10.3928/01477447-20090101-19.

13. Zhang A, Ficklscherer A, Pietschmann M, Jansson V, Müller P. Apoptosis and necrosis-inducing cell toxicity of ropivacaine, bupivacaine and triamcinolone in fibroblasts, tenocytes and human mesenchymal stem cells. *Sports Orthop Traumatol.* 2016;32(2):201. https://doi.org/10.1016/j.orthtr.2016.03.019.

14. Iwasaki K, Sudo H, Yamada K, Ito M, Iwasaki N. Cytotoxic effects of the radiocontrast agent iotrolan and anesthetic agents bupivacaine and lidocaine in three dimensional cultures of human intervertebral disc nucleus pulposus cells: identification of the apoptotic pathways. *PloS One.* 2014;9(3). https://doi.org/10.1371/journal.pone.0092442.

15. Dregalla RC, Lyons NF, Reischling PD, Centeno CJ. Amide-type local anesthetics and human mesenchymal stem cells: clinical implications for stem cell therapy. *Stem Cells Transl Med.* 2014;3(3):365–374. https://doi.org/10.5966/sctm.2013-0058.

16. Grishko V, Xu M, Wilson G, Pearsall 4th AW. Apoptosis and mitochondrial dysfunction in human chondrocytes following exposure to lidocaine, bupivacaine, and ropivacaine. *J Bone Jt Surg Am.* 2010;92(3). https://doi.org/10.1016/j.spinee.2010.05.024, 609–18. *Spine J* 2010;10(7):653.

17. Piper SL, Kim HT. Comparison of ropivacaine and bupivacaine toxicity in human articular chondrocytes. *J Bone Jt Surg.* 2008;90(5):986–991. https://doi.org/10.2106/JBJS.G.01033.

18. Breu A, et al. Cytotoxicity of local anesthetics on human mesenchymal stem cells in Vitro. *Arthroscopy.* 2013; 29(10):1676–1684.

19. Rao AJ, Johnston TR, Harris AH, Smith RL, Costouros JG. Inhibition of chondrocyte and synovial cell death after exposure to commonly used anesthetics. *Am J Sports Med.* 2013;42(1):50–58. https://doi.org/10.1177/0363546513507426.

20. McAlindon TE, LaValley MP, Harvey WF, et al. Effect of intra-articular triamcinolone vs saline on knee cartilage volume and pain in patients with knee osteoarthritis: a randomized clinical trial. *J Am Med Assoc.* 2017;317(19): 1967–1975. https://doi.org/10.1001/jama.2017.5283.

21. Kilincoglu V, Yeter A, Servet E, Kangal M, Yildirim M. Short term results comparison of intraarticular platelet-rich plasma (prp) and hyaluronic acid (ha) applications in early stage of knee osteoarthritis. *Int J Clin Exp Med.* 2015;8:18807–18812.

22. Sinno H, Prakash S. Complements and the wound healing cascade: an updated review. *Plast Surg Int.* 2013;2013:7. Article ID 146764.

23. Giusti I, Rughetti A, D'Ascenzo S, et al. Identification of an optimal concentration of platelet gel for promoting angiogenesis in human endothelial cells. *Transfusion.* 2009; 49(4):771–778.

24. Hauser RA, Lackner JB, Steilen-Matias D, Harris DK. A systematic review of dextrose prolotherapy for chronic musculoskeletal pain. *Clin Med Insights Arthritis Musculoskelet Disord.* 2016;9:139–159. https://doi.org/10.4137/CMAMD.S39160.

25. Peister A, Mellad JA, Larson BL, Hall BM, Gibson LF, Prockop DJ. Adult stem cells from bone marrow (MSCs) isolated from different strains of inbred mice vary in surface epitopes, rates of proliferation, and differentiation potential. *Blood.* 2004;103(5):1662–1668.

26. Golpanian S, Wolf A, Hatzistergos KE, Hare JM. Rebuilding the damaged heart: mesenchymal stem cells, cell-based therapy, and engineered heart tissue. *Physiol Rev.* 2016;96(3):1127−1168. https://doi.org/10.1152/physrev.00019.2015.

27. Mazini L, Rochette L, Amine M, Malka G. Regenerative capacity of adipose derived stem cells (ADSCs), comparison with mesenchymal stem cells (MSCs). *Int J Mol Sci.* 2019; 20(10):2523. https://doi.org/10.3390/ijms20102523.

28. Reeves KD. Randomized prospective double-blind placebo-controlled study of dextrose prolotherapy for knee osteoarthritis with or without ACL laxity. *Alternative Ther.* 2000;6:68−80.

29. Dumais R, et al. Effect of RIT on function and pain in patients with knee osteoarthritis: a randomized crossover study. *Pain Med.* 2012;13:990−999.

30. Rabago D, Zgierska A, Fortney L, et al. Hypertonic dextrose injections (prolotherapy) for knee osteoarthritis: an uncontrolled study with one-year follow-up. *J Alternative Compl Med.* 2012;18(4):408−414.

31. Rabago D, Patterson JJ, Mundt M, et al. Dextrose prolotherapy for knee osteoarthritis: a randomized controlled trial. *Ann Fam Med.* 2013;11(3):229−237.

32. Rabago D, Mundt M, Zgierska A, et al. Hypertonic dextrose injection (Prolotherapy) for knee osteoarthritis: long term outcomes. *Compl Ther Med.* 2015;23: 388−395.

33. Sit RWS, Chung VCH, Reeves KD, et al. Hypertonic dextrose injections (prolotherapy) in the treatment of symptomatic knee osteoarthritis: a systematic review and meta-analysis. *Sci Rep.* 2016;6.

34. Louw WF, et al. Treatment of temporomandibular dysfunction with hypertonic dextrose injection (prolotherapy): a randomized controlled trial with long-term partial crossover. *Mayo Clin Proc.* 2019;94(5):820−832.

35. Murrell G. Understanding tendinopathies. *Br J Sports Med.* 2002;36(6):392−393.

36. Khan KM, Cook JL, Bonar F, Harcourt P, Astrom M. Histopathology of common tendinopathies. Update and implications for clinical management. *Sports Med.* 1999;27(6): 393−408.

37. Guillodo Y, Madouas G, Simon T, Le Dauphin H, Saraux A. Platelet-rich plasma (PRP) treatment of sports-related severe acute hamstring injuries. *Muscles Ligaments Tendons J.* 2016;5(4):284−288.

38. Ben-Nafa W, Munro W. The effect of corticosteroid versus platelet-rich plasma injection therapies for the management of lateral epicondylitis: a systematic review. *SICOT J.* 2018;4:11. https://doi.org/10.1051/sicotj/2017062.

39. Ferrero G, Fabbro E, Orlandi D, et al. Ultrasound-guided injection of platelet-rich plasma in chronic achilles and patellar tendinopathy. *J Ultrasound.* 2012;15(4): 260−266. https://doi.org/10.1016/j.jus.2012.09.006.

40. Reurink G, Goudswaard GJ, Moen MH, et al. Dutch HIT-study Investigators.Rationale, secondary outcome scores and 1-year follow-up of a randomised trial of platelet-rich plasma injections in acute hamstring muscle injury:

41. Zanon G, Combi F, Combi A, Perticarini L, Sammarchi L, Benazzo F. Platelet-rich plasma in the treatment of acute hamstring injuries in professional football players. *Joints.* 2016;4(1):17−23.

42. Zayni R, Thaunat M, Fayard JM, et al. Platelet-rich plasma as a treatment for chronic patellar tendinopathy: comparison of a single versus two consecutive injections. *Muscles Ligaments Tendons J.* 2015;5(2):92−98.

43. Gonnade N, Bajpayee A, Elhence A, et al. Regenerative efficacy of therapeutic quality platelet-rich plasma injections versus phonophoresis with kinesiotaping for the treatment of chronic plantar fasciitis: a prospective randomized pilot study. *Asian J Transfus Sci.* 2018;12(2):105−111.

44. Centeno CJ, Pitts J, Al-Sayegh H, Freeman MD. Anterior cruciate ligament tears treated with percutaneous injection of autologous bone marrow nucleated cells: a case series. *J Pain Res.* 2015;8:437−447. https://doi.org/10.2147/JPR.S86244.

45. Vahdatpour B, Kianimehr L, Moradi A, Haghighat S. Beneficial effects of platelet-rich plasma on improvement of pain severity and physical disability in patients with plantar fasciitis: a randomized trial. *Adv Biomed Res.* 2016;5:179. https://doi.org/10.4103/2277-9175.192731.

46. Cusi M, Saunders J, Hungerford T, et al. The use of prolotherapy in the sacroiliac joint. *Br J Sports Med.* 2010;44(2): 100−104.

47. Kim WM, Lee HG, Jeong CW, Kim CM, Yoon MH. A randomized controlled trial of intra-articular prolotherapy versus steroid injection for sacroiliac joint pain. *J Alternative Compl Med.* 2010;16(12): 1285−1290. https://doi.org/10.1089/acm.2010.0031.

48. Yelland MJ, Glasziou PP, Bogduk N, Schluter PJ, McKernon M. Prolotherapy injections, saline injections, and exercises for chronic low-back pain: a randomized trial. *Spine.* 2004;29(1):9−16.

49. Klein RG. A randomized double-blind trial of dextrose-glycerine-phenol injections for chronic, low back pain. *J Spinal Disord.* 1993;6(1):23−33.

50. Dechow E, Davies RK, Carr AJ, Thompson PW. A randomized, double-blind, placebo-controlled trial of sclerosing injections in patients with chronic low back pain. *Rheumatology.* 1999;38(12):1255−1259.

51. Kim K-H, Park J-Y, Park H-S, et al. Which iodinated contrast media is the least cytotoxic to human disc cells? *Spine J.* 2015;15(5):1021−1027. https://doi.org/10.1016/j.spinee.2015.01.015.

52. Chee AV, Ren J, Lenart BA, Chen E-Y, Zhang Y, An HS. Cytotoxicity of local anesthetics and nonionic contrast agents on bovine intervertebral disc cells cultured in a three-dimensional culture system. *Spine J.* 2014;14(3): 491−498. https://doi.org/10.1016/j.spinee.2013.06.095.

53. Oznam K, Sirin DY, Yilmaz I, et al. Iopromide- and gadopentetic acid-derived preparates used in MR arthrography may be harmful to chondrocytes. *J Orthop Surg Res.* 2017;12(1). https://doi.org/10.1186/s13018-017-0600-5.

CHAPTER 18

Future Research in Pain

MAURO ZAPPATERRA, MD, PHD • UDAI NANDA, DO

INTRODUCTION

In previous decades, pain research has been relatively stagnant and with limited funding. In 2011, only 1% of the $30 billion National Institutes of Health (NIH) budget was devoted to pain research.[1] An integral piece in the framework of pain research was added in 2009 with the Congressional Mandate and National Pain Care Policy Act, which set out plans for the Secretary of Health and Human Services to meet with the National Academy of Medicine (previously known as Institute of Medicine) for a conference on pain.

In 2011, the NIH and National Academy of Medicine (NAM) published *Relieving Pain in America: A Blueprint for Transforming Prevention, Care, Education, and Research*.[2] This effort helped guide the development of the *National Pain Strategy: A Comprehensive Population Health-Level Strategy for Pain*, released by the US Department of Health and Human Services (HHS) and the Interagency Pain Research Coordinating Committee (IPRCC) 5 years later.[3] The National Pain Strategy promoted providing individualized, patient-centered, interdisciplinary care to people experiencing pain. In addition, the Federal Pain Research Strategy was developed to expand upon the goals of the National Pain Strategy.

The Federal Pain Research Strategy was released in 2017 and helped to identify and prioritize a long-term strategic plan for the federal pain research agenda.[4] In 2018, the NIH established the initiative Helping to End Addiction Long-Term (HEAL), which included the efforts of multiple agencies to promote and fund research for managing pain in the context of the national opioid public health crisis.[5]

Pain continues to have a substantial impact on patients, their environment, and the healthcare system.[6] Globally, the estimated prevalence of chronic pain in adults is 20%.[7,8] In the United States, an estimated 50 million (20.4%) adults have chronic pain, with 19.6 million (8.0%) of adults having high-impact chronic pain that interferes with work or life most days or every day.[9]

Total annual costs for chronic pain in the United States are estimated at $560–$635 billion. This figure is greater than six of the most costly major diagnoses: cardiovascular diseases ($309 billion); neoplasms ($243 billion); injury and poisoning ($205 billion); endocrine, nutritional, and metabolic diseases ($127 billion); digestive system diseases ($112 billion); and respiratory system diseases ($112 billion).[10,11] Interestingly, the per-person cost of pain is less than the other conditions, but because pain affects a larger number of individuals the total costs are higher.[10]

To address the extensive ongoing burden of pain, it is imperative to thoughtfully consider all management options. This chapter focuses on future directions in pain research but does not claim to be an exhaustive list, as the goal of ongoing research is to develop new contributions to the field and continually improve the management available to those suffering from pain.

BROAD RESEARCH PROPOSALS

The International Association for the Study of Pain defines pain as "an unpleasant sensory and emotional experience associated with actual or potential tissue damage, or described in terms of such damage." Prompted by this definition, future research will tackle the treatment of pain by attempting to better understand the sensory inputs, the emotional inputs, as well as the whole of the person's experience. A person's experience is personal and subjective, and therefore, future research will look into individualized treatment options.

The goal will be to treat acute or chronic pain with a plan that addresses the numerous issues that contribute to pain and affect the patient's functioning. Research

Pain Care Essentials and Innovations. https://doi.org/10.1016/B978-0-323-72216-2.00018-1

will attempt to address novel nociceptive and neuro-pathic signaling mechanisms at the point where the pain originates, as well as transduction pathways along the peripheral and central nervous system and cortical areas responsible for perceiving and responding to the signals that create an individual experience of pain.[1,12,13] It will be important to understand the transition from acute to chronic pain, as well as develop interventions that prevent chronic pain from developing.

There will be a need to increase our knowledge of peripheral and central signaling mechanisms at the molecular level, with a better understanding of receptors, downstream activators, and transcription factors, as well as pathways involved in the pathophysiology of pain. This will also include a better understanding of individualized pain responses based on gender, genetics, epigenetic changes, as well as pharmacogenomic interactions. Improved animal models and high-throughput screening technologies will be needed to quickly screen small molecules for improved pharmacotherapy.

In addition, improved assays will be developed to elucidate drug interactions and drug metabolism based on an individual's genetic makeup. Furthermore, functional MRIs will be used to evaluate pain in real time, to better understand how brain regions change with pain, which brain regions impact pain processing, and which emotional and cognitive factors can influence pain and alter pain perception and, therefore, the pain experience.

Research will also be aimed at attempting to identify objective measures of pain. This includes biomarkers that may be present in the brain, blood, or tissues, so that researchers can objectively evaluate pain treatment. In addition, research will focus on the identification of pain phenotypes, including descriptions of pain, such as shooting, stabbing, pricking, or burning, and use of specific treatments for different pain phenotypes as a means of attempting to correlate these phenotypes with genotypes.[1]

MULTIDISCIPLINARY TREATMENTS

Pain is a physical, social, psychological, and spiritual experience. Numerous individualized treatments have been used to address the various aspects of the pain experience, including but not limited to the following: education, exercise (strength training and stretching), acupuncture, physical therapy, occupational therapy, aquatherapy, massage, chiropractic therapy, osteopathic therapy, craniosacral therapy, relaxation training,

guided imagery, homeopathy, energy medicine, hypnosis, meditation/mindfulness, sleep hygiene, breathing techniques, yoga, Pilates, tai chi, cognitive behavioral therapy, acceptance and commitment therapy, biofeedback, nutraceuticals, and medications.

The pain experience is complex, and the etiology is multifactorial. With multiple factors and pathways contributing to the pain signal and modulating the experience, multiple targets are needed to treat the pain. This would therefore not only include the possibility of multiple pharmaceuticals but also multiple treatment modalities. It is generally accepted that pain management and pain treatment will be a team-based care model that is integrated, interdisciplinary, coordinated, and patient-centered.[14] It will address the multiple dimensions of pain from a physical, social, psychological, and spiritual perspective. However, there is still a lack of data for long-term sustainability of effects and overlapping pain conditions and psychosocial factors, as well as for which modalities should be combined in an interdisciplinary model, and at which intervals or doses.[13,15]

Research will be performed to determine which modalities should be combined, at what time in the healing process, and at what dose and frequency.[13,14] Given the multifactorial nature of pain, it is unlikely that the same treatment modality, or combination of modalities, could be used for everyone. Interdisciplinary treatment modalities will need to be individualized, as treatment is not a one-size-fits-all paradigm; therefore, research will need to be performed to help identify which patients will respond to which particular combination of modalities and interventions. This has the potential of dramatically improving the treatment of pain.

In addition, oftentimes, nonpharmacological treatment modalities are not available to patients, either due to access issues or insurance coverage. Future research will help expand healthcare and increase access to treatment options through technologies such as telehealth and digital platforms. This may include educational or instructional videos, podcasts, and live telehealth appointments with health professionals in individual or group settings. More research will be performed using treatment apps on smartphones and web portals on computers and by monitoring progress with direct patient-to-provider communication and alerts. This may help improve patient compliance, increase monitoring that may decrease emergency room or hospital visits, and help advance interdisciplinary treatment models that can be provided long distance through technology.

NOVEL PHARMACEUTICALS

The topic of pharmaceuticals is broad and includes medications that have previously been used, are currently being used, or are being considered for future use in treating pain. Here we concentrate on pharmaceuticals and pharmacological targets in the treatment of pain that are in various stages of discovery and development. The discovery, development, and implementation of potential pharmaceutical treatments involve many factors, including the significant roles of the various pharmaceutical regulatory agencies and organizations worldwide; for example, the regulations of the US Food and Drug Administration. While some of the pharmaceuticals and their targets listed below are currently used in practice and are being evaluated for improvements, others are in more experimental stages of development. Clinical trials for the novel pharmaceuticals discussed below and currently registered on https://ClinicalTrials.gov are highlighted in Table 18.1.

TABLE 18.1

Clinical Trials Registered on https://ClinicalTrials.gov for Novel Pharmaceuticals and Mechanisms Discussed Above.

Drug Name	ClinicalTrials.gov Identifier	Mechanism/Target	Condition or Disease	Phase	Recruitment Status
PF-04457845	NCT00981357	Fatty acid amino hydrolase inhibitor	Pain, knee osteoarthritis	2	Completed
Lacosamide	NCT00220337	Voltage-gated sodium channels antagonist	Painful diabetic neuropathy	3	Completed
Lacosamide	NCT00546351	Voltage-gated sodium channels antagonist	Painful distal diabetic neuropathy	3	Completed
Eslicarbazepine acetate (ESL)	NCT00980746	Voltage-gated sodium channels antagonist	Painful diabetic neuropathy	2	Completed
Eslicarbazepine acetate (ESL)	NCT01129960	Voltage-gated sodium channels antagonist	Painful diabetic neuropathy	3	Terminated
Rufinamide	NCT02095899	Voltage-gated sodium channels antagonist	Postthoracotomy pain syndrome	2	Terminated
Tetrodotoxin (TTX)	NCT00725114	Voltage-gated sodium channels antagonist	Moderate to severe inadequately controlled cancer-related pain	3	Completed
Pregabalin	NCT01529190	Voltage-gated calcium channels antagonist	Pain intensity and interleukin-6 levels in living donor kidney	2	Completed
Ethosuximide	NCT02100046	Voltage-gated calcium channels antagonist	Peripheral neuropathic pain	2	Completed
Ziconotide	NCT00002160	Voltage-gated calcium channels antagonist	Chronic pain in cancer and AIDS	2	Completed
Ziconotide	NCT03942848	Voltage-gated calcium channels antagonist	Severe refractory neuropathic pain	3	Not yet recruiting
Flupirtine	NCT01450865	Voltage-gated potassium channel agonist	Pain, neuronal change	1	Completed
SB705498	NCT00461682	TRPV1 receptor antagonist	Rectal pain	2	Terminated
SB705498	NCT00281684	TRPV1 receptor antagonist	Dental pain	2	Completed

Continued

TABLE 18.1
Clinical Trials Registered on https://ClinicalTrials.gov for Novel Pharmaceuticals and Mechanisms Discussed Above.—cont'd

Drug Name	ClinicalTrials.gov Identifier	Mechanism/Target	Condition or Disease	Phase	Recruitment Status
Ketamine	NCT02729805	TRPV1 and TRPA1 receptor gene expression	Chronic pain, mastectomy	4	Active, not recruiting
Resiniferatoxin	NCT03226574	TRPV1 receptor agonist	Intractable cancer pain	1	Recruiting
Resiniferatoxin	NCT03542838	TRPV1 receptor agonist	Pain, knee osteoarthritis	1	Recruiting
Resiniferatoxin	NCT04044742	TRPV1 receptor agonist	Pain, knee osteoarthritis	3	Recruiting
GZ389988	NCT02424942	Tropomyosin-related kinase a (TrkA) inhibitor	Pain, knee osteoarthritis	1	Completed
Oxytocin	NCT02100956	Oxytocin receptor	Neuropathic pain	2	Recruiting
Oxytocin	NCT03060031	Oxytocin receptor	Pain, social influence effects on pain	1	Completed
Oxytocin	NCT03011307	Oxytocin receptor	Postoperative pain (hip surgery)	2	Recruiting

Fatty Acid Amino Hydrolase

Fatty acid amino hydrolase (FAAH) is an intracellular membrane-bound enzyme that hydrolyzes the endocannabinoid N-arachidonylethanolamide (AEA, or anandamide) and other fatty acid amides. AEA acts as an agonist at cannabinoid receptors, and by inhibiting FAAH, its physiologic effects can be prolonged.[16] Some researchers suggest that it is possible to both utilize the cannabinoid system in the treatment of pain and limit the undesirable side effects reported with administration of exogenous cannabinoids by targeting the endocannabinoid system.[17]

One example of the effect of the endocannabinoid system and AEA can be seen by looking at a microdeletion in a novel FAAH pseudogene (FAAH-OUT), identified in a patient with high AEA concentrations and pain insensitivity.[18] Both pharmacologic and genetic targeting of FAAH have been studied in relation to multiple medical conditions, including pain.

Pharmacologic studies have yielded a wide range of results. A prior Phase I trial had unfortunate outcomes, when an acute neurologic disorder developed in healthy volunteers.[19] Subsequent use of FAAH inhibitors for treating pain and other medical disorders has shown more promise, however. Another Phase I trial evaluating an FAAH inhibitor and peripheral neuropathic pain demonstrated a more favorable safety profile but no significant difference in primary endpoint versus placebo; however, it did so within subgroup analysis.[20] More promise has been shown in Phase II trials evaluating FAAH inhibitors with cannabis use disorder and as a possible treatment for posttraumatic stress disorder.[21,22]

In addition to further FAAH inhibitor trials, gene-editing techniques are also being considered. One such study explored how utilizing CRISPR interference (CRISPRi) to enable gene repression at the FAAH-OUT promoter reduces FAAH-OUT and FAAH expression.[23] This highlights how CRISPRi and gene-editing techniques targeting FAAH-OUT may be developed as novel therapies in the treatment of pain.

Voltage-Gated Sodium Channels

Voltage-gated sodium channels (VGSCs) have nine identified subtypes ($Na_v1.1–Na_v1.9$), each with unique properties and tissue distributions.[24] They play an integral role in membrane excitability and the propagation of action potentials. Although many VGSCs may have a role in pain, three are most strongly associated: $Na_v1.7$, $Na_v1.8$, and $Na_v1.9$.[25] In particular, $Na_v1.7$ has demonstrated properties that make it a target of interest in the treatment of pain. $Na_v1.7$ channel gain of function mutations are linked to severe pain, and loss of function mutations are linked to pain insensitivity.[26,27] In three related families demonstrating a congenital inability to perceive pain but intact ability to perceive other sensory modalities, a mutation was found in gene SCN9A, the gene encoding the alpha subunit of $Na_v1.7$.[28]

Clinical trials thus far exploring novel $Na_v1.7$ channel inhibitors have shown good safety but inconsistent clinical efficacy. Although results were less promising in subjects with pain due to trigeminal neuralgia[29] and diabetic neuropathy,[30] lacosamide, with a mechanism involving $Na_v1.3$, $Na_v1.7$, and $Na_v1.8$, had a significant effect on pain, general well-being, and sleep quality in subjects with $Na_v1.7$-related small-fiber neuropathy.[31] In addition, tetrodotoxin, a neurotoxin produced by the pufferfish that primarily blocks $Na_v1.7$, has shown a favorable risk-benefit profile in the treatment of uncontrolled moderate to severe cancer-related pain. There have been numerous clinical trials with ongoing studies underway.[32]

Voltage-Gated Calcium Channels

Voltage-gated calcium channels (VGCCs) play an important role in regulating signal transduction and initiating multiple physiologic events.[33] The two major classes of VGCC include high voltage-activated (L, P/Q, N, R types) and low voltage-activated (T type). L, N, and T type VGCCs have been studied regarding their influence on pain.

L type VGCCs (Ca_v1) are primarily located postsynaptically and regulate neuronal firing and gene expression in a number of physiologic processes, including pain. With application to the dorsal horn, they were found to alter short-term pain sensitization, inflammation-induced hyperexcitability, and neuropathy-induced allodynia.[34]

N type VGCCs ($Ca_v2.2$), located presynaptically, play a large role in neurotransmitter release.[35] They are concentrated in dorsal root ganglia and the dorsal horn and have currently accepted medical use in the treatment of pain. Ziconotide (SNX-111) is a synthetic form of the peptide ω-conotoxin MVIIA (ω-MVIIA), which is found in Conus magus snail venom.[36] Ziconotide has limited permeability across the blood-brain barrier and must be administered intrathecally. Potential limitations include side effect profile and mode of administration.

Various studies have been conducted in an effort to utilize the N type VGCC with an orally administered medication. Phase II trials evaluating a novel oral VGCC inhibitor with lumbosacral radiculopathy and postherpetic neuralgia did not meet their primary endpoint and were discontinued.[37] Adjustments to

the structure of these agents and their mode of action are currently being evaluated with electrophysiology experiments.[38]

T type VGCCs (Ca_v3), located presynaptically, have a role in excitatory synaptic transmission and have multiple locations, including reticular thalamic neurons, cortical pyramidal neurons, the dorsal root ganglia, and the dorsal horn of the spinal cord.[39,40] Various subtypes have been implicated in multiple neurologic disorders, ranging from epilepsy[41] to various chronic pain states,[42] with a notably large impact on the initiation and maintenance of neuropathic pain.

A few examples of currently utilized pharmaceutical agents that target T type VGCC and their indications include ethosuximide (epilepsy), valproic acid (epilepsy, bipolar disorder), zonisamide (epilepsy), and nimodipine (hypertension).[38] A Phase II trial evaluated the safety profile and analgesic efficacy of a novel selective T type $Ca_v3.2$ VGCC blocker in subjects with neuropathic pain. The novel agent was compared with pregabalin and a placebo and was found to lack analgesic efficacy, with mild to moderate side effects reported.[43]

Another study compared ethosuximide with an inactive control in subjects with nondiabetic peripheral neuropathic pain but was stopped due to adverse events reported in the treatment group.[44] A double-blind, placebo-controlled, randomized study of a novel orally available triple T-type Ca^{2+} channel blocker (blocking $Ca_v3.1$, $Ca_v3.2$, $Ca_v3.3$) was found to have good tolerability after a single administration in healthy male subjects. Its tolerability, along with pharmacokinetic and pharmacodynamic properties, warrants further studies of multiple doses.[45]

Potassium Channels

Potassium channels play a role in repolarization/hyperpolarization of the neuronal membrane, which can limit action potential propagation and firing rate.[46] Potassium channels are described as the most widely distributed and diverse group of ion channels in neurons[42] and are organized into four subgroups: voltage-gated (VGKC, or K_v), two-pore (K_{2P}), calcium-activated (K_{Ca}), and inward-rectifying (K_{ir}).[47] One illustration of the potential impact of potassium channels may be found in Isaacs Syndrome (acquired neuromyotonia), an antibody-mediated potassium channel disorder (channelopathy). Autoantibodies target VGKC and decrease the voltage-gated outward potassium current, causing peripheral motor nerve hyperexcitability.[48]

VGKC complex autoantibodies have more recently been identified as being involved in the hyperexcitability of nociceptive pathways and development of chronic pain.[49] As a decrease in potassium channel expression/current density can contribute to the development of chronic pain, therapeutically targeting the opening of potassium channels may promote analgesia.[50] The results of an animal study showed that the drug riluzole prevented the chronic neuropathy that is often associated with the use of the chemotherapy agent oxaliplatin. The two-pore potassium channel TREK-1 was identified as playing a central role in the riluzole-induced antineuropathic effect.[51]

Transient Receptor Potential Channels

Transient receptor potential channels (TRP channels) are a group of cation channels that play a role in the response to various external stimuli, including light, sound, chemical, temperature, and touch.[52] There are seven subfamilies of TRP channels in total, some of which play a large role in nociception. The two most often implicated in pain are the transient receptor potential ankyrin 1 (TRPA1) and transient receptor potential vanilloid 1 (TRPV1) channels.[53] TRPA1 and TRPV1 are coexpressed in a number of nociceptive sensory nerves, and their function is at times interlinked.[54,55]

TRPA1 is the only member of the TRPA subfamily. The classic TRPA1 agonist was identified as mustard oil (active component allyl isothiocyanate), which is also present in wasabi and horseradish.[50] There have been multiple agonists identified over time, with TRPA1 being identified as a potential therapeutic target in the treatment of pain.

The wide range of toxins that target TRPA1 have unique mechanisms to be considered. Crotalphine is the venom isolated from the South American rattlesnake *Crotalus durissus* terrificus that has been shown to provide significant analgesia in inflammatory, neuropathic, and cancer pain models.[56] An animal study found that picomolar concentrations of administered crotalphine resulted in analgesia. By selectively acting as partial agonists at TRPA1 channels, they led to prolonged desensitization of the channel, causing the analgesic effect.[57] An alternate mechanism was utilized while incorporating the wasabi receptor toxin (WaTx) isolated from the Black Rock scorpion. WaTx binding was found to stabilize the TRPA1 in an open state and diminish calcium permeability. This did produce pain and pain hypersensitivity but did not cause neurogenic inflammation.[58] This suggests that WaTx as a potential treatment in limiting the neurogenic inflammation component to TRPA1-mediated pain, while preserving its acute protective role in chemical nociception.[54]

TRPV1 is one of the six members in the vanilloid TRP subfamily. TRPV1 is the only member that is actually activated by vanilloids, with its classic agonist identified as capsaicin, the active component in chili peppers.[50] It was then established that heat greater than 43°C and pH less than 5.9 also activates the channel.[50]

Over time, many exogenous and endogenous agonists, as well as endogenous modulators, have been identified. One exogenous agonist that has been investigated extensively is resiniferatoxin (RTX). RTX is derived from the *Euphorbia resinifera* plant and has been reported to be the most potent among all synthetic and endogenous TRPV1 agonists.[59] RTX acts by producing prolonged channel opening and calcium influx, causing cytotoxicity to the TRPV1-positive pain fibers or cell bodies.[55] In addition, its mechanism has been referred to as "molecular neurosurgery," or selective neuroablation, as it spares motor, proprioceptive, and other somatosensory function.[55]

An animal study evaluating pain in the postsurgical period found that a targeted injection of RTX reduced evoked and nonevoked pain-related behaviors in subjects over the duration of postsurgical recovery.[60] Animal studies with intrathecal administration of RTX on subjects with cancer pain showed promising results and have led to Phase I clinical trials in humans. In Phase I clinical trials, changes in pain assessed with the numeric rating scale (NRS) were not statistically significant at the doses of RTX tested. There are ongoing studies evaluating the safety and efficacy of higher administered doses of intrathecal RTX in subjects with severe refractory pain due to advanced cancer.[61]

Tropomyosin-Related Kinases

Tropomyosin-related kinases (Trk), a family of receptor tyrosine kinases, have three isomers—TrkA, TrkB, and TrkC—that are expressed in neurons.[62] These isomers are each activated by complementary neurotrophins: nerve growth factor (NGF) binds to TrkA; brain-derived neurotrophic factor (BDNF) binds to TrkB; and neurotrophin-3 (NT-3) binds to TrkC.[63] All three Trk receptors have been implicated in neuropathic pain,[59] while also being evaluated for their role in other types of pain.

TrkA receptors have been targeted as a potential therapeutic target for the treatment of pain. The neurotrophin NGF has roles in early neural development and in adults and contributes to neural plasticity, hypersensitization to noxious stimuli, and the signaling of pain.[64] Increased levels of NGF have been associated with acute and chronic pain states.[65]

The humanized anti-NGF monoclonal antibody tanezumab has been studied in a variety of clinical scenarios. Two randomized, double-blind, placebo-controlled, Phase I studies were conducted to evaluate safety, tolerability, and analgesic efficacy of tanezumab.[60] Statistically significant improvements in tanezumab-associated analgesia in doses greater than or equal to 100 micrograms/kg were seen in a study evaluating knee pain secondary to osteoarthritis; however, no statistically significant improvements were noted in the study evaluating patients undergoing bunionectomy.[60]

A notable Phase III clinical trial included subjects with hip or knee osteoarthritis randomly placed in groups, with one taking 2.5 mg tanezumab every 8 weeks, another taking 5 mg tanezumab every 8 weeks, and a third taking daily NSAIDs. Results suggested that tanezumab has some analgesic efficacy for hip or knee osteoarthritis but is associated with increased rates of rapidly progressive osteoarthritis and total joint replacement.[66] Phase III clinical trials are also underway evaluating tanezumab and chronic low back pain.[67]

TrkB receptors and the neurotrophin BDNF have roles in both central and peripheral pain mechanisms.[68] BDNF supports neuronal growth and is upregulated in the central nervous system in chronic pain states.[64] The peripheral role of TrkB and BDNF in pain is increasingly being studied. TrkB receptors in the synovial tissue have been associated with increased levels of osteoarthritic knee pain. An animal study employing rodent models of osteoarthritis compared intraarticular injections of exogenous BDNF and TrkB-Fc chimera (proposed to sequester endogenous BDNF). Findings supported the hypothesis that BDNF and TrkB receptors play a role in the maintenance of chronic pain due to peripheral joint osteoarthritis and are a potential therapeutic target.[64]

TrkC receptors and the neurotrophin NT-3 have been shown to modulate pain responses with a variety of proposed mechanisms. In animal studies, NT-3 and TrkC receptors had modulatory effects on neuropathic pain via their impact at the dorsal root ganglia.[69]

Oxytocin

Oxytocin is a nonapeptide hormone that is primarily synthesized in the hypothalamus, transported to the posterior pituitary gland, and subsequently released into peripheral circulation.[70] There is great diversity in the physiologic roles oxytocin plays, ranging from lactation to social attachment.[71] Regarding pain transmission, oxytocin plays a role at peripheral, spinal, and supraspinal levels.[67] The exact mechanism is evolving over time, with reports that oxytocin has analgesic effects via the central endogenous opioid system,[72] while others suggest that the combined actions of oxytocin, GABA, and TRPV1 contribute to oxytocin's analgesic effects.[67]

Various modes of oxytocin administration have been studied for therapeutic treatment of pain. A Phase I safety assessment of intrathecal oxytocin was conducted in a dose-escalating manner.[73] One subject in the study experienced focal neurologic symptoms and transient cardiovascular depression; however, overall, the study did not demonstrate a high incidence of effects on blood pressure, heart rate, QT interval, serum sodium, or neurologic symptoms. The intrathecal oxytocin administered was not found to produce analgesia when acute noxious heat stimuli were introduced to healthy subjects.[69] A placebo-controlled, double-blind, within participants, crossover investigation evaluated the effect of intranasal oxytocin administration on acute cold pressor pain. Subjects receiving a 40-IU dose of intranasal oxytocin reported lower pain intensity, unpleasantness, and pain descriptors after a cold pressor task versus placebo.[74]

Mammalian Target of Rapamycin Pathway

The mammalian target of rapamycin (mTOR) pathway plays an integral role in cell growth and proliferation. There are two complexes: mTOR complex 1 (mTORC1) and mTOR complex 2 (mTORC2). mTORC1 is switched on by oncogenic signaling pathways and can be hyperactive in many forms of cancer.[75] Its most established current role as a therapeutic target is demonstrated by mTOR inhibitors, which are FDA approved for the treatment of cancer.

The mTOR pathway is also being investigated for its potential role in pain. This includes the development and maintenance of chronic pain, opioid-induced tolerance, and opioid-induced hyperalgesia.[76] Microinjections of rapamycin (mTORC1 inhibitor) to the insular cortex of rats after sciatic nerve lesion caused an increase in pain threshold and reduction in mechanical hypersensitivity.[77] A retrospective review evaluated three cases of patients with neurofibromatosis 1 and painful plexiform neurofibromas. Administration of the immunosuppressive agent and mTOR inhibitor sirolimus not only stabilized the cancerous mass but also resulted in alleviation of pain symptoms.[78] These examples highlight that mTOR inhibitors being utilized in the treatment of certain cancers may be a potential treatment for chronic pain.[74]

Janus Kinase/Signal Transducer and Activator of Transcription 3 Signaling Pathway

The Janus kinase/signal transducer and activator of transcription 3 signaling pathway (JAK/STAT3 pathway) has a large number of roles in the body, including embryonic development, stem cell maintenance, hematopoiesis, and inflammatory responses. Signals are transduced via cytokines, interleukins, and growth factors acting through transmembrane receptor families.[79] An FDA-approved JAK/STAT inhibitor, tofacitinib, is utilized in the treatment of rheumatoid arthritis. The JAK/STAT pathway also has an established role in certain cancers.[75]

The JAK/STAT3 pathway has been found to have a potential role in the treatment of pain. Ligustrazine is an active ingredient in the Chinese medicine Ligusticum chuanxiong Hort and has been used in the treatment of cardiovascular disease.[80] Its role in pain is also becoming more established. In a rat model of sciatic nerve chronic constriction injury, ligustrazine decreased neuropathic pain via JAK/STAT3 pathway inhibition.[81]

NONINVASIVE NEUROMODULATION

The field of brain neuromodulation includes both invasive and noninvasive stimulation to artificially stimulate or inhibit brain regions involved in specific brain signaling, leading to enhanced neuroplasticity. Examples of invasive brain stimulation are deep brain stimulation and motor cortex stimulation; both have shown to be beneficial in reducing pain, but they also have limitations of cost and greater potential complications.[82] As a result, noninvasive forms of brain neuromodulation are also being studied, including transcranial magnetic stimulation (TMS), transcranial direct current stimulation (tDCS), and transcranial ultrasound (TUS).

TMS is increasingly being studied as a noninvasive form of neurostimulation for treating neurologic disorders impacting brain function and as a noninvasive neurostimulation treatment for pain. It was first utilized in 1985 and employs electromagnetic induction to reach neighboring cells.[83] Application can be in the form of single or multiple stimulation pulses. Repetitive TMS (rTMS) utilizes a repetition of multiple pulses rapidly applied and is the primary form of TMS in therapeutic use.[78] The frequency of rTMS also plays a role on the subject's physiologic response to treatment. High-frequency rTMS (5 Hz or faster) usually increases excitability, whereas low-frequency rTMS (approximately 1 Hz) usually decreases excitability.

One example of the use of rTMS in the treatment of pain involves diabetic neuropathic pain. In a study, high-frequency rTMS was applied to subjects in two groups with diabetic neuropathy: insulin-dependent and noninsulin-dependent. Visual analog scale for pain and nerve conduction studies had significant improvements in both subject groups when comparing values prior to and following rTMS treatment. Notably, there were sustained analgesic effects in a portion of subjects who completed extended follow-up of 5 weeks.[84] The proposed mechanism for the reduction in pain following rTMS treatment was attributed to enhanced cortical plasticity and inhibition of pain-processing pathways.[80]

Another study of high-frequency rTMS in subjects with painful diabetic neuropathy highlighted an interesting response.[85] Cortical inhibition was decreased in diabetic patients with neuropathic pain versus in diabetic patients without neuropathic pain. It was suggested that rTMS strengthened the defective intracortical inhibition and subsequently improved neuropathic pain symptoms.[81]

tDCS is another noninvasive technique that utilizes an electrical current conducted to the brain through electrodes on the scalp. The application of the electrical current is used to modulate brain activity, induce neuroplasticity, and thereby modify brain function.[86] Animal studies in rats showed that electrical currents induced cortical activation or inhibition that was stable after the end of stimulation and led to intracellular modifications similar to long-term potentiation and long-term depression[87]; therefore, it can both excite and inhibit brain activity, and the results can be long lasting.[88]

tDCS has been investigated for the treatment of numerous conditions, including drug addiction, major depression, attention deficit hyperactivity disorder, schizophrenia, Alzheimer's disease, and disorders of consciousness. It has also been investigated as a treatment for neuropathic pain from spinal cord injuries, multiple sclerosis, trigeminal neuralgia, poststroke pain syndrome, and amputation, and has had promising short-term results when compared with a placebo.[89,90] It is also currently being investigated for treatment of carpal tunnel syndrome to assess improvement in pain and function.[91] tDCS is being compared with trans-spinal DCS for chronic pelvic pain due to endometriosis, assessing the differences between cortical modulation and spinal modulation.[92]

There are some advantages of tDCS over TMS, in that tDCS is relatively cheaper, portable, and user-friendly.[84] tDCS is also considered safer, as TMS has been associated with seizures; furthermore, tDCS has been postulated to have longer-lasting effects on cortical activity.[84]

Combining tDCS with other techniques and modalities, such as MRI, TMS, or TUS, is currently under investigation, as combinatorial modalities may have an increased potential for targeting the current, and therefore, increased cortical modulation. High-definition tDCS is being developed for improved stimulation of cortical regions.

As noted, TUS is another modality that is currently under investigation for the treatment of pain. Brain activity can be modulated using ultrasound as measured with fMRI and EEG.[93] To date, the brain targets that have been modulated include the motor cortex, somatosensory cortex, thalamus, caudate, and visual cortex, and the majority of studies have been performed on healthy volunteers assessing perception and behavior.[94] One study specifically looked at ultrasound stimulation over the posterior frontal cortex, contralateral to the most pain in patients with chronic pain, and showed reduced pain and improved mood compared to sham controls.[95]

TUS is believed to be safe, with minimal side effects. The most common reported side effects are neck pain, headache, sleepiness, muscle twitch, and itchiness, all of which were temporary. However, both short- and long-term safety studies need to be performed in humans. Compared with TMS and tDCS, TUS could be superior, due to increased spatial resolution and depth perception.[96,94] TUS can target superficial and deep cortical tissues as well as subcortical targets.[97] In addition, although all the modalities can lead to modulation of brain activity, only TUS has been investigated for its ability to ablate tissues.

TUS is currently FDA approved for thalamotomy, as a treatment for medication refractory essential tremor. A feasibility study currently underway assesses thalamotomy for the treatment of chronic trigeminal neuropathic pain,[98] as well as TUS thalamotomy for neuropathic pain due to lumbar radiculopathy, spinal cord injury, or phantom limb pain.[99] Investigations of combinatorial noninvasive modulation are also underway to assess TUS plus tDCS for painful diabetic neuropathy,[100] and the effects of pain perception and functional limitations in chronic low back pain and knee osteoarthritis.[101,102]

TUS is also being combined with magnetic resonance (MR) for focusing the ultrasound to the appropriate cortical area. Interestingly, ultrasound is not only being investigated transcranially for the treatment of pain but peripherally as well. Current research is underway assessing MR-guided ultrasound for pain relief in residual limb neuromas in amputees, bone metastasis, facet arthropathy, as well as osteoarthritis of the knee, hip, and hand.[103,104]

Future research will need to elucidate the mechanism of action for TMS, tDCS, and TUS. It will need to optimize treatment parameters, including location of treatment, dosing, frequency, intensity, and duration. Lastly, it will need to assess both short- and long-term safety and effects of cortical structural changes.

GENE THERAPY

Gene therapy utilizes a vector to deliver the intracellular instructions from a therapeutic gene to target cells.[105] The target cells subsequently express the encoded peptides and proteins to produce the desired substance at their site of action.[106] The potential benefits of gene therapy and pain are being investigated.

To investigate a treatment for neuropathic pain induced by spinal nerve transection in mice, a gene therapy was engineered using lentiviral vectors targeting dorsal root ganglion tissues. This was found to silence TNF-alpha and relieve neuropathic pain.[107] Another animal study evaluated intraarticular administration of an adeno-associated virus (AAV) vector, targeting genes encoding matrix metalloproteinase 13 (MMP13), Interleukin-1 (Il-1), and nerve growth factor (NGF) in a surgically induced osteoarthritis mouse model.[108] Although osteoarthritic pain improved, articular cartilage destruction and osteophyte growth increased.[95]

Gene therapy has many potential advantages, warranting exploration into new viral vectors and signaling pathways. These advantages include the longevity of benefits, potentially reducing the need for frequent medication dosing, and the increased specificity for target tissues, potentially limiting side effects experienced from the many systemic pharmaceutical treatments we currently use in the treatment of pain.[25]

CONCLUSION

An increase in dedicated initiatives for pain research is creating an important structure to explore promising advances in the field. New research is being directed at improving our understanding, assessment, and treatment of pain processes. As each person's experience of pain is unique, identifying ways to further individualize treatment will be essential. This includes not only developing novel techniques and technologies but also understanding their roles alone, in combination, and in unique individuals.

Novel treatments are being discovered all the time, with only a small number able to be discussed in this chapter. Multiple resources should be reviewed to recognize the diverse perspectives being applied to pain research and for updates in the field. Awareness of ongoing advances can be fostered via many avenues. These include reviewing clinical trials, exploring newly funded initiatives, and meeting with peers in the field. As pain continues to have a widely detrimental impact on patients, their environment, and the healthcare system, the current expansion in pain research provides an exciting opportunity for truly consequential advances for the future of pain management.

REFERENCES

1. Worley SL. New directions in the treatment of chronic pain: national pain strategy will guide prevention, management, and research. *P T*. 2016;41(2):107–114.
2. Institute of Medicine (US), Committee on Advancing Pain Research, Care, and Education. *Relieving Pain in America: A Blueprint for Transforming Prevention, Care, Education, and Research*. Washington (DC): National Academies Press (US); 2011. Available from:https://www.ncbi.nlm.nih.gov/books/NBK91497/.
3. Department of Health and Human Services UG.*National Pain Strategy: a Comprehensive Population Health Strategy for Pain*. Available at: https://iprcc.nih.gov/docs/HHS National_Pain_Strategy.pdf.
4. The Interagency Pain Research Coordinating Committee. *FPRS Research Recommendations*. 2018. Available at: https://iprcc.nih.gov/sites/default/files/iprcc/FPRS_ Research_Recommendations_Final_508C.pdf.
5. Collins FS, Koroshetz WJ, Volkow ND. Helping to end addiction over the long-term: the research plan for the NIH HEAL initiative. *J Am Med Assoc*. 2018;320(2):129–130.
6. Dueñas M, Ojeda B, Salazar A, Mico JA, Failde I. A review of chronic pain impact on patients, their social environment and the health care system. *J Pain Res*. 2016;9:457–467.
7. Moore RA, Derry S, Taylor RS, Straube S, Phillips CJ. The costs and consequences of adequately managed chronic non-cancer pain and chronic neuropathic pain. *Pain Pract*. 2013;14(1):79–94.
8. Goldberg DS, Mcgee SJ. Pain as a global public health priority. *BMC Publ Health*. 2011;11:770.
9. Dahlhamer J, Lucas J, Zelaya C, et al. Prevalence of chronic pain and high-impact chronic pain among adults — United States, 2016. *Morb Mortal Wkly Rep*. 2018;67(36):1001–1006.
10. Gaskin DJ, Richard P. The economic costs of pain in the United States. *J Pain*. 2012;13(8):715–724.
11. *National Heart, Lung, and Blood Institute: FactBook Fiscal Year 2010*. Bethesda, MD: U.S. Dept. of Health and Human Services, National Heart, Lung, and Blood Institute; 2011.
12. Perez J, Koltzenburg M, Mantyh P. New directions in chronic pain: what might the future hold? *Can J Pain*. 2019. https://doi.org/10.1080/24740527.2019.1591804.
13. Thorp SL, Suchy T, Vadivelu N, Helander EM, Urman RD, Kaye AD. Functional connectivity alterations: novel therapy and future implications in chronic pain management. *Pain Physician*. 2018;21(3):E207–E214.
14. Department of Health and Human Services USA. *Pain Management Best Practices Inter-Agency Task Force Report*. May 2019.
15. Skelly AC, Chou RR, Dettori JA, et al. *Noninvasive Non-pharmacological Treatment for Chronic Pain: A Systematic Review*. November 2018. https://doi.org/10.23970/ahrqepccer209.
16. Bhuniya D, Kharul RK, Hajare A, et al. Discovery and evaluation of novel FAAH inhibitors in neuropathic pain model. *Bioorg Med Chem Lett*. 2019;29(2):238–243.
17. Ahn K, Smith SE, Liimatta MB, et al. Mechanistic and pharmacological characterization of PF-04457845: a highly potent and selective fatty acid amide hydrolase inhibitor that reduces inflammatory and noninflammatory pain. *J Pharmacol Exp Therapeut*. 2011;338(1):114–124.
18. Habib AM, Okorokov AL, Hill MN, et al. Microdeletion in a FAAH pseudogene identified in a patient with high anandamide concentrations and pain insensitivity. *Br J Anaesth*. 2019;123(2):e249–e253.
19. Kerbrat A, Ferré JC, Fillatre P, et al. Acute neurologic disorder from an inhibitor of fatty acid amide hydrolase *N Engl J Med*. 2016;375(18):1717–1725.
20. Schaffler K, Yassen A, Reeh P, Passier P. A randomized, double-blind, placebo- and active comparator-controlled phase I study of analgesic/antihyperalgesic properties of ASP8477, a fatty acid amide hydrolase inhibitor, in healthy female subjects. *Pain Med*. 2018; 19(6):1206–1218.
21. Mayo LM, Asratian A, Lindé, et al. Elevated anandamide, enhanced recall of fear extinction, and attenuated stress responses following inhibition of fatty acid amide hydrolase (FAAH): a randomized, controlled experimental medicine trial. *Biol Psychiatr*. 2020;87(6):538–547.
22. D'souza DC, Cortes-briones J, Creatura G, et al. Efficacy and safety of a fatty acid amide hydrolase inhibitor (PF-04457845) in the treatment of cannabis withdrawal and dependence in men: a double-blind, placebo-controlled, parallel group, phase 2a single-site randomised controlled trial. *Lancet Psychiatry*. 2019;6(1):35–45.
23. Mikaeili H, Yeung C, Habib AM, et al. CRISPR interference at the FAAH-OUT genomic region reduces FAAH expression. *BioRxiv;* 2019. Cold Spring Harbor Laboratory www.biorxiv.org/content/10.1101/633396v1.
24. Knezevic NN, Yekkirala A, Yaksh TL. Basic/translational development of forthcoming opioid- and nonopioid-targeted pain therapeutics. *Anesth Analg*. 2017;125(5):1714–1732.

25. Kaye AD, Cornett EM, Hart B, et al. Novel pharmacological nonopioid therapies in chronic pain. *Curr Pain Headache Rep.* 2018;22(4):31.

26. Huang J, Mis MA, Tanaka B, et al. Atypical changes in DRG neuron excitability and complex pain phenotype associated with a Na1.7 mutation that massively hyperpolarizes activation. *Sci Rep.* 2018;8(1):1811.

27. Dib-hajj SD, Waxman SG. Sodium channels in human pain disorders: genetics and pharmacogenomics. *Annu Rev Neurosci.* 2019;42:87−106.

28. Cox JJ, Reimann F, Nicholas AK, et al. An SCN9A channelopathy causes congenital inability to experience pain. *Nature.* 2006;444(7121):894−898.

29. Zakrzewska JM, Palmer J, Morisset V, et al. Safety and efficacy of a Nav1.7 selective sodium channel blocker in patients with trigeminal neuralgia: a double-blind, placebo-controlled, randomised withdrawal phase 2a trial. *Lancet Neurol.* 2017;16(4):291−300.

30. Mcdonnell A, Collins S, Ali Z, et al. Efficacy of the Nav1.7 blocker PF-05089771 in a randomised, placebo-controlled, double-blind clinical study in subjects with painful diabetic peripheral neuropathy. *Pain.* 2018; 159(8):1465−1476.

31. De greef BTA, Hoeijmakers JGJ, Geerts M, et al. Lacosamide in patients with Nav1.7 mutations-related small fibre neuropathy: a randomized controlled trial. *Brain.* 2019;142(2):263−275.

32. Hagen NA, Cantin L, Constant J, et al. Tetrodotoxin for moderate to severe cancer-related pain: a multicentre, randomized, double-blind, placebo-controlled, parallel-design trial. *Pain Res Manag.* 2017;2017:7212713.

33. Catterall WA. Voltage-gated calcium channels. *Cold Spring Harb Perspect Biol.* 2011;3(8):a003947.

34. Roca-lapirot O, Radwani H, Aby F, Nagy F, Landry M, Fossat P. Calcium signalling through L-type calcium channels: role in pathophysiology of spinal nociceptive transmission. *Br J Pharmacol.* 2018;175(12): 2362−2374.

35. Su SC, Seo J, Pan JQ, et al. Regulation of N-type voltage-gated calcium channels and presynaptic function by cyclin-dependent kinase 5. *Neuron.* 2012;75(4): 675−687.

36. Mcgivern JG. Ziconotide: a review of its pharmacology and use in the treatment of pain. *Neuropsychiatric Dis Treat.* 2007;3(1):69−85.

37. Sałat K, Kowalczyk P, Gryzło B, Jakubowska A, Kulig K. New investigational drugs for the treatment of neuropathic pain. *Expet Opin Invest Drugs.* 2014;23(8): 1093−1104.

38. Gleeson EC, Graham JE, Spiller S, et al. Inhibition of N-type calcium channels by fluorophenoxyanilide derivatives. *Mar Drugs.* 2015;13(4):2030−2045.

39. Jacus MO, Uebele VN, Renger JJ, Todorovic SM. Presynaptic Cav3.2 channels regulate excitatory neurotransmission in nociceptive dorsal horn neurons. *J Neurosci.* 2012; 32(27):9374−9382.

40. Mckay BE, Mcrory JE, Molineux ML, et al. Ca(V)3 T-type calcium channel isoforms differentially distribute to somatic and dendritic compartments in rat central neurons. *Eur J Neurosci.* 2006;24(9):2581−2594.

41. Weiss N, Zamponi GW. T-type calcium channels: from molecule to therapeutic opportunities. *Int J Biochem Cell Biol.* 2019;108:34−39.

42. Bourinet E, Altier C, Hildebrand ME, Trang T, Salter MW, Zamponi GW. Calcium-permeable ion channels in pain signaling. *Physiol Rev.* 2014;94(1):81−140.

43. Ziegler D, Duan WR, An G, Thomas JW, Nothaft W. A randomized double-blind, placebo-, and active-controlled study of T-type calcium channel blocker ABT-639 in patients with diabetic peripheral neuropathic pain. *Pain.* 2015;156(10):2013−2020.

44. Kerckhove N, Pereira B, Soriot-thomas S, et al. Efficacy and safety of a T-type calcium channel blocker in patients with neuropathic pain: a proof-of-concept, randomized, double-blind and controlled trial. *Eur J Pain.* 2018; 22(7):1321−1330.

45. Richard M, Kaufmann P, Kornberger R, Dingemanse J. First-in-man study of ACT-709478, a novel selective triple T-type calcium channel blocker. *Epilepsia.* 2019;60(5): 968−978.

46. Tsantoulas C, Mcmahon SB. Opening paths to novel analgesics: the role of potassium channels in chronic pain. *Trends Neurosci.* 2014;37(3):146−158.

47. Ocaña M, Cendán CM, Cobos EJ, Entrena JM, Baeyens JM. Potassium channels and pain: present realities and future opportunities. *Eur J Pharmacol.* 2004; 500(1−3):203−219.

48. Arimura K, Sonoda Y, Watanabe O, et al. Isaacs' syndrome as a potassium channelopathy of the nerve. *Muscle Nerve Suppl.* 2002;11. S55−8.

49. Klein CJ, Lennon VA, Aston PA, Mckeon A, Pittock SJ. Chronic pain as a manifestation of potassium channel-complex autoimmunity. *Neurology.* 2012;79(11): 1136−1144.

50. Du X, Gamper N. Potassium channels in peripheral pain pathways: expression, function and therapeutic potential. *Curr Neuropharmacol.* 2013;11(6):621−640.

51. Poupon L, Lamoine S, Pereira V, et al. Targeting the TREK-1 potassium channel via riluzole to eliminate the neuropathic and depressive-like effects of oxaliplatin. *Neuropharmacology.* 2018;140:43−61.

52. Venkatachalam K, Montell C. TRP channels. *Annu Rev Biochem.* 2007;76:387−417.

53. Jardín I, López JJ, Diez R, et al. TRPs in pain sensation. *Front Physiol.* 2017;8:392.

54. Fernandes ES, Fernandes MA, Keeble JE. The functions of TRPA1 and TRPV1: moving away from sensory nerves. *Br J Pharmacol.* 2012;166(2):510−521.

55. Story GM, Peier AM, Reeve AJ, et al. ANKTM1, a TRP-like channel expressed in nociceptive neurons, is activated by cold temperatures. *Cell.* 2003;112(6):819−829.

56. Maatuf Y, Geron M, Priel A. The role of toxins in the pursuit for novel analgesics. *Toxins.* 2019;11(2).

57. Bressan E, Touska F, Vetter I, et al. Crotalphine desensitizes TRPA1 ion channels to alleviate inflammatory hyperalgesia. *Pain.* 2016;157(11):2504−2516.

58. Lin king JV, Emrick JJ, Kelly MJS, et al. A cell-penetrating scorpion toxin enables mode-specific modulation of TRPA1 and pain. *Cell*. 2019;178(6), 1362–1374.e16.

59. Brown DC. Resiniferatoxin: the evolution of the "molecular scalpel" for chronic pain relief. *Pharmaceuticals*. 2016;9(3).

60. Raithel SJ, Sapio MR, Lapaglia DM, Iadarola MJ, Mannes AJ. Transcriptional changes in dorsal spinal cord persist after surgical incision despite preemptive analgesia with peripheral resiniferatoxin. *Anesthesiology*. 2018;128(3):620–635.

61. Heiss J, Iadarola M, Cantor F, Oughourli A, Smith R, Mannes A. (364) A Phase I study of the intrathecal administration of resiniferatoxin for treating severe refractory pain associated with advanced cancer. *J Pain*. 2014; 15(4). https://doi.org/10.1016/j.jpain.2014.01.275.

62. Shirahashi H, Toriihara E, Suenaga Y, et al. The discovery of novel 3-aryl-indazole derivatives as peripherally restricted pan-Trk inhibitors for the treatment of pain. *Bioorg Med Chem Lett*. 2019;29(16):2320–2326.

63. Khan N, Smith MT. Neurotrophins and neuropathic pain: role in pathobiology. *Molecules*. 2015;20(6): 10657–10688.

64. Walicke PA, Hefti F, Bales R, et al. First-in-human randomized clinical trials of the safety and efficacy of tanezumab for treatment of chronic knee osteoarthritis pain or acute bunionectomy pain. *Pain Rep*. 2018;3(3):e653.

65. Mantyh PW, Koltzenburg M, Mendell LM, Tive L, Shelton DL. Antagonism of nerve growth factor-TrkA signaling and the relief of pain. *Anesthesiology*. 2011; 115(1):189–204.

66. Katz JN. Tanezumab for painful osteoarthritis. *J Am Med Assoc*. 2019;322(1):30–32.

67. Webb MP, Helander EM, Menard BL, Urman RD, Kaye AD. Tanezumab: a selective humanized mAb for chronic lower back pain. *Therapeut Clin Risk Manag*. 2018;14:361–367.

68. Gowler PRW, Li L, Woodhams SG, et al. Peripheral brain derived neurotrophic factor contributes to chronic osteoarthritis joint pain. *Pain*. 2019.

69. Tender GC, Kaye AD, Li YY, Cui JG. Neurotrophin-3 and tyrosine kinase C have modulatory effects on neuropathic pain in the rat dorsal root ganglia. *Neurosurgery*. 2011;68(4):1048–1055.

70. Tracy LM, Georgiou-karistianis N, Gibson SJ, Giummarra MJ. Oxytocin and the modulation of pain experience: implications for chronic pain management. *Neurosci Biobehav Rev*. 2015;55:53–67.

71. Gonzalez-hernandez A, Charlet A. Oxytocin, GABA, and TRPV1, the analgesic triad? *Front Mol Neurosci*. 2018;11: 398.

72. Han Y, Yu LC. Involvement of oxytocin and its receptor in nociceptive modulation in the central nucleus of amygdala of rats. *Neurosci Lett*. 2009;454(1):101–104.

73. Eisenach JC, Tong C, Curry R. Phase 1 safety assessment of intrathecal oxytocin. *Anesthesiology*. 2015;122(2): 407–413.

74. Rash JA, Campbell TS. The effect of intranasal oxytocin administration on acute cold pressor pain: a placebo-controlled, double-blind, within-participants crossover investigation. *Psychosom Med*. 2014;76(6):422–429.

75. Xie J, Wang X, Proud CG. mTOR inhibitors in cancer therapy. *F1000Res*. 2016;5.

76. Lutz BM, Nia S, Xiong M, Tao YX, Bekker A. mTOR, a new potential target for chronic pain and opioid-induced tolerance and hyperalgesia. *Mol Pain*. 2015;11:32.

77. Kwon M, Han J, Kim UJ, et al. Inhibition of mammalian target of rapamycin (mTOR) signaling in the insular cortex alleviates neuropathic pain after peripheral nerve injury. *Front Mol Neurosci*. 2017;10:79.

78. Hua C, Zehou O, Ducassou S, et al. Sirolimus improves pain in NF1 patients with severe plexiform neurofibromas. *Pediatrics*. 2014;133(6):e1792–e1797.

79. Thomas SJ, Snowden JA, Zeidler MP, Danson SJ. The role of JAK/STAT signalling in the pathogenesis, prognosis and treatment of solid tumours. *Br J Cancer*. 2015; 113(3):365–371.

80. Wang H, Zhang W, Cheng Y, et al. Design, synthesis and biological evaluation of ligustrazine-flavonoid derivatives as potential anti-tumor agents. *Molecules*. 2018; 23(9).

81. Wang S, Li A, Guo S. Ligustrazine attenuates neuropathic pain by inhibition of JAK/STAT3 pathway in a rat model of chronic constriction injury. *Pharmazie*. 2016;71(7): 408–412.

82. Klein MM, Treister R, Raij T, et al. Transcranial magnetic stimulation of the brain: guidelines for pain treatment research. *Pain*. 2015;156(9):1601–1614.

83. Barker AT, Jalinous R, Freeston IL. Non-invasive magnetic stimulation of human motor cortex. *Lancet*. 1985; 1(8437):1106–1107.

84. Abdelkader AA, Gohary AME, Mourad HS, Salmawy DAE. Repetitive TMS in treatment of resistant diabetic neuropathic pain. *Egypt J Neurol Psychiatr Neurosurg*. 2019;55(1). https://doi.org/10.1186/s41983-019-0075-x.

85. Han Y, Lee CH, Min KW, Han KA, Choi HS, Kang YJ. Effects of repetitive high frequency motor cortex transcranial magnetic stimulation and cortical disinhibition in diabetic patients with neuropathic pain: acase control study. *Clin Pain*. 2019;18(1):1–7.

86. Stagg CJ, Nitsche MA. Physiological basis of transcranial direct current stimulation. *Neuroscientist*. 2011;17(1): 37–53. https://doi.org/10.1177/1073858410386614.

87. Nitsche MA, Cohen LG, Wassermann EM, et al. Transcranial direct current stimulation: state of the art 2008. *Brain Stimul*. 2008;1(3):206–223. https://doi.org/10.1016/j.brs.2008.06.004.

88. Zhao H, Qiao L, Fan D, et al. Modulation of brain activity with noninvasive transcranial direct current stimulation (tDCS): clinical applications and safety concerns. *Front Psychol*. 2017;8. https://doi.org/10.3389/fpsyg.2017.00685.

89. David MCMM, Moraes AAD, Costa MLD, Franco CIF. Transcranial direct current stimulation in the modulation of neuropathic pain: a systematic review. *Neurol Res.* 2018;40(7):557−565. https://doi.org/10.1080/01616412.2018.1453190.

90. Ngernyam N, Jensen MP. Transcranial direct current stimulation in neuropathic pain. *J Pain Relief.* 2014. https://doi.org/10.4172/2167-0846.s3-001.

91. *Effects of Cerebral & Peripheral Electrical Stimulation on Pain and Function in CTS.* https://clinicaltrials.gov/ct2/show/NCT04092088. Accessed 6 October 2019.

92. *tDCS Versus tsDCS for Endometriosis-Related Chronic Pelvic Pain Treatment.* https://clinicaltrials.gov/ct2/show/NCT02958423. Accessed 6 October 2019.

93. Wang P, Zhang J, Yu J, Smith C, Feng W. Brain modulatory effects by low-intensity transcranial ultrasound stimulation (TUS): asystematic review on both animal and human studies. *Front Neurosci.* 2019;13. https://doi.org/10.3389/fnins.2019.00696.

94. Biase LD, Falato E, Lazzaro VD. Transcranial focused ultrasound (tFUS) and transcranial unfocused ultrasound (tUS) neuromodulation: from theoretical principles to stimulation practices. *Front Neurol.* 2019;10. https://doi.org/10.3389/fneur.2019.00549.

95. Hameroff S, Trakas M, Duffield C, et al. Transcranial ultrasound (TUS) effects on mental states: a Pilot study. *Brain Stimul.* 2013;6(3):409−415. https://doi.org/10.1016/j.brs.2012.05.002.

96. Lee EJ, Fomenko A, Lozano AM. Magnetic resonance-guided focused ultrasound :current status and future perspectives in thermal ablation and blood-brain barrier opening. *J Korean Neurosurg Soc.* 2019;62(1):10−26. https://doi.org/10.3340/jkns.2018.0180.

97. Legon W, Bansal P, Tyshynsky R, Ai L, Mueller JK. *Transcranial Focused Ultrasound Neuromodulation of the Human Primary Motor Cortex.* August 2018. https://doi.org/10.1101/234666.

98. *Feasibility Study of ExAblate Thalamotomy for Treatment of Chronic Trigeminal Neuropathic Pain.* https://clinicaltrials.gov/ct2/show/NCT03309813. Accessed 6 October 2019.

99. *MR Guided Focused Ultrasound for Treatment of Neuropathic Pain.* https://clinicaltrials.gov/ct2/show/NCT03111277. Accessed 6 October 2019.

100. *Optimization of NIBS for Diabetic Neuropathy Neuropathic Pain.* https://clinicaltrials.gov/ct2/show/NCT03625752. Accessed 6 October 2019.

101. *Effects of tDCS and tUS on Pain Perception in OA of the Knee.* https://clinicaltrials.gov/ct2/show/NCT02723929. Accessed 6 October 2019.

102. *Effects of tDCS and TUS on the Perception of Pain and Functional Limitations Due to Non-Specific Chronic Low Back Pain.* https://clinicaltrials.gov/ct2/show/NCT02954432. Accessed 6 October 2019.

103. *Focused Ultrasound Treatment of Stump Neuromas for the Relief of Chronic Post-Amputation Neuropathic Pain.* https://clinicaltrials.gov/ct2/show/NCT03255395. Accessed 6 October 2019.

104. Namba H, Kawasaki M, Izumi M, Ushida T, Takemasa R, Ikeuchi M. Effects of MRgFUS treatment on musculoskeletal pain: comparison between bone metastasis and chronic knee/lumbar osteoarthritis. *Pain Res Manag.* 2019;2019:1−7. https://doi.org/10.1155/2019/4867904.

105. Rubanyi GM. *Gene Therapy-Basic Principles and the Road from Bench to Bedside.Pharmaceutical Sciences Encyclopedia.* John Wiley and Sons, Inc.; 2010.

106. Pleticha J, Maus TP, Beutler AS. Future directions in pain management: integrating anatomically selective delivery techniques withnovel molecularly selective agents. *Mayo Clin Proc.* 2016;91(4):522−533.

107. Ogawa N, Kawai H, Terashima T, et al. Gene therapy for neuropathic pain by silencing of TNF-αexpression with lentiviral vectors targeting the dorsal root ganglion in mice. *PloS One.* 2014;9(3).

108. Zhao L, Huang J, Fan Y, et al. Exploration of CRISPR/Cas9-based gene editing as therapy for osteoarthritis. *Ann Rheum Dis.* 2019;78(5):676−682.

Index

Note: Page numbers followed by "t" indicate tables, "f" indicate figures and "b" indicate boxes.

Printed and bound by CPI Group (UK) Ltd, Croydon, CR0 4YY

03/10/2024

01040300-0006